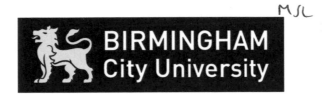

Small Parts and Superficial Structures

Editor

NIRVIKAR DAHIYA

ULTRASOUND CLINICS

www.ultrasound.theclinics.com

Consulting Editor
VIKRAM S. DOGRA

July 2014 • Volume 9 • Number 3

ELSEVIER

1600 John F. Kennedy Boulevard • Suite 1800 • Philadelphia, Pennsylvania, 19103-2899

http://www.theclinics.com

ULTRASOUND CLINICS Volume 9, Number 3
July 2014 ISSN 1556-858X, ISBN-13: 978-0-323-31174-8

Editor: John Vassallo
Developmental Editor: Stephanie Carter

Ultrasound Clinics (ISSN 1556-858X) is published quarterly by Elsevier, Inc., 360 Park Avenue South, New York, NY 10010-1710. Months of publication are January, April, July, and October. Business and editorial offices: 1600 John F. Kennedy Boulevard, Suite 1800, Philadelphia, Pennsylvania 19103-2899. Accounting and circulation offices: 6277 Sea Harbor Drive, Orlando, FL 32887-4800. Periodicals postage paid at New York, NY, and additional mailing offices. Subscription prices are $270 per year for (US individuals), $327 per year for (US institutions), $130 per year for (US students and residents), $305 per year for (Canadian individuals), $369 per year for (Canadian institutions), $325 per year for (international individuals), $369 per year for (international institutions), and $155 per year for (Canadian and foreign students/residents). To receive student/resident rate, orders must be accompanied by name of affiliated institution, date of term, and the signature of program/residency coordinator on institution letterhead. Orders will be billed at individual rate until proof of status is received. Foreign air speed delivery is included in all Clinics subscription prices. All prices are subject to change without notice. **POSTMASTER:** Send address changes to *Ultrasound Clinics,* Elsevier Health Sciences Division, Subscription Customer Service, 3251 Riverport Lane, Maryland Heights, MO 63043. **Customer Service (orders, claims, online, change of address): Telephone: 1-800-654-2452 (U.S. and Canada); 314-447-8871 (outside U.S. and Canada). Fax: 314-447-8029. E-mail: journalscustomerservice-usa@elsevier.com (for print support); journalsonlinesupport-usa@elsevier.com (for online support).**

Reprints: For copies of 100 or more, of articles in this publication, please contact the Commercial Reprints Department, Elsevier Inc., 360 Park Avenue South, New York, NY 10010-1710. Tel.: +1-212-633-3874; Fax: +1-212-633-3820; E-mail: reprints@elsevier.com.

Contributors

CONSULTING EDITOR

VIKRAM S. DOGRA, MD
Professor of Radiology, Urology, and
Biomedical Engineering; Associate Chair for
Education and Research; Director of
Ultrasound; Department of Imaging Sciences,
University of Rochester School of Medicine,
Rochester, New York

EDITOR

NIRVIKAR DAHIYA, MD
Assistant Professor, Department of Radiology,
Mayo Clinic, Phoenix, Arizona

AUTHORS

BIANCA BIGNOTTI, MD
Resident of Radiology, Radiology Department,
DISSAL, Università di Genova, Genova, Italy

BORIS BRKLJAČIĆ, MD, PhD
Professor of Radiology, University of
Zagreb School of Medicine; Breast Unit,
Department of Diagnostic and Interventional
Radiology, University Hospital "Dubrava,"
Zagreb, Croatia

JARED S. BURLISON, MD, PhD
Department of Radiology, The University of
New Mexico, Albuquerque, New Mexico

NIRVIKAR DAHIYA, MD
Assistant Professor, Department of Radiology,
Mayo Clinic, Phoenix, Arizona

DIANA GAITINI, MD
Clinical Professor, Director, Unit of Ultrasound,
Department of Medical Imaging, Rambam
Health Care Center and Bruce Rappaport
Faculty of Medicine, Israel Institute of
Technology, Haifa, Israel

GORDANA IVANAC, MD, PhD
Assistant Professor of Radiology, University of
Zagreb School of Medicine; Breast Unit,

Department of Diagnostic and Interventional
Radiology, University Hospital "Dubrava,"
Zagreb, Croatia

BRADLEY K. LAMPRICH, MD
Assistant Professor, Department of
Radiological Sciences, University of Oklahoma
Health Sciences Center, Oklahoma City,
Oklahoma

DANIEL LONDON, MD
Head of the Ultrasonography Unit; Radiology
Department, Barzilai Medical Center,
Ashkelon; Faculty of Medicine, Ben Gurion
University of the Negev, Beer Sheva, Israel

CARLO MARTINOLI, MD
Associate Professor of Radiology, Radiology
Department, DISSAL, Università di Genova,
Genova, Italy

VINCENT M. MELLNICK, MD
Assistant Professor, Mallinckrodt Institute of
Radiology, Washington University School of
Medicine, St Louis, Missouri

CHRISTINE O. MENIAS, MD
Professor, Department of Radiology, Mayo
Clinic, Phoenix, Arizona

WILLIAM D. MIDDLETON, MD, FACR
Professor of Radiology, Mallinckrodt Institute
of Radiology, Washington University School of
Medicine, St Louis, Missouri

ODED NAHLIELI, DMD
Faculty of Medicine, Ben Gurion University
of the Negev, Beer Sheva; Professor and
Chairman, Department of Oral and
Maxillofacial Surgery, Barzilai Medical Center,
Ashkelon, Israel

DANIEL B. NISSMAN, MD, MPH, MSEE
Clinical Assistant Professor, Musculoskeletal
Imaging Section, Department of Radiology,
University of North Carolina School of
Medicine, Chapel Hill, North Carolina

MAITRAY D. PATEL, MD
Associate Professor, Department of Radiology,
Mayo Clinic, Phoenix, Arizona

KATHRYN A. ROBINSON, MD
Assistant Professor of Radiology, Mallinckrodt
Institute of Radiology, Washington University
School of Medicine, St Louis, Missouri

ALBERTO TAGLIAFICO, MD
Radiologist, Assistant Professor of Human
Anatomy; Department of Experimental

Medicine, DIMES, Università di Genova,
Genova, Italy

**S. BOOPATHY VIJAYARAGHAVAN, MD,
DMRD**
Consultant Diagnostic Radiologist,
Sonoscan Ultrasonic Scan Centre,
Coimbatore, Tamil Nadu, India

JASON M. WAGNER, MD
Assistant Professor, Department of
Radiological Sciences, University of Oklahoma
Health Sciences Center, Oklahoma City,
Oklahoma

HANS-PETER WESKOTT, MD
Head of Central Ultrasound Department,
Klinikum Siloah, KRH, Hannover,
Germany

MICHAEL R. WILLIAMSON, MD
Professor, Department of Radiology,
The University of New Mexico, Albuquerque,
New Mexico

SANSHAN YIN, MD
Department of Ultrasound, Key Laboratory of
Carcinogenesis and Translational Research,
Peking University Cancer Hospital & Institute,
Beijing, People's Republic of China

Contents

Sonography of the Salivary Glands   313

Daniel London and Oded Nahlieli

Among the various imaging modalities, sonography is considered first-line imaging for the evaluation of the salivary glands. This article describes an ultrasound investigation of the parotid gland, the submandibular gland, and the sublingual gland.

Ultrasonographic Evaluation of the Thyroid   325

Kathryn A. Robinson and William D. Middleton

This article reviews the ultrasonographic evaluation of the thyroid. The normal thyroid anatomy is described, in addition to the imaging appearance of benign and malignant thyroid disease and diffuse thyroid disease. Selection of thyroid nodules for fine-needle aspiration biopsy is discussed.

Parathyroid Sonography   339

Vincent M. Mellnick and William D. Middleton

Hyperparathyroidism can lead to symptoms related to hypercalcemia. Evaluation of the parathyroid glands with sonography requires knowledge of the classic and variant appearances of parathyroid lesions as well as the range of anatomic locations. The accuracy of ultrasonography in characterizing parathyroid disease is augmented by correlation with scintigraphy; although neither sonography nor scintigraphy excels in detecting multigland disease or after failed resection, they are still used in those settings with varying sensitivities. Because of the increasing use of minimally invasive techniques, ultrasonography and ultrasound-guided fine-needle aspiration play a crucial role in preoperative characterization of abnormal parathyroid glands.

Ultrasonography in the Assessment of Lymph Node Disease   351

Hans-Peter Weskott and Sanshan Yin

 Videos of color Doppler and B-flow examinations accompany this article

Ultrasonography has become the first-line imaging modality in patients with inflammatory or malignant diseases for the evaluation of peripheral and abdominal lymph node (LN) status. A typical reactive LN has an oval shape, with even thickness of its preserved cortex and regular vessel architecture. LN metastases are mostly round and hypoechoic to cystic; an echogenic hilum is missed and the vessel architecture is chaotic. Ultrasound-guided biopsies are in most cases successful in defining LN characteristics. The use of contrast agents is advantageous in the detection of tissue perfusion, thus confirming the effect of chemotherapy or radiation therapy.

adjacent to the femoral vein. Indirect hernias move obliquely from superiolaterally near the anterior superior iliac spine in an inferior medial direction toward the pubic symphysis. Direct hernias move from posterior to anterior in the medial part of the lower quadrants of the abdomen. Umbilical hernias occur anywhere within 2 to 3 cm of the center of the umbilicus.

ULTRASOUND CLINICS

PROGRAM OBJECTIVE
The goal of the *Ultrasound Clinics* is to keep practicing radiologists and radiology residents up to date with current clinical practice in ultrasound by providing timely articles reviewing the state of the art in patient care.

TARGET AUDIENCE
Practicing radiologists, radiology residents and other healthcare professionals who provide care based on radiologic findings.

LEARNING OBJECTIVES
Upon completion of this activity, participants will be able to:
1. Review sonography of testis.
2. Discuss ultrasound of lumps and bumps; tendons; breast; and peripheral nerves.
3. Describe ultrasound in assessment of lymph node disease.

ACCREDITATION
The Elsevier Office of Continuing Medical Education (EOCME) is accredited by the Accreditation Council for Continuing Medical Education (ACCME) to provide continuing medical education for physicians.

The EOCME designates this enduring material for a maximum of 15 *AMA PRA Category 1 Credit*(s)™. Physicians should claim only the credit commensurate with the extent of their participation in the activity.

All other health care professionals requesting continuing education credit for this enduring material will be issued a certificate of participation.

DISCLOSURE OF CONFLICTS OF INTEREST
The EOCME assesses conflict of interest with its instructors, faculty, planners, and other individuals who are in a position to control the content of CME activities. All relevant conflicts of interest that are identified are thoroughly vetted by EOCME for fair balance, scientific objectivity, and patient care recommendations. EOCME is committed to providing its learners with CME activities that promote improvements or quality in healthcare and not a specific proprietary business or a commercial interest.

The planning committee, staff, authors and editors listed below have identified no financial relationships or relationships to products or devices they or their spouse/life partner have with commercial interest related to the content of this CME activity:

Bianca Bignotti, MD; Boris Brkljačić, MD, PhD; Jared S. Burlison, MD, PhD; Stephanie Carter; Nirvikar Dahiya, MD; Joseph Daniel; Vikram S. Dogra, MD; Diana Gaitini, MD; Kristen Helm; Brynne Hunter; Gordana Ivanac, MD, PhD, Bradley K. Lamprich, MD; Sandy Lavery; Daniel London, MD; Carlo Martinoli, MD; Jill McNair; Vincent M. Mellnick, MD; Christine O. Menias, MD; William D. Middleton, MD, FACR; Oded Nahlieli, DMD; Daniel B. Nissman, MD, MPH, MSEE; Maitray D. Patel, MD; Kathryn A. Robinson, MD; Alberto Tagliafico, MD; John Vassallo; S. Boopathy Vijayaraghavan, MD, DMRD; Jason M. Wagner, MD; Hans-Peter Weskott, MD; Michael R. Williamson, MD; Sanshan Yin, MD.

The planning committee, staff, authors and editors listed below have identified financial relationships or relationships to products or devices they or their spouse/life partner have with commercial interest related to the content of this CME activity:

UNAPPROVED/OFF-LABEL USE DISCLOSURE
The EOCME requires CME faculty to disclose to the participants:
1. When products or procedures being discussed are off-label, unlabelled, experimental, and/or investigational (not US Food and Drug Administration (FDA) approved); and
2. Any limitations on the information presented, such as data that are preliminary or that represent ongoing research, interim analyses, and/or unsupported opinions. Faculty may discuss information about pharmaceutical agents that is outside of FDA-approved labelling. This information is intended solely for CME and is not intended to promote off-label use of these medications. If you have any questions, contact the medical affairs department of the manufacturer for the most recent prescribing information.

TO ENROLL
To enroll in the *Ultrasounds Clinic* Continuing Medical Education program, call customer service at 1-800-654-2452 or sign up online at http://www.theclinics.com/home/cme. The CME program is available to subscribers for an additional annual fee of USD 212.

METHOD OF PARTICIPATION
In order to claim credit, participants must complete the following:
1. Complete enrolment as indicated above.
2. Read the activity.
3. Complete the CME Test and Evaluation. Participants must achieve a score of 70% on the test. All CME Tests and Evaluations must be completed online.

CME INQUIRIES/SPECIAL NEEDS
For all CME inquiries or special needs, please contact elsevierCME@elsevier.com.

Erratum

An error was made in the April 2014 issue of *Ultrasound Clinics,* Vol. 9, No. 2, on page 206. The **Fig. 14** legend reads, "Skull with soft tissue swelling (arrow);" however, the arrow is pointing to the skull fracture, rather than the swelling. Please see the replacement image included here, with the arrow pointing at the swelling as originally intended.

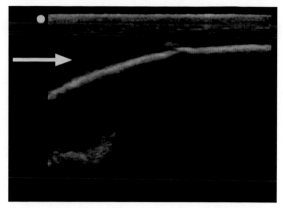

Fig. 14. Skull with soft tissue swelling (*arrow*).

Ultrasound Clin 9 (2014) xi
http://dx.doi.org/10.1016/j.cult.2014.04.001
1556-858X/14/$ – see front matter © 2014 Elsevier Inc. All rights reserved.

Preface
Small Parts and Superficial Structures

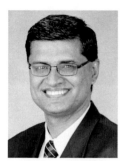

Nirvikar Dahiya, MD
Editor

One of the strengths of ultrasound is its excellent resolution when imaging superficial structures. The introduction of high-frequency transducers has dramatically changed the diagnostic landscape over the last few years. Today, we are routinely using 18-MHz transducers to look at small tendons and nerves. Evaluation of thyroid, parathyroids, salivary glands, breast, and scrotum has undergone a significant transformation and characterization of lesions within these structures is much improved in accuracy. Soft tissue evaluations, where patients present with palpable lumps and bumps, are a part of our routine practice in current times. Addition of dynamic imaging has helped in the musculoskeletal imaging and for the diagnosis of hernias. Contrast imaging has further changed the terrain of lymph node imaging.

Putting together an issue with such diverse topics is a challenging task. However, I am proud to say that in this issue a motivated and inspiring group of authors has come together and contributed excellent articles dealing with all of the above situations. Where needed, quality videos are provided to effectively convey a teaching point. The range of pathologies covered in this issue makes it a single valuable resource for anyone who does small-parts ultrasound.

I hope you will find something relevant to your practice in this issue and that it leads to an improvement in patient care. After all, that is our mission—to improve patient care and to make it better than before.

Nirvikar Dahiya, MD
Department of Radiology
Mayo Clinic
5777 East Mayo Boulevard
Phoenix, AZ 85054, USA

E-mail address:
nirvikardahiya@yahoo.com

Ultrasound Clin 9 (2014) xiii
http://dx.doi.org/10.1016/j.cult.2014.03.010
1556-858X/14/$ – see front matter © 2014 Elsevier Inc. All rights reserved.

Sonography of the Salivary Glands

Daniel London, MD[a,b,*], Oded Nahlieli, DMD[b,c]

KEYWORDS

- Sonography • Salivary glands • Parotid gland • Submandibular gland • Sublingual gland • Calculi
- Tumor • Inflammation

KEY POINTS

- The salivary glands are superficially located and can be investigated by sonography in detail.
- It is important to scan each gland in a systematic manner.
- The salivary glands can be affected by inflammatory, benign, and malignant pathology that can be detected by sonography.
- The salivary glands can have congenital anatomic abnormalities and can contain calculi that are also detected by sonography.
- The learning objective is to obtain deep knowledge about structure of healthy glands, applicable sonographic technique, pathologic changes, and differential diagnosis of the pathologies.

PHYSICS AND INSTRUMENTATION

Ultrasound is a high-frequency acoustic wave using frequencies outside the normal hearing range (20 Hz–20 kHz). Most equipment for head and neck and maxillofacial use is set at 8 MHz (8 million/cycles per second) or higher. This contrasts with ultrasound equipment used for general surgery or obstetrics, which works at 5 to 6 MHz, allowing a greater depth of tissue penetration but reduced resolution. Probes generating frequencies up to 20 MHz and, in the case of ultrasound biometrics, up to 50 MHz, are now also used for salivary gland imaging. These allow resolution of very small structures. Three large salivary glands (the parotid gland, the submandibular gland, and the sublingual gland) are arranged in pairs and easily accessible to sonographic diagnosis, including high-frequency linear probes (8–18 MHz), because of their superficial location.[1]

Nowadays the use of high-end ultrasound devices features a sonographic image like in an anatomy book. Resolution and penetration depth of ultrasound depends on the deployed frequency. The higher the frequency, the better the resolution but the penetration is worsened.[2] For imaging of the salivary glands linear arrays with 7.5 MHz (5.0–13.5 MHz)[3,4] are most useful. **Box 1** outlines scanning sequence.

Under normal conditions, the three large salivary glands exhibit similar homogeneous intermediate echogenicity with sharp borders.[5–7] Small salivary glands become accessible to sonographic diagnosis only when pathologic lesions are present (eg, tumorous or neoplastic gland enlargement). The indications for sonographic examination include swelling or enlargement in the region of the salivary glands, and pain.[8,9] Examination by ultrasound (**Box 2**) enables the sonographer to verify whether masses are localized in, or merely

None of the authors has conflict of interest with the submission.

No financial support was received for this submission.

[a] Radiology Department, Barzilai Medical Center, Ashkelon 78306, Israel; [b] Faculty of Medicine, Ben Gurion University of the Negev, Beer Sheva, Israel; [c] Department of Oral and Maxillofacial Surgery, Barzilai Medical Center, Rehov Haistadrut 2, Ashkelon 78306, Israel

* Corresponding author.

E-mail address: dlondon@barzi.health.gov.il

Ultrasound Clin 9 (2014) 313–323

http://dx.doi.org/10.1016/j.cult.2014.03.007

Box 1
Scanning sequence

- It is important to scan the gland in a systematic manner.
- Initially a wide window is used, particularly to visualize the gland itself.
- Subsequently concentrate at any solid lesions and other pathology.

Box 3
Parotid gland scanning procedure

- The supine position
- Transverse and longitudinal scans over the mandibular angle
- Cover the preauricular, infra-auricular, retro-auricular, and cervical regions
- Examine the gland bilaterally because some diseases may occur bilaterally

---

adjacent to, the inspected salivary gland. This distinction often cannot be made solely based on clinical examination.[10]

HOW TO SCAN (PROTOCOLS)
The Parotid Gland

The parotid gland can be easily assessed with the patient's head turned sideways and hyperextended. A summary of scanning procedures is found in **Box 3**.

First, the transverse section is scanned, proceeding from the angle of the jaw up to a point slightly above the tragus. Next, the longitudinal section is scanned. The ultrasound probe must be adequately adapted to the surface of the skin by applying a sufficient amount of gel, particularly in the region of the angle of the jaw.[1,7,11]

The Submandibular Gland

If the patient's head is moderately extended, the submandibular gland can be sonographically examined without any problems.[1,7,11] First, in the midline of the neck, the ultrasound scanner is moved in transverse orientation from the hyoid up to the horizontal ramus of the mandible. Occasionally, both submandibular glands can be imaged simultaneously. Next, by shifting the scanner to one side, parallel to the horizontal ramus of the mandible, a clear image of the respective

---

Box 2
Components to ultrasound examination

- Topographic examination, to assess the shape and location of any abnormality
- Quantitative assessment, to assess reflectivity, attenuation, and structure of any abnormality within the salivary gland
- Kinetic evaluation, to assess the mobility of abnormal structures (calculi, foreign bodies) within the salivary gland
- Doppler, elastography

---

submandibular gland can be obtained. The gel contact of the scanner to the skin has to be ensured here.

The Sublingual Gland

The examination of the sublingual gland involves no essential differences in procedure compared with the examination of the submandibular gland. The scanner is placed on the skin in a transverse plane in the median line immediately below the mandible, thus allowing visualization of both sublingual glands. It is important to note that all the averaged scans should be within 0.2 mm of each other, and any outliers carefully assessed and discarded and rescanned if necessary.

ANATOMY
Refresh Your Gray's Anatomy

The parotid glands consist of a prismatic body and two extensions: the anterior portion resting on the deep masseter muscle and the deeper extension, which reaches the lateral wall of the pharynx passing between the prestyloid muscles and the stylomandibular ligament.

The submandibular glands are located in the submandibular space beneath the floor of the mouth and they have a mesial extension called the "hook." Wharton excretory duct arises from this extension running at the base of the lingual frenulum to open into the sublingual caruncle.

The sublingual glands are a group of glands situated in the sublingual space, surrounded by the lingual fossa, the floor of the mouth, and the mylohyoid muscle.

Normal Anatomy by Ultrasound

The parotid gland
The parotid glands, which are the largest of the salivary glands, are enclosed by a separate fascia that penetrates the glands thereby forming changeable lobes. In a transverse section, the parotid gland presents as a sharply bordered,

homogeneous organ with intermediate echogenicity (**Fig. 1**). The gland can be clearly distinguished from subcutaneous fatty tissue. The anterior parts of the gland ride on the masseter muscle and can be differentiated from the buccal fatty tissue, which exhibits lower echogenicity, by the contraction and relaxation of the masticatory muscles.[12,13] The posterior part of the gland is located in the retromandibular fossa clearly demarcated anteriorly by the ascending ramus of the mandible and posteriorly by the sternocleidomastoid muscle and the mastoid. Mediocaudal to the lower pole of the parotid gland, the posterior belly of the digastric muscle and the internal carotid artery can be discerned.[14] It is important to remember that a small portion of the parotid gland may be hidden by the acoustic shadow of the mandible.

In and around the gland can be found the internal jugular vein and the retromandibular vein, which is located in the glandular parenchyma, can be visualized, particularly in a longitudinal section. In transverse planes distal to the retromandibular vein, the styloid process is projected into the glandular parenchyma and should not be confused with a sialolith. The facial nerve is not normally visible. With modern high-resolution scanners, it is occasionally possible to obtain a sonographic image of the main efferent duct.[15,16]

The submandibular gland

The submandibular gland extends cranially up to the mandible and the mylohyoid muscle and has a close relationship to the anterior belly of the digastric muscle. The submandibular gland surrounds the posterior border of the mylohyoid muscle in an arc and often reaches ventromedially as far as the sublingual gland. An echopaque structure with posterior shadowing is often projected into the hilar region of the submandibular gland. Here, one must differentiate between parts of the hyoid and sialoliths of the submandibular gland, both of which can show comparable image characteristics.[2,7] The sonographic image characteristics of the submandibular gland comprise an intermediately echogenic feature with a regular reflection pattern, corresponding in appearance to the parenchymal echo pattern of the parotid gland (**Fig. 2**).

In and around the gland the sonographically easily discernible facial artery and facial vein run across the gland. The course of the efferent glandular duct can occasionally be visualized with the aid of high-resolution ultrasound scanners, even if there is no obstruction of the duct. If parts of the hyoid are in question, displacements can be observed during swallowing motions.

The sublingual gland

Visualization of the sublingual gland can at times be difficult to achieve. The sublingual gland is located under the mucosa in the floor of the mouth, below the tip of the tongue, close to the lingual frenulum. The dorsal glands frequently touch the submandibular gland.

The gland is bounded ventrally and medially by the geniohyoid and genioglossus muscles, and caudolaterally by the mandible. The short efferent duct normally cannot be imaged. Accumulation of saliva can be detected in and around the sublingual gland forming a ranula (**Fig 3**).

PATHOLOGIC FINDINGS

Box 4 provides a brief list of salivatory gland pathologies.

Acute Sialadenitis

Because we have to deal with paired organs it is valuable to compare both glands in one picture. The findings are attributed to the edematose inflammation swelling of the organ and to the increased fluid content of the parenchyma

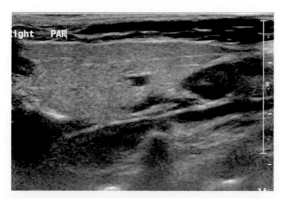

Fig. 1. Normal parotid gland.

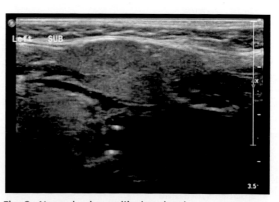

Fig. 2. Normal submandibular gland.

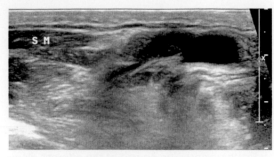

Fig. 3. Sublingual ranula.

transformed by the inflammation process. We usually see the following[3,9,13]:

- A diffuse enlargement of the entire afflicted gland
- The organ can be reliably demarcated from adjacent structures
- The parenchymal pattern appears loosely connected, inhomogeneous, roughly textured, and more hypoechogenic
- Circumscript hypoechogenic masses can be detected as a concomitant inflammatory reaction of the intraglandular lymph nodes
- Liquefication zones (as signs of abscess formation) appear hypoechogenic to echo-free with hyperechogenic border wall and distinct distal signal enhancement
- Roughly patterned hyperechogenic echoes at the center of such liquefaction foci can correspond to necrotic tissue contributions

Chronic Sialadenitis

The sonographic image is highly dependent on the duration and the degree of inflammation of the glandular parenchyma. As in the case of acute sialadenitis, a conclusive distinction between the various pathogenic forms of chronic sialadenitis cannot be made using sonography. We usually see the following:

- A distinctive increase in the roughness of the echo texture
- The internal structure appears inhomogeneous, probably as a consequence of scarred parenchyma fibrosis

---

Box 4
Salivary gland pathologies

- Inflammations
- Calculi
- Benign lesions
- Malignant tumors
- Sjögren syndrome

- Small cystic echo-free domains are formed that correspond to circumscript duct ectasias (**Fig. 4**)[17,18]
- Occasionally, intraglandular concrements become visible as echopaque structures with distal shadowing

Differential diagnosis is important with the following situations:

1. Patients suffering from Sjögren syndrome show sonographically enlarged, inhomogeneously structured, hypoechogenic salivary glands. Numerous hypoechogenic circumscript masses are detected intraparenchymatously that may correspond to cystic duct extensions on the one hand or enlarged intraglandular lymph nodes on the other hand. Sonographically the structure of the salivary glands appears "cloudy."[19]
2. Epitheloid cell sialadenitis (Heerfordt syndrome) is sonographically characterized by an echo-rich structure interrupted by numerous enlarged lymph nodes, which appear as hypoechogenic tumors.[20]
3. Küttner tumor of the submandibular gland occurs like an echo-poor formation within parts of the submandibular gland and can easily be mistaken as an adenoma.[21]
4. Ultrasound can detect alterations after radiotherapy. The echohomogenous pattern disappears after radiation and a more hypoechogenic and sometimes irregular pattern appears as a sign of loss of function.
5. Other secondary pathologic changes (edema, infections, and soft tissue tumors) around the salivary glands can be distinguished easily from a primary salivary gland pathology.

Parotid Abscess

The abscessual evolution of the inflammation is characterized by hypoanechoic lesion with irregular margins. We usually see the following[22–24]:

- A hypoanechoic lesion, with irregular margins
- Peripheral hypervascularity detected on color Doppler examination
- If partially necrotic, lymph nodes with anechoic areas of necrosis
- In case with fistula, fistula reaches the skin tissue, surrounded by edema

An important signal of abscess is the appearance of vessels with a linear and reasonably regular path that subsequently becomes more irregular and characterized by numerous anastomoses, which can be highlighted by the increase in intensity of the color Doppler signal. In the abscessual

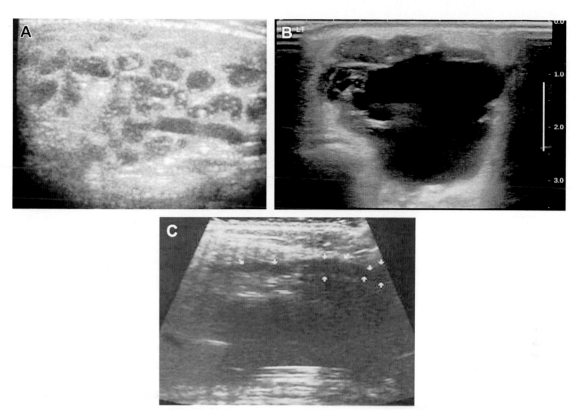

Fig. 4. (*A*) Parotid chronic sialoadenitis. (*B*) Parotid gland sialocele. (*C*) Stensen duct dilatation (*arrows*).

forms, the color Doppler signal has a peripheral typology, because in this case the vessels entwine in the area that is peripheral to the abscess.

Lymph Node Enlargements

Lymph nodes can be found within the parotid gland but only around the submandibular gland because of the embryologic development. In the parotid gland a group of small lymph nodes (3–5 mm) is located along the course of the retromandibular vein. These lymph nodes drain lymph from the eustachian tube, the external auditory canal, and the deep regions of the face. The intraglandular and extraglandular lymph nodes do not exceed 9 mm in diameter under physiologic conditions.

In the ultrasound image of a sonographically unremarkable glandular parenchyma, mostly multiple hypoechogenic masses that are essentially free from any distal signal enhancement can be discerned. No reliable evidence can be derived from sonography that would permit a conclusive differential diagnosis between benign and malignant lymph node enlargements.[25]

A reliable distinction between reactive lymphadenitis (**Fig. 5**), a non-Hodgkin lymphoma (**Fig. 6**), a MALT lymphoma, or intraglandular metastatic

spread is not possible based on sonographic findings.[26] Clinical signs, number, arrangement, and sometimes texture of the nodes may lead to the diagnosis but do not resemble histology. Like in lymph node enlargements of the neck, some authors mention the so-called "hilus" as a sign of reactive lymphadenitis.[27]

Cystic Tumors

Congenital or acquired cysts of the salivary glands are normally filled with a transparent liquid. We usually see an echo-free tumor and sharp borders

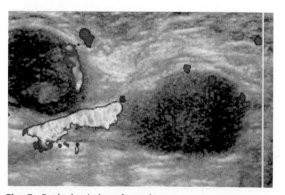

Fig. 5. Pathologic lymph node.

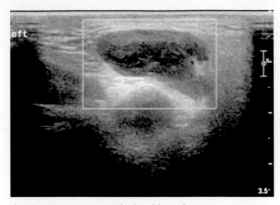

Fig. 6. Primary parotid gland lymphoma.

with distal acoustic enhancement (**Fig. 7**).[14,28] It is important to note that if cystic tumors are sonographically detected in both parotid glands, and if the patient's history corresponds, lymphoepithelial cysts caused by HIV infection should be suspected.[29]

Sialolithiasis

Whereas the distal shadowing feature is generally detectable, the reflection may at times be only indistinct or lacking. This phenomenon is the result of the reflected ultrasound component not reaching the transducer, but being dispersed out of the image plane. We usually see an echopaque reflection with distinct distal shadowing (**Fig. 8**)[30] and dilation of the efferent ducts.

Stones of the parotid duct contain organic components and should be visualized with more effort. Sometimes only a distinct echopaque reflex without distal shadowing may be detected. However, in many of these cases dilation of the efferent ducts of the salivary glands can be considered as a further indirect indication of a stone disorder if a

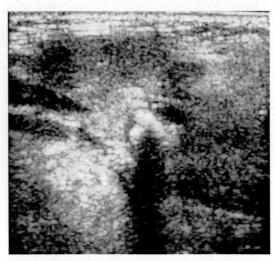

Fig. 8. Submandibular intraglandular sialolithiasis.

concrement cannot be reliably identified.[17] Nonetheless, a duct dilation can also be caused by constrictions in the connective tissue (eg, as observed after an inadequately performed incision of a duct or after acute inflammation). Concrements located in the region of the large salivary glands can be reliably detected by sonography from a diameter of 1.5 to 2 mm upward.[31]

It is important to note that exact determination of the position of sialoliths (intraglandular, extraglandular, intraductal) has great significance.[25] Differential diagnosis is important with air within the ducts, as in the case of pneumoparotitis, foreign bodies, angiolithiasis, and calcified lymph nodes or arteriovenous malformations (**Fig. 9**). Remember, because of its limited sensitivity and limited negative predictive value, sonography does not allow reliable exclusion of small salivary gland calculi. Further diagnostic investigations are needed to detect calculi in patients with normal sonographic findings and suspected lithiasis.[32]

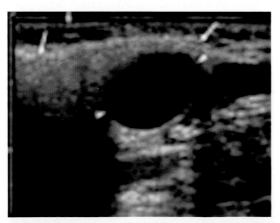

Fig. 7. Salivary gland cyst (*arrows* denote parotid gland; *arrowheads* denote cyst).

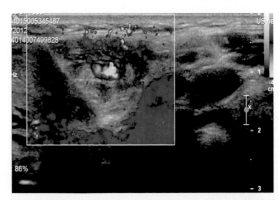

Fig. 9. Salivary gland arteriovenous malformation.

Sialadenosis (Sialosis)

All large salivary glands can be simultaneously affected by sialadenosis. Sialadenosis is a noninflammatory condition characterized by bilateral enlargement of the salivary glands, most often the parotid glands. We usually see that[13,33] the glands appear indistinctly enlarged and can be demarcated from surrounding structures only with difficulty, the echostructure appears homogeneously hyperechogenic, and no tumor-like lesions are present in sialadenosis.[4] In some cases the parotid gland is so enlarged that ultrasound examination requires a low-frequency probe for the evaluation of the deep portion.

Benign Epithelial Tumors of the Salivary Glands

A clearly defined border between the surrounding salivary gland tissue and the tumor itself is a characteristic feature of a benign salivary gland tumor.[34] Because sonography is unable to visualize nerves, it is not possible to establish reliably the relationship of parotid tumors to the facial nerve.

Pleomorphic adenomas exhibit a homogeneous/hypoechogenic texture. However, inhomogeneous structures with solid and cystic contributions also may occasionally be discernible. Distal acoustic enhancement is the rule in these cases (Fig. 10).

Monomorphic adenomas (adenolymphomas) can also appear sonographically homogeneous and hypoechogenic, as in the case of pleomorphic adenomas.[4,29] If proportion of cystic structures is high, an adenolymphoma can also present itself completely echo-free with extended distal enhancement. Sometimes septa can be identified within the tumor.

The remaining, less common types of benign tumors of the salivary glands (eg, basal cell adenomas, oncocytomas, lymphoepithelial lesions) show similarly unspecific sonomorphologic features.[35]

A conclusive sonographic identification and differentiation between the diverse types of benign tumors of the salivary glands is not possible at the present time, even though a substantial cystic proportion tends to indicate an adenolymphoma, and a general absence of cystic areas points toward a ploomorphic adenoma. To a certain degree, parotid tumors can be assigned to the "superficial" or "deep" portion of the gland.

Benign Nonepithelial Tumors of the Salivary Glands

Lymphangiomas and hemangiomas (Figs. 11 and 12) show similar sonomorphologic characteristics, making their clear differentiation impossible. At examination, loosely connected alveolar structural patterns composed partially of hypoechogenic and hyperechogenic areas can be detected. Sonography allows one to assess the depth of penetration and the extension of this mass into the respective salivary gland and into the periglandular soft tissue regions.[25]

Intraglandular and extraglandular lipomas (Fig. 13) appear as sharply demarcated, ovoid masses with hypoechogenic, homogeneous reflection patterns. A lipoma shows a more hypoechogenic reflection pattern than the remaining parenchyma of the salivary gland, but its echo texture is more hyperechogenic than that of the other types of intraglandular tumors and exhibits a linear, hyperechogenic feathery texture.

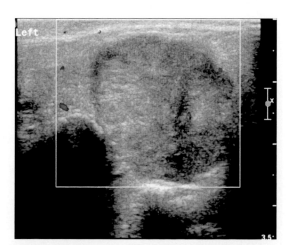

Fig. 10. Parotid gland pleomorphic adenoma.

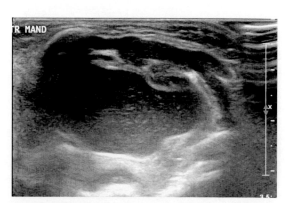

Fig. 11. Intraglandular lymphangioma.

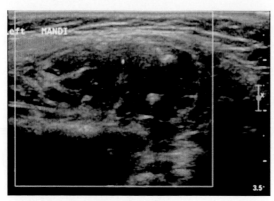

Fig. 12. Submandibular hemangioma.

Malignant Tumors of the Salivary Glands

We usually see an unclear margin and an inhomogeneous echo texture. It is possible to describe the relation between invasive tumor growth and the surrounding tissue. It is impossible to detect malignant invasion of the facial nerve. The most common malignant salivary gland tumors are mucoepidermoid carcinoma, adenocystic carcinoma, carcinoma arising in pleomorphic adenoma, and metastasis from distant origin (Fig 14).[36]

However, these sonographic indications are sometimes absent, so that in the preoperative stage a definite statement as to the benign or malignant character of tumor development cannot be made with ultimate certainty. If malignancy is suspected by ultrasound and fine-needle aspiration, it may be helpful to classify the tumor more adequately in the preoperative stage.[37]

It is important to note that if the tumor margins cannot be precisely imaged by sonography, especially when the tumor has reached bone or deep

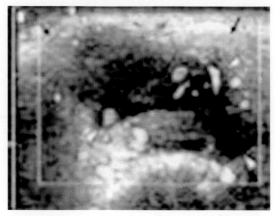

Fig. 14. Metastatic melanoma in the parotid gland (*arrows* denote parotid gland; *arrowheads* denote metastasis).

structures, diagnostic imaging of the patient should be expanded to include computed tomography and/or magnetic resonance imaging examinations at all costs.

Sjögren Syndrome

Sjögren syndrome appears when lymphocytes invade and destroy the exocrine glands. It is the second most common autoimmune syndrome after rheumatoid arthritis that affects the salivary glands in 40% to 80% of the cases. This results in a higher incidence of lymphomas in the parotid glands and salivary calculi. We usually see the following[1,4,13]:

- In the early stage, sonography is normal
- Later there is enlargement of the glands and widespread structural irregularities
- The gland is inhomogeneous
- In a more advanced stage sonography shows sialectasis and marked hypervascularity on color Doppler ultrasound

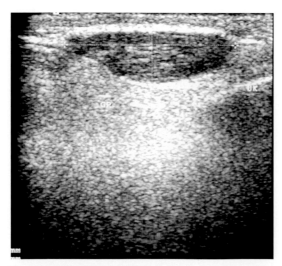

Fig. 13. Well-defined lipoma.

The intraoperative role of sonography became important after minimally invasive surgical techniques were implemented into salivary gland surgery. During the operation, if endoscopic observation of the surgical field is impossible, sonography guidance can be used to

- Indicate an exact position of the stone (Fig 15)

- Indicate an exact position of the stricture

- Monitor sialocele elimination and precise Botox filling (Fig 16)

- Monitor cerebral palsy drooling treatment with precise Botox injections

- Monitor fine-needle biopsy in cases of parotid tumors

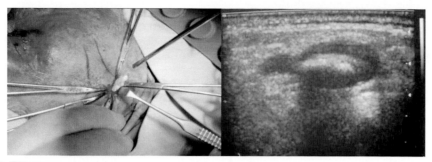

Fig. 15. Minimally invasive procedure with ultrasonographic guidance.

Color Doppler Sonography of Salivary Glands

The regular B-scan is a well-established tool in diagnosing diseases of salivary glands. In tumors located in the salivary glands it is of great interest to noninvasively acquire clinical information, such as growth and invasiveness, and to establish an accurate diagnosis before surgery. Before the benefits of sophisticated ultrasound work-up were available, this was performed on a regular basis by correlating simple sonomorphologic criteria, such as the echo-free regions, with specific histologic entities.[14] Over the last few years color Doppler sonography has become a well established part of ear-nose-throat head and neck surgery and the maxillofacial surgery diagnostic armamentarium, particularly in the framework of preoperative assessment of tumors and cervical lymph nodes.[7,38–42]

Color-Coded Duplex Sonography

Color-coded duplex sonography (**Box 5**) is a combination of B-scan sonography, a pulsed Doppler system, and the color-coded representation of perfused areas. The main principle of color-coded duplex sonography is a shift of transducer-emitted frequency, which is caused by reflection from the floating erythrocytes. The speed and direction at which the erythrocytes approach and move away from the transducer provides the information necessary for the function of the duplex sonography.[25]

The option of using Doppler signal-enhancing agents to achieve improved visualization of tumor vascularization has provided new possibilities for characterizing masses. Analysis of microvascularization and time-dependent changes after administration of Doppler signal-enhancing agent and also elastography are promising new tools to determine whether these changes are typical of certain types of salivary gland tumors (**Fig. 17**).[45–47]

The referring physician needs to know the following:

- Sonography yields a high sensitivity in the diagnosis of inflammation and provides a valid contribution to the clinical investigation.

- Sonography is mandatory as a first-line examination, and in many cases it provides a differential diagnosis with a high diagnostic confidence.

- Tuberculosis can involve the salivary glands by dissemination through the blood circulation or the lymphatic system. The patient presents with acute onset of sialadenitis causing pain and diffuse swelling with a subacute evolution mimicking a neoplastic lesion.

- Glands affected by chronic inflammation are characterized by sialectasis and reduced salivary secretion. That leads to parenchymal damage, often in the presence of calculi and ductal stenosis.

- HIV parotitis shows painless swelling of both parotid glands. The sonography shows multiple small hypoechoic areas, which are a sign of lymphoid infiltration or a characteristic pattern with multiple large bilateral cysts that may contain calcifications.

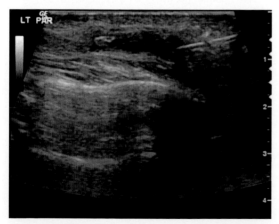

Fig. 16. Therapeutic intraglandular Botox injection.

<table>
Box 5
Color-coded duplex sonography

- The direction of the blood flow is normally coded in colors
- Qualitatively the color distribution gives information about the vascularization of tumor masses
- Quantitatively the blood flow and circulation resistance can be assessed
- No unequivocal differences between the investigated tumor groups (eg, adenolymphomas, pleomorphic adenomas, and squamous cell carcinomas of the parotid gland)
- Increased vascularization in malignant parotid tumors compared with benign parotid tumors[43,44]
</table>

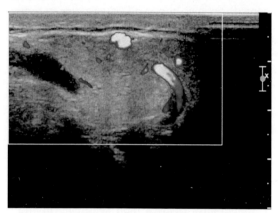

Fig. 17. Salivary gland power Doppler analysis.

SUMMARY

Sonography has established itself as the primary imaging technique in the diagnosis of salivary gland diseases. A sonographic examination is generally sufficient to diagnose sialolithiasis. If chronic sialadenitis or sialadenosis is suspected and if sonographic findings turn out to be insufficient, a conventional sialography may be required in specific cases. Histologic clarification is imperative once the presence of a mass has been established. In the event that the extension and relationship of the tumor to its surroundings cannot be determined sonographically, a subsequent computed tomography or magnetic resonance imaging examination should be performed.

REFERENCES

1. Mancuso AA, Hanafee WN. Head and neck radiology. Philadelphia: Lippincott Williams & Wilkins; 2011.
2. Alyas F, Lewis K, Williams M, et al. Diseases of submandibular gland as demonstrated using high resolution ultrasound. Br J Radiol 2005;78:362–9. http://dx.doi.org/10.1259/bjr/93120352.
3. Gritzmann N, Koischwitz D. Ultrasound of the neck. J Otolaryngol 1993;22:315–20.
4. Iro H, Uttenweiler V, Zenk J. Kopf-Hals-Sonographie. Berlin: Springer Verlag; 2000.
5. Nitsche N, Iro H. Ultraschalldiagnostik in der Hals-Nasen-Ohrenheilkunde - Möglichkeiten und Grenzen Teil 1. Otorhinolaryngol Nova 1992;2:135–46.
6. Baatenburg de Jong RJ, Rongen RJ. Guidelines for the use of ultrasound in the head and neck. ORL J Otorhinolaryngol Relat Spec 1993;55:309–12.
7. Liyanage SH, Spencer SP, Hogarth KM, et al. Imaging of salivary glands. Imaging 2007;19:14–27. http://dx.doi.org/10.1259/imaging/67453895.
8. Dewes W, Gritzmann N, Hirschner A, et al. High resolution small parts sonography (7.5 MHz) of the head and neck region. Radiologe 1996;36:12–21 [in German].
9. Zengel P, Schrötzlmair F, Reichel C, et al. Sonography: the leading diagnostic tool for diseases of the salivary glands. Semin Ultrasound CT MR 2013;34(3):196–203. http://dx.doi.org/10.1053/j.sult.2012.11.012.
10. Gosepath K, Hinni M, Mann W. The state of the art of ultrasonography in the head and neck. Ann Otolaryngol Chir Cervicofac 1994;111:1–5.
11. Peter B. Ultrasound diagnosis of face and neck organs. Schweiz Rundsch Med Prax 2001;90:687–91 [in German].
12. Emshoff R, Bertram S, Strobl H. Ultrasonographic cross-sectional characteristics of muscles of the head and neck. Oral Surg Oral Med Oral Pathol Oral Radiol Endod 1999;87:93–106.
13. Orlandi MA, Pistorio V, Guerra PA. Ultrasound in sialadenitis. J Ultrasound 2013;16(1):3–9. http://dx.doi.org/10.1007/s40477-013-0002-4.
14. Neiman HL, Phillips JF, Jaques DA, et al. Ultrasound of the parotid gland. J Clin Ultrasound 1976;4:11–3.
15. Bruneton JN, Mourou MY. Ultrasound in salivary gland disease. ORL J Otorhinolaryngol Relat Spec 1993;55:284–9.
16. Nitsche N, Iro H. Ultraschalldiagnostik in der Hals-Nasen-Ohren-Heilkunde: Möglichkeiten und Grenzen Teil 2. Otorhinolaryngol Nova 1992;2:178–94.
17. Ching AS, Ahuja AT, King AD, et al. Comparison of the sonographic features of acalculous and calculous submandibular sialadenitis. J Clin Ultrasound 2001;29:332–8.
18. Rubaltelli L, Sponga T, Candiani F, et al. Infantile recurrent sialectatic parotitis: the role of sonography and sialography in diagnosis and follow-up. Br J Radiol 1987;60:1211–4.
19. Schwerk WB, Schroeder HG, Eichhorn T. High-resolution real-time sonography in salivary gland

diseases. I: inflammatory diseases. HNO 1985;33:505–10 [in German].

20. Fischer T, Muhler M, Beyersdorff D, et al. Use of state-of-the-art ultrasound techniques in diagnosing sarcoidosis of the salivary glands (Heerfordt's syndrome). HNO 2003;51:394–9 [in German].

21. Ahuja AT, Richards PS, Wong KT, et al. Kuttner tumour (chronic sclerosing sialadenitis) of the submandibular gland: sonographic appearances. Ultrasound Med Biol 2003;29:913–9.

22. Tan VE, Goh BS. Parotis abscess: a five-year review - clinical presentation, diagnosis and management. J Laryngol Otol 2007;121:872–9. http://dx.doi.org/10.1017/S0022215106004166.

23. Kishore R, Ramachandran K, Ngoma C, et al. Unusual complication of parotid abscess. J Laryngol Otol 2004;118:388–90. http://dx.doi.org/10.1258/002221504323086642.

24. Viselner G, van der Byl GG, Maira A, et al. Parotid abscess: mini-pictorial essay. J Ultrasound 2013;16(1):11–5. http://dx.doi.org/10.1007/s40477-013-0006-0.

25. Brown J, Greess H, Zenk J, et al. Diagnostic and imaging methods. In: Nahlieli O, Iro H, McGurk M, et al, editors. Modern management preserving the salivary glands. Herzliya (Israel): Isradon; 2007. p. 34–55.

26. Yasumoto M, Yoshimura R, Sunaba K, et al. Sonographic appearances of malignant lymphoma of the salivary glands. J Clin Ultrasound 2001;29:491–8.

27. Evans RM, Ahuja A, Metreweli C. The linear echogenic hilus in cervical lymphadenopathy: a sign of benignity or malignancy? Clin Radiol 1993;47:262–4.

28. Teymoortash A, Kulkens C, Werner JA, et al. Sonographic features of a submandibular epidermoid cyst. Ultraschall Med 2003;24:261–3 [in German].

29. Schroeder HG, Schwerk WB, Eichhorn T. High-resolution real-time sonography in salivary gland diseases. II: salivary gland tumors. HNO 1985;33:511–6 [in German].

30. Yoshimura Y, Inoue Y, Odagawa T. Sonographic examination of sialolithiasis. J Oral Maxillofac Surg 1989;47:907–12.

31. Födra C, Kaarmann H, Iro H. Sonography and plain roentgen image in diagnosis of salivary calculi: experimental studies. HNO 1992;40:259–65 [in German].

32. Terraz S, Poletti PA, Dulguerov P, et al. How reliable is sonography in the assessment of sialolithiasis? AJR Am J Roentgenol 2013;201(1):W104–9. http://dx.doi.org/10.2214/AJR.12.9383.

33. Scully C, Bagán JV, Eveson JW, et al. Sialosis: 35 cases of persistent parotid swelling from two countries. Br J Oral Maxillofac Surg 2008;46:468–72. http://dx.doi.org/10.1016/j.bjoms.2008.01.014.

34. Daghfous MH, Oueslati B, Ben Jaafar M, et al. The role of ultrasonography in the study of tumors of the salivary glands. Tunis Med 1987;65:495–8 [in French].

35. Goto TK, Shimizu M, Kobayashi I, et al. Lymphoepithelial lesion of the parotid gland. Dentomaxillofac Radiol 2002;31:198–203.

36. El-Khateeb SM, Abou-Khalaf AE, Farid MM, et al. A prospective study of three diagnostic sonographic methods in differentiation between benign and malignant salivary gland tumours. Dentomaxillofac Radiol 2011;40:476–85.

37. Cho HW, Kim J, Choi J, et al. Sonographically guided fine-needle aspiration biopsy of major salivary gland masses: a review of 245 cases. AJR Am J Roentgenol 2011;196:1160–3.

38. Leuwer RM, Westhofen M, Schade G. Color duplex echography in head and neck cancer. Am J Otolaryngol 1997;18:254–7.

39. Schreiber J, Mann W, Lieb W. Color duplex ultrasound measurement of lymph node perfusion: a contribution to diagnosis of cervical metastasis. Laryngorhinootologie 1993;72:187–92.

40. Steinkamp HJ, Mueffelmann M, Böck JC, et al. Differential diagnosis of lymph node lesions: a semiquantitative approach with colour Doppler ultrasound. Br J Radiol 1998;71:828–33.

41. Steinkamp JH, Maurer J, Cornehl M, et al. Recurrent cervical lymphadenopathy: differential diagnosis with color-duplex sonography. Eur Arch Otorhinolaryngol 1994;251:404–9.

42. Benzel W, Zenk J, Iro H. Farbdopplersonographische untersuchungen von parotistumoren. HNO 1995;43:25–30.

43. Martinoli C, Derchi LE, Solbiati L, et al. Color Doppler sonography of salivary glands. Am J Roentgenol 1994;163:933–41.

44. Schick S, Steiner E, Gahleitner A, et al. Differentiation of benign and malignant tumors of the parotid gland: value of pulsed Doppler and colour Doppler sonography. Eur Radiol 1998;8:1462–7.

45. Steinhart H, Zenk J, Sprang K, et al. Contrast-enhanced colour Doppler sonography of parotid gland tumors. Eur Arch Otorhinolaryngol 2003;260:344–8.

46. Rickert D, Jecker P, Metzler V, et al. Color coded duplex sonography of the cervical lymph nodes: improved differential diagnostic assessment after administration of the signal enhancer SH U 508 A (Levovist). Eur Arch Otorhinolaryngol 2000;257:453–8.

47. Angerer F, Zenk J, Iro H, et al. Use of a portable ultrasound system in the perisurgical assessment of head and neck patients. HNO 2013;61(10):866–71. http://dx.doi.org/10.1007/s00106-013-2727-y.

Ultrasonographic Evaluation of the Thyroid

Kathryn A. Robinson, MD*, William D. Middleton, MD

KEYWORDS

- Thyroid • Thyroid ultrasonography • Thyroid nodule evaluation • Fine-needle aspiration
- Diffuse thyroid disease

KEY POINTS

- Normal thyroid anatomy.
- Benign and malignant thyroid disease.
- Selection of nodules for fine-needle aspiration.
- Diffuse thyroid disease.

INSTRUMENTATION AND TECHNIQUE

Evaluation of the thyroid gland is best achieved with a linear transducer of high frequency, such as 7 to 18 MHz. Most current linear transducers provide high spatial resolution of 0.7 to 1.0 mm with deep penetration of up to 5 cm.[1] The patient is placed supine on a stretcher, and a towel or pillow is rolled behind the lower cervical spine to extend the neck as much as possible. The thyroid gland must be examined thoroughly in both longitudinal and transverse planes. In addition, the examination should include an evaluation of the lateral and central neck compartments for abnormal lymph nodes, Levels II to VII.[2] This evaluation is achieved by scanning laterally in the region of the carotid artery and jugular vein, superiorly to detect submandibular and upper central neck adenopathy, and inferiorly to visualize supraclavicular and lower central neck adenopathy.

ANATOMY

The thyroid gland is located in the anteroinferior neck, infrahyoid compartment. It is made up of 2 lobes located on either side of the trachea. The lobes are connected by a thin isthmus that crosses anterior to the trachea, at the lower third of the gland. A minority of patients have a small pyramidal lobe arising superiorly from the isthmus and lying in front of the thyroid cartilage. The thyroid gland is bordered by thin strap muscles (sternohyoid, sternothyroid, and omohyoid) anteriorly, sternocleidomastoid muscles more laterally, and longus colli muscles posteriorly. The common carotid arteries are located lateral to each thyroid lobe, and the jugular veins are anterior and lateral to the carotids. In many patients the esophagus is seen posterior to the thyroid and trachea, on the left side more commonly than the right. It is identified by the typical target appearance of bowel in the transverse plane, and peristaltic movement when the patient swallows.

The normal thyroid gland has a homogeneous medium- to high-level echogenicity and is hyperechoic relative the adjacent muscles. The thin hyperechoic line that surrounds the thyroid lobe is the thyroid capsule. The normal thyroid lobe measures 4 to 6 cm in length and 1.3 to 1.8 cm in anterior posterior and transverse diameter. The normal isthmus measures up to 3 mm in thickness (**Fig. 1**).[1,3] Thyroid gland demonstrates scattered, readily detectable internal blood flow with color or power Doppler (**Fig. 2**).

Thyroid is enlarged when the transverse or anteroposterior diameter is greater than 2 cm or when the parenchyma extends anterior to the carotid artery. The superior thyroidal artery and vein are

The authors have nothing to disclose.
Mallinckrodt Institute of Radiology, Washington University School of Medicine, 510 South Kingshighway Boulevard, St Louis, MO 63110, USA
* Corresponding author.
E-mail address: robinsonk@mir.wustl.edu

Ultrasound Clin 9 (2014) 325–337
http://dx.doi.org/10.1016/j.cult.2014.02.003

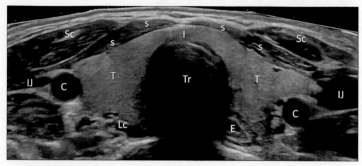

Fig. 1. Normal thyroid. Transverse extended-field-of-view scan of the neck shows the normal right and left lobes of the thyroid (T) located on either side of the trachea (Tr). The common carotid arteries (C) and the internal jugular vein (IJ) are seen lateral to the carotid. The overlying strap muscles (S) are immediately anterior to the thyroid, and the sternocleidomastoid muscles (Sc) are anterolateral to the thyroid. The isthmus (I) of the thyroid is anterior to the trachea. The longus colli muscle (Lc) is seen posteriorly on the right, and the esophagus (E) is seen posterior to left thyroid.

found at the upper pole of each lobe, the inferior thyroidal vein is found at the lower pole, and the inferior thyroidal artery is located posterior to the lower third of each lobe (**Fig. 3**). The recurrent laryngeal nerve and the inferior thyroidal artery pass in the angle between the trachea, esophagus, and thyroid lobe.

Histologically each lobe of the thyroid gland consists of numerous follicles that constitute the structural and functional unit of the gland. Each

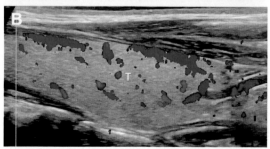

Fig. 2. Normal thyroid. (*A*) Longitudinal view of the thyroid (T) shows the lenticular shape of the thyroid and hyperechogenicity of the thyroid compared with the overlying strap muscles (S) and the sterno-cleidomastoid muscles (Sc). The longus colli muscle (Lc) is seen posteriorly. (*B*) Longitudinal color Doppler view of the thyroid (T) shows normal flow throughout the thyroid gland.

follicle consists of a single layer of cuboidal epithelial cells constituting the follicular epithelium, enclosing a central lumen containing a colloid substance rich in thyroglobulin. The shape of the normal follicles ranges from round to oval, and they show considerable variation based on the degree of gland activity. Thyroid follicles are composed of 2 endocrine cell populations: follicular cells, responsible for secreting T3 and T4 hormones that control basal metabolism; and C cells or parafollicular cells, mainly known for producing calcitonin, a hypocalcemic and hypophosphatemic hormone (**Fig. 4**).

CONGENITAL THYROID ABNORMALITIES

Congenital abnormalities of the thyroid gland include thyroid ectopia, hypoplasia, or aplasia. Ectopic thyroid is a rare entity resulting from abnormal development of the thyroid gland during embryogenesis. It is typically found in a midline suprahyoid position between the foramen cecum of the tongue and the epiglottis. Alternatively, ectopic tissue can be found sublingually, intratracheally, paralaryngeally, laterally within the neck, or in distant places such as the mediastinum and subdiaphragmatic organs. Ultrasonography plays little role in the evaluation of thyroid ectopia. Instead, nuclear medicine scans are more commonly used to detect ectopic thyroid tissue. By contrast, hypoplastic and aplastic thyroid are easily evaluated with ultrasonography.

Thyroglossal duct cysts, which are cysts of epithelial remnants of thyroglossal duct, are the most common form of congenital cyst in the neck. During embryologic development, as the thyroid migrates from the foramen cecum of tongue to the lower neck along a path through the tongue, hyoid bone, and neck muscles, it

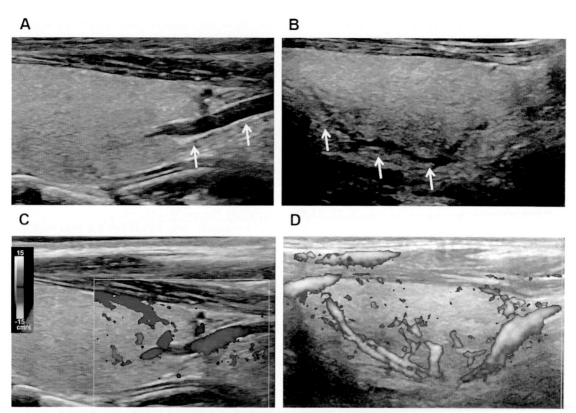

Fig. 3. Major blood of vessels of the thyroid gland. Longitudinal view of the thyroid shows (*A*) inferior thyroid vein at the inferior pole of the thyroid (*arrows*) and (*B*) inferior thyroidal thyroid artery along the posterior surface of the thyroid (*arrows*). (*C*) Color and (*D*) power Doppler images illustrating the same.

leaves an epithelial tract called the thyroglossal duct. This duct normally involutes in the eighth week of fetal life. Thyroid cells may remain in the thyroglossal duct in 5% of cases. Despite the embryogenesis, thyroid tissue is usually not detected pathologically in resected specimens.[3] Thyroglossal duct cysts are typically located in the midline between the thyroid gland and the hyoid bone. Fewer than 20% are suprahyoid. On sonography, thyroglossal duct cysts appear as a

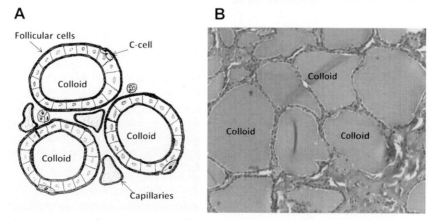

Fig. 4. Histologic components of the normal thyroid gland. (*A*) Diagram of the thyroid follicles. Each follicle consists of a simple layer of cuboidal epithelial cells, the follicular epithelium enclosing a central lumen containing colloid. C cells are sparse and typically not distinguishable from follicular cells. (*B*) Hematoxylin and eosin stain shows follicular epithelium enclosing a central lumen containing colloid. ([*B*] *Courtesy of* R. Chernock, MD, Washington University School of Medicine, St Louis, MO).

cystic lesion with low-level internal reflectors, and usually do not appear as simple cysts (**Fig. 5**).

NODULAR THYROID DISEASE

Thyroid nodules are extremely common and are found in 4% to 8% of adults via palpation,[4] 10% to 41% by ultrasonography,[5–8] and 50% of autopsy studies in patients with clinically normal thyroid.[9] The prevalence of nodules increases with age, and the percentage of patients with nodules is approximately equal to the age in years minus 10.[3]

The overwhelming majority of thyroid nodules are benign and the incidence of malignancy is low, at 3% to 5%.[10] The incidence of thyroid cancer for patients with thyroid nodules selected for fine-needle aspiration (FNA) is 9% to 13 %, no matter how many nodules are present on ultrasonography.[11–13] Based on American Cancer Society estimates, in 2013 there were 60,220 new cases of thyroid cancer and 1850 deaths from thyroid cancer. Thyroid cancer accounts for 3.6% of all new cancer cases and 0.3% of all cancer deaths.[14] Risk factors for thyroid cancer include family history of thyroid cancer, history of head and neck radiation, male gender, age younger than 30 or older than 60 years, and multiple endocrine neoplasia (MEN) type II.

Over the past several decades the incidence of thyroid cancer has increased, with an annual estimated rate of increase of 3% in the past decade.[15,16] Although increasing incidence along with stable overall mortality has been attributed to increased detection of small subclinical cancers rather than an increase in the true occurrence of thyroid cancer,[15] an analysis at the National Cancer Institute's Surveillance Epidemiology and End Results (STEER) database found an increase in the rates of differentiated thyroid cancer of all sizes including tumors greater than 4 cm, suggesting that increased detection is not the sole explanation.[17] The clinical challenge is to distinguish the few clinically significant malignant nodules from the many benign ones, and to identify those patients for whom surgical excision is indicated.

Benign Nodules

Thyroid hyperplasia accounts for approximately 80% of nodular thyroid disease. Its etiology is related to iodine deficiency, familial causes, and idiopathic or poor utilization of iodine from medications. When hyperplasia results in an enlarged gland it is called a goiter. Women are 3 times more likely than men to have the disease, and the peak age of patients with goiter is between 35 and 50 years. Histologically the initial stage is cellular hyperplasia of the thyroid acini, which progresses to formation of micronodules and macronodules. Hyperplastic nodules often undergo liquefactive degeneration with accumulation of blood, serous fluid, or colloid substance. Pathologically nodules are designated as hyperplastic, adenomatous, or colloid. Sonographically these nodules demonstrate a common appearance, frequently with cystic components. When cystic components are predominant, they are usually associated with multiple internal septations and mural nodules. Bright internal punctate echogenic foci, often with comet-tail artifact on ultrasonography, indicate inspissated colloid. Less frequently a hypoechoic sponge-like or honeycomb pattern is seen. Hyperplastic nodules demonstrate variable echogenicity, including hypoechoic, isoechoic, or hyperechoic relative to the normal thyroid parenchyma (**Fig. 6**).

Benign follicular adenoma

Benign follicular adenomas represent 5% to 10% of all nodular disease of the thyroid. Most patients have no thyroid dysfunction. A small minority of follicular adenomas will cause symptomatic hyperthyroidism. Benign follicular adenoma is a true thyroid neoplasm of follicular-cell differentiation that

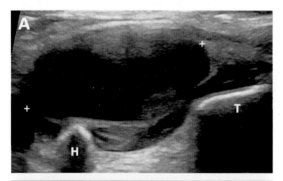

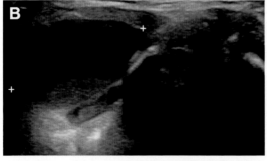

Fig. 5. Thyroglossal duct cyst. (*A*) Longitudinal and (*B*) transverse views of the midline of the neck in the suprathyroid region show a complex cystic lesion with low-level internal echoes consistent with a thyroglossal duct cyst (*cursors*). H, hyoid bone; T, thyroid cartilage.

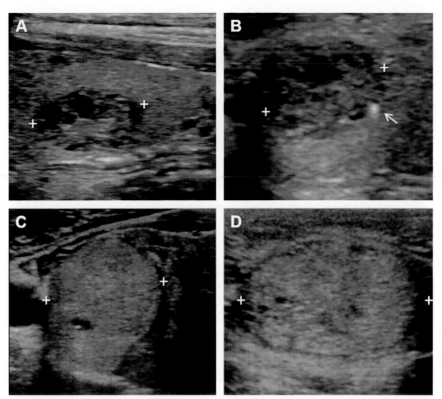

Fig. 6. Nodular hyperplasia (*cursors*) in different patients. (*A, B*) Hypoechoic predominantly solid nodules with multiple small internal cystic spaces; this is the typical appearance of small lesions. Arrow in *B* shows an additional finding of inspissated colloid, which casts a comet-tail artifact. (*C, D*) Transverse and longitudinal images of a large, hyperechoic solid nodule with minimal internal cystic spaces and a peripheral hypoechoic halo. This nodule simulates a follicular neoplasm.

consists of microfollicular architecture with follicles lined by cuboidal epithelial cells. Subtypes include fetal adenoma, Hurthle cell adenoma, and embryonal adenoma, based on character and pattern of cell proliferation. Follicular adenomas are distinguished from follicular carcinomas based only on vascular or capsular invasion, features identified by histologic rather than cytologic analysis. Therefore, FNA biopsy results of a follicular lesion are generally followed by surgical resection. Sonographically, benign follicular adenomas are typically solid and range from hypoechoic to hyperechoic. These adenomas are well marginated and often have a peripheral smooth hypoechoic halo. Well-defined cystic spaces occur in a minority of these nodules (**Fig. 7**).

Malignant Nodules

Most thyroid cancers are derived from follicular epithelium[18] and are well differentiated. Histopathologic classification of these tumors comprises papillary carcinoma 75% to 80%, follicular carcinoma 10% to 20%, medullary carcinoma 3% to 5%, and anaplastic carcinoma 1% to 2%.[4] Malignancy of other origin, including lymphoma (1%–2%) and metastatic disease (0.5%–1%) (lung, breast, renal, gastrointestinal, or melanoma), is an uncommon cause of thyroid carcinoma.[19]

Papillary thyroid carcinoma occurs more frequently in women than in men and typically presents in the 20- to 55-year-old age group. It accounts for 75% to 80% of thyroid malignancies. Lymphatic dissemination is much more common than hematogenous spread, and cervical lymph node metastases are often present at the time of diagnosis. Papillary thyroid carcinoma has an excellent prognosis, and the presence of metastatic cervical lymph nodes has little effect on the prognosis. Papillary carcinoma is multicentric within the thyroid gland in at least 20% of cases.[20] Microcalcifications, which result from deposition of calcium salts in psammoma bodies, are common in papillary carcinoma and are one of the most specific features of thyroid malignancy.[11,21] Microcalcifications and cystic degenerative areas

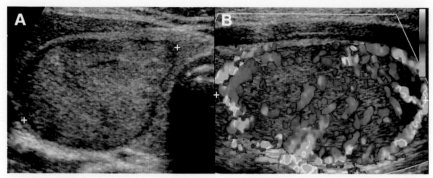

Fig. 7. Follicular adenoma. (A) Transverse view shows a solid hypoechoic nodule with thin peripheral hypoechoic halo (*cursors*). (B) Longitudinal color Doppler view of the same nodule shows hypervascularity of the nodule (*cursors*).

in lymph nodes are also very typical of papillary carcinoma. Of note, inspissated colloid, which is very common in nodular hyperplasia, can be confused with microcalcification. Sonographic features of papillary thyroid carcinoma include solid hypoechoic mass, tiny echogenic foci caused by microcalcifications (±posterior acoustic shadowing), nodular margins, a taller than wide shape, and cervical lymph node metastasis, which may contain microcalcifications or cystic components (**Fig. 8**).

Follicular carcinoma is the second type of well-differentiated thyroid cancer, accounting for approximately 10% to 20% of thyroid malignancies. It is more common in women in the sixth decade of life, and is divided into minimally and widely invasive forms. Follicular carcinoma tends to spread hematogenously rather than via lymphatics, especially to bone, brain, lung, and liver. Metastases to neck nodes are rare in follicular carcinoma. As already stated, follicular carcinoma overlaps in appearance with follicular adenoma,

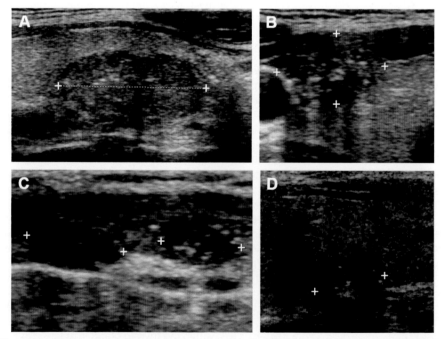

Fig. 8. Papillary thyroid cancer in different patients. (A) Longitudinal view of the thyroid shows a solid, hypoechoic lesion with lobulated borders and microcalcifications (*cursors*). (B) Transverse view shows a solid, hypoechoic lesion with indistinct margins and microcalcifications (*cursors*). (C) Longitudinal view of the isthmus shows 2 lesions (*cursors*). The lesion on the left is very hypoechoic to nearly anechoic, and the lesion to the right has microcalcifications. (D) Longitudinal view of the inferior thyroid shows a very hypoechoic solid lesion with internal calcifications (*cursors*).

and it is not possible to distinguish these lesions with sonography or FNA. However, in a retrospective review of thyroid follicular lesions, Sillery and colleagues[22] showed that larger lesion size, lack of sonographic halo, hypoechoic appearance, and absence of cystic change favored a diagnosis of follicular carcinoma (**Fig. 9**). Increased patient age and male sex were also associated with malignancy.

Medullary carcinoma is derived from parafollicular or C cells, and typically secretes calcitonin; therefore, serum calcitonin can be used as a tumor marker. It accounts for 5% of thyroid malignancies. Whereas up to 25% are hereditary (familial medullary thyroid cancer, MEN IIA and MEN IIB), most cases (75%) are sporadic.[23] Medullary carcinoma demonstrates more aggressive behavior than the differentiated carcinomas, and is characterized by early lymphatic spread, distant hematogenous metastasis to the liver, lungs, and bones, and a 10-year survival of 75% to 80%.[23] It does not respond to chemotherapy and radiation therapy. Sonographically, medullary carcinoma has features that overlap with papillary carcinomas, including hypoechoic solid mass with microcalcifications in both primary tumor and nodal metastasis (**Fig. 10**). In one study, however, medullary carcinoma differed from papillary carcinoma in that the former was larger, and had a more homogeneous echotexture and increased frequency of cystic changes.[24]

Anaplastic carcinoma is a highly aggressive, undifferentiated carcinoma that is derived from thyroid follicular epithelium. It accounts for less than 1% to 2% of thyroid malignancies. Anaplastic carcinoma is rarely seen in patients younger than 60 years, is more common in women, and has a dismal prognosis. At presentation these lesions are typically large, with a mean reported size of 7 to 8 cm. More than 50% of patients will have extrathyroidal tumor extension and/or metastasis to

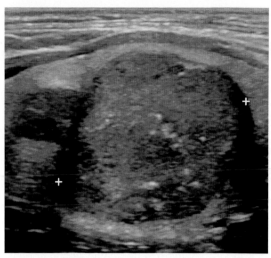

Fig. 10. Medullary thyroid cancer. Longitudinal view shows a solid, hypoechoic nodule with internal calcifications (*cursors*), an appearance very similar that of papillary thyroid cancer.

lymph nodes or distant metastases at the time of diagnosis (**Fig. 11**).[23]

Primary thyroid lymphoma represents less than 5% of thyroid malignancy, and can occur as a manifestation of generalized lymphoma or as a primary abnormality. It is mostly of the non-Hodgkin variety and usually affects elderly women. Chronic lymphocytic thyroiditis or Hashimoto thyroiditis is found in more than 90% of cases of thyroid lymphoma.[25] On sonography, thyroid lymphoma is usually a large, solid, hypoechoic mass that infiltrates much of the thyroid parenchyma (**Fig. 12**).

Metastases to the thyroid are infrequent, occurring late in the course of neoplastic disease, most commonly from lung, breast, and renal cancers.

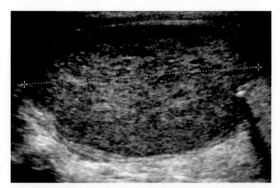

Fig. 9. Follicular cancer. Longitudinal view shows a large, solid, heterogeneous, hypoechoic nodule replacing most of the thyroid gland (*cursors*).

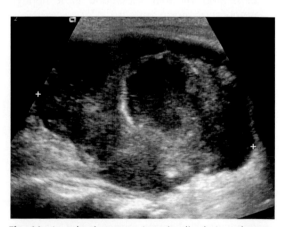

Fig. 11. Anaplastic cancer. Longitudinal view shows a large, lobulated, primarily solid hypoechoic mass replacing the entire thyroid gland. There is a central cystic component (*cursors*).

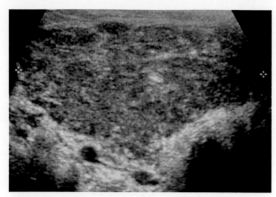

Fig. 12. Lymphoma. Transverse view shows a markedly enlarged heterogeneous, hypoechoic thyroid (*cursors*).

On sonography there is no characteristic appearance, but metastases should be considered when a solitary nodule is identified in a patient with known extrathyroidal malignancy.

Distinguishing Benign from Malignant Nodules

Although considerable overlap exists in the sonographic appearance of benign and malignant disease, there are sonographic findings that favor one or the other.

Sonographic findings that favor benign disease include:

- Simple cysts
- Nodule with predominantly cystic components
- Cystic nodules with internal echogenic foci with posterior reverberation "comet-tail" artifacts
- Nodules containing multiple cystic spaces separated by thin septations in a honeycomb/spongiform pattern.[21,26,27]

Sonographic findings that favor malignancy include:

- Entirely solid with marked hypoechogenicity compared with the strap muscles
- Microcalcifications or peripheral calcifications
- Thick irregular halo; irregular lobulated margins
- More tall than wide (anteroposterior dimension on both longitudinal or transverse views)
- Refractive shadows from the edge of a solid hypoechoic lesion
- Direct tumor invasion of adjacent soft tissues
- Associated lymph nodes that appear malignant, especially if they contain microcalcifications or cystic areas of necrosis.[21,26,27]

Checklist for evaluating sonographic features of a thyroid nodule include:

1. Internal consistency
   a. Solid
   b. Mixed solid and cystic
   c. Purely cystic
2. Echogenicity relative to the adjacent thyroid parenchyma
   a. Hypoechoic
   b. Isoechoic
   c. Hyperechoic
3. Margin
   a. Smooth
   b. Irregular or lobulated
   c. Poorly defined
4. Presence and pattern of calcification
   a. Microcalcification
   b. Macrocalcification
   c. Peripheral calcification
5. Peripheral hypoechoic halo
   a. Thin and smooth
   b. Thick and irregular
6. Presence and distribution of blood flow signal
   a. No blood flow
   b. Presence of blood flow
      i. Peripheral
      ii. Central

Sonographic findings that favor benign disease include: simple cysts; nodule with predominantly cystic components; cystic nodules with internal echogenic foci with posterior reverberation "comet-tail" artifacts; and nodules containing multiple cystic spaces separated by thin septations in a honeycomb/spongiform pattern.[21,26,27]

Sonographic findings that favor malignancy include: entirely solid with marked hypoechogenicity compared with the strap muscles; microcalcifications or peripheral calcifications; thick irregular halo; irregular lobulated margins; more tall than wide (anteroposterior dimension on both longitudinal or transverse views); refractive shadows from the edge of a solid hypoechoic lesion; direct tumor invasion of adjacent soft tissues; and associated lymph nodes that appear malignant, especially if they contain microcalcifications or cystic areas of necrosis.[21,26,27]

GUIDELINES FOR FINE-NEEDLE ASPIRATION OF THYROID NODULES

FNA biopsy of thyroid nodules is a safe and minimally invasive procedure performed to obtain cytologic evaluation of nodules. It is the most accurate and cost-effective method for the diagnostic evaluation of thyroid nodules. Ultrasound-guided FNA has a sensitivity of 77% to 98%, specificity of

71% to 100%, false-negative rate of 0% to 5%, false-positive rate of 0% to 5.7%, and overall accuracy of 69% to 97%.[28]

At present there are multiple guidelines for thyroid FNA:

1. The Society of Radiologists in Ultrasound suggest that FNA should be considered for a nodule 1 cm or bigger at the largest diameter if microcalcifications are present, and for a nodule 1.5 cm or larger if the nodule is almost entirely solid or there are coarse calcifications within the nodule.[4]
2. The American Association of Clinical Endocrinologists recommends FNA even for nodules smaller than 1 cm whenever clinical information and sonographic features arouse suspicion about the presence of malignancy or for all hypoechoic nodules larger than 1 cm with irregular margin, increased vascularity, tall configuration, or microcalcifications.[29]
3. American Thyroid Association (ATA) guidelines recommend biopsy in high-risk patients if a nodule is larger than 5 mm with suspicious features. In low-risk patients ATA recommends biopsy of: nodules larger than 1 cm if microcalcifications are present, or if the nodule is solid and hypoechoic; isoechoic to hyperechoic nodules from 1 to 1.5 cm in size; mixed cystic and solid nodules with suspicious features between 1.5 and 2 cm in size, or without suspicious sonographic features if it is larger than 2 cm; a spongiform nodule larger than 2 cm; and abnormal cervical lymph nodes (**Table 1**).[30]
4. The Korean Task Force recommends biopsy for all nodules with features suspicious for malignancy. If the nodule is smaller than 5 mm, FNA biopsy is selected based on risk factors of the patient and experience of the clinician.[31]

Although size is a common criterion used by many guidelines in the identification of thyroid nodules for biopsy, many investigators have demonstrated that nodule size is not predictive of malignancy.[4,11,21,32] In fact, sonographic features of nodules are more useful than nodule size in identifying nodules that are likely to be malignant. Kwak and colleagues[33] analyzed sonographic features of thyroid nodules associated with significant risk of thyroid carcinoma: solid component, hypoechogenicity/marked hypoechogenicity, microlobulated or irregular margins, microcalcifications, and taller than wide shape. As the number of suspicious imaging features increased, the probability and risk of malignancy within a nodule increased. The risk of malignancy was 3.3% in patients with 1 suspicious

Table 1
Revised American Thyroid Association guidelines indicating sonographic and clinical features of nodules with recommended nodule threshold size for fine-needle aspiration

US/Clinical Features	Size for FNA (mm)	
High-risk history[a]		
Malignant US features[b]	>5	(Rec A)
No malignant US features	>5	(Rec I)
Abnormal lymph nodes	All (or node)	(Rec A)
Microcalcifications	≥10	(Rec B)
Solid nodule		
Hypoechoic	>10	(Rec B)
Isoechoic/hyperechoic	≥10–15	(Rec C)
Mixed solid and cystic		
With malignant US features	≥10–15	(Rec B)
Without malignant US features	≥20	(Rec C)
Spongiform	≥20	(Rec C)
Cyst	No FNA	(Rec E)

Recommendations: A, strongly recommends; B, recommends based on fair evidence; C, recommends based on expert opinion; E, recommends against, based on fair evidence; I, recommends neither for nor against, insufficient evidence.

Abbreviations: FNA, fine-needle aspiration; Rec, recommendation; US, ultrasonographic.

[a] Family history, radiotherapy as a child, radiation exposure as a child, hemithyroidectomy + presence of carcinoma, positive on positron emission tomography scan, risk of medullary thyroid cancer.

[b] Microcalcifications, hypoechoic, increased vascularity, infiltrative margins, taller than wide.

Adapted from Cooper DS, Doherty G, Haugen BR, et al. Revised American Thyroid Association management guideline for patients with thyroid nodules and differentiated thyroid cancer. Thyroid 2009;19:1167–214.

sonographic feature and 87.5% in patients with all 5 suspicious sonographic features.

It is particularly important when evaluating patients with multiple thyroid nodules for FNA to carefully evaluate the sonographic features of each nodule and not merely target the dominant nodule. Recent literature indicates that patients with multiple thyroid nodules have the same risk of malignancy as patients with solitary thyroid nodule.[11,34] Moreover, Frates and colleagues[4,35] reported that in cases of multiple thyroid nodules, the likelihood of an individual thyroid nodule being cancerous is decreased, but the likelihood of thyroid cancer does not differ between patients with a solitary nodule and patients with multiple nodules. Therefore, in the presence of multiple thyroid nodules, adequate evaluation warrants a meticulous search for suspicious sonographic features.

CYTOLOGIC FINDINGS AND FOLLOW-UP STRATEGIES
The Thyroid Bethesda System

In 2009, the Bethesda System for Reporting Thyroid Cytopathology was created out of the need for a unified system for interpretation of thyroid FNA. Project participants created a framework that would facilitate communication among various physicians, facilitate cytologic-histologic correlation for thyroid disease, facilitate research, and allow easy and reliable sharing of data from different laboratories. The terminology framework produced was based on a literature search dating back to 1995 and formal interdisciplinary discussions. The Bethesda System recommends that each cytopathology report begin with 1 of 6 general diagnostic categories. Each of the categories has an implied cancer risk that links it to an appropriate clinical management guideline (Table 2).[36,37]

The physician must understand the cytopathologic findings before selecting an appropriate follow-up strategy for the patient. An FNA biopsy specimen is either diagnostic or nondiagnostic. Criteria for cytologic adequacy include the presence of at least 6 follicular cell groups, each containing 10 to 15 cells derived from at least 2 aspirates of a nodule.[30] A nondiagnostic cytology is usually the result of a smear that contains too few cells to allow a diagnosis. This problem typically results from excessive blood, necrotic material, or debris obscuring cellular details or from poor fixation, preparation, or staining.[38] Nondiagnostic finding is usually listed as "cellular insufficiency," "unsatisfactory," or "inadequate" in the report. Nondiagnostic results range from approximately 5% to 15%. A diagnostic cytologic finding is characterized as malignant, indeterminate (follicular or Hurthle cell neoplasm, or possible papillary carcinoma), or benign.

Malignant findings
Most malignant nodules are papillary thyroid carcinoma. If an FNA biopsy specimen indicates malignancy, surgery is recommended.[30]

Indeterminate findings
Indeterminate findings include follicular and Hurthle cell neoplasms and findings suggestive of papillary thyroid carcinoma. As stated earlier, FNA cannot be used to distinguish a benign follicular neoplasm from a malignant neoplasm. Thyroid scintigraphy with radioactive iodine may be helpful. If a concordant autonomously functioning nodule is not seen, lobectomy or total thyroidectomy should be considered. If the cytologic diagnosis is "suspicious for papillary carcinoma" or "Hurthle cell neoplasm," lobectomy or total thyroidectomy is recommended, depending on the lesion size and other risk factors.[30]

Benign findings
Most benign thyroid nodules are nonneoplastic, adenomatoid nodules with a variable amount of colloid, or an increased number of follicular epithelial cells or lymphocytic thyroiditis. If an FNA biopsy specimen is benign, further immediate diagnostic studies or treatment are not routinely required.[30] A repeat FNA biopsy should be considered if there is discordance between imaging and cytologic findings.[28] Some investigators proposed a 3-month interval between the initial FNA and repeat FNA to avoid problems in cytologic interpretation that may be posed by

---

Table 2
The Bethesda System for reporting cytopathology illustrating the diagnostic category, implied risk of malignancy, and recommended clinical management

Diagnostic Category	Risk of Malignancy (%)	Usual Management
Nondiagnostic or unsatisfactory	1–4	Repeat FNA with ultrasonography
Benign	0–3	Follow
Atypia or follicular lesion of undetermined significance	~5–15	Repeat FNA
Follicular neoplasm or suspicious for a follicular neoplasm	15–30	Surgical lobectomy
Suspicious for malignancy	60–75	Lobectomy or total thyroidectomy
Malignant	97–99	Total thyroidectomy

Adapted from Cibas ES, Ali SZ. The Bethesda System for reporting thyroid cytopathology. Thyroid 2009;19:1159–65.

reparative cellular atypia.[39,40] Others have demonstrated that the diagnostic yield and accuracy of repeat FNA is independent of the time interval between procedures, but may be related to the original FNA diagnosis.[41] Repeat biopsy of nodules with previously benign cytology should be considered when there has been significant interval growth, defined as a greater than 50% increase in estimated nodule volume over a period of 1 year.

DIFFUSE THYROID DISEASE

There are several thyroid diseases characterized by diffuse thyroid involvement. Most common are subacute thyroiditis, Hashimoto thyroiditis, and Graves disease.

Hashimoto thyroiditis, also known as chronic autoimmune lymphocytic thyroiditis, results from an autoimmune-mediated destruction of the thyroid gland. It typically affects middle-aged women. Patients may be euthyroid initially, but generally become hypothyroid owing to replacement of functioning thyroid tissue caused by infiltration of lymphocytes and plasma cells. The diagnosis is often made serologically. Hashimoto thyroiditis is the most common cause of hypothyroidism in the United States. There is a slight increased risk for thyroid lymphoma in patients with Hashimoto thyroiditis. On sonography, the thyroid gland is normal in size or enlarged, hypoechoic, diffusely heterogeneous, with thin echogenic fibrous septations that may cause a multilobulated or micronodular appearance. Often there is hypervascularity. Not infrequently, cervical lymphadenopathy is present. In addition to diffuse involvement, Hashimoto thyroiditis can produce focal nodules that have a highly variable sonographic appearance. These nodules may occur with background parenchymal changes that are typical of diffuse Hashimoto thyroiditis, or may occur with relatively normal background parenchyma (**Fig. 13**).[42]

Graves disease is the most common cause of hyperthyroidism. It is more common in young women but can occur in persons of any age. It is an autoimmune disease in which the body produces antibodies to the receptor for thyroid-stimulating hormone as well as thyroglobulin and/or the thyroid hormones, resulting in hyperthyroidism. In most cases the diagnosis is made with clinical signs and a blood test. On sonography, findings include gland enlargement, decreased echogenicity, occasional heterogeneity, and hypervascularity (**Fig. 14**). The sonographic appearance of Graves disease and Hashimoto thyroiditis often overlap.

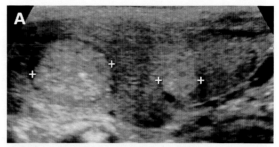
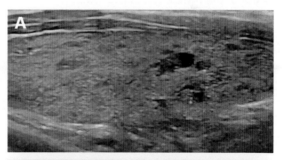

Fig. 13. Hashimoto thyroiditis. (*A*) Longitudinal view shows a slightly hypoechoic, heterogeneous thyroid gland with discrete hyperechoic nodules (*cursors*). (*B*) Color Doppler shows marked hypervascularity throughout the thyroid gland. Fine-needle aspiration of the dominant nodule confirmed that it was due to Hashimoto thyroiditis.

Subacute granulomatous thyroiditis, also known as de Quervain thyroiditis, is an uncommon cause of hyperthyroidism and affects women more often than men. It is presumed to be caused by a viral

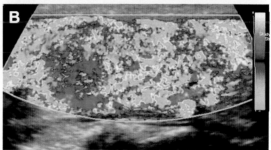
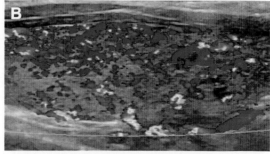

Fig. 14. Graves disease. (*A*) Longitudinal view shows a hypoechoic gland. (*B*) Color Doppler images shows diffuse hypervascularity of the gland.

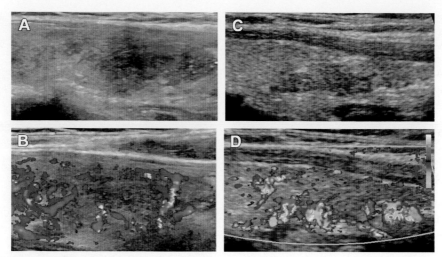

Fig. 15. Subacute thyroiditis. (*A*) Longitudinal and (*B*) color Doppler views show poorly marginated regions of decreased echogenicity in the inferior gland with decreased blood flow in this area. (*C, D*) follow-up imaging 4 months later shows interval decrease in size of the involved area.

infection or postviral inflammatory process, typically 2 to 8 weeks following an upper respiratory infection. Patients often present with an enlarged, painful thyroid gland. The involvement may be diffuse or focal. Hyperthyroidism is typical at presentation, followed by euthyroidism, hypothyroidism, and, ultimately, restoration of normal thyroid function. On sonography there is a poorly marginated area or areas of decreased echogenicity in the involved regions of the thyroid. There may be normal or decreased vascularity owing to diffuse edema of the thyroid gland (**Fig. 15**).

REFERENCES

1. Solbiati L, Charboneau W, Reading CC, et al. The thyroid gland. In: Rumack CM, Wilson SR, Charboneau JW, et al, editors. Diagnostic ultrasound. 4th edition. Philadelphia: Elsevier Mosby, Inc; 2011.

2. Som PM, Curtin HD, Mancuso AA. Imaging-based classification of neck metastatic adenopathy. AJR Am J Roentgenol 2000;174:837–84.

3. Middleton WD, Kurtz AB, Hertzberg BS. Neck and chest. In: Thrall JH, editor. Ultrasound: the requisites. 2nd edition. St Louis (MO): Mosby; 2004.

4. Frates MC, Benson CB, Charboneau JW, et al. Management of thyroid nodules detected at US: Society of Radiologist in Ultrasound consensus conference statement. Radiology 2005;237:794–800.

5. Wiest PW, Hartshorne MF, Inskip PD, et al. Thyroid palpation versus high-resolution thyroid ultrasonography in the detection of nodules. J Ultrasound Med 1998;17:487–96.

6. Carrol BA. Asymptomatic thyroid nodule: incidental sonographic detection. AJR Am J Roentgenol 1982;138:499–501.

7. Brander A, Vlikinkoski F, Nickels J, et al. Thyroid gland: US screening in a random adult population. Radiology 1991;181:683–7.

8. Bruneton JN, Balu-Maestro C, Marcy PY, et al. Very high frequency (13 MHZ) ultrasonographic examination of the normal neck: detection of normal lymph nodes and thyroid nodules. J Ultrasound Med 1994;13:87–90.

9. Mortensen JD, Woolner LB, Bennett WA. Gross and microscopic findings in clinically normal thyroid glands. J Clin Endocrinol Metab 1955;15:1270–80.

10. Bonavita JA, Mayo J, Babb J, et al. Pattern recognition of benign nodules at ultrasound of the thyroid: which nodules can be left alone? AJR Am J Roentgenol 2009;193:207–13.

11. Papini E, Guglielmi R, Bianchini A, et al. Risk of malignancy in nonpalpable thyroid nodules: predictive value of ultrasound and color-Doppler features. J Clin Endocrinol Metab 2002;897:1941–6.

12. Hegedus L, Bonnema SJ, Bennedbaek FN. Management of simple nodular goiter: current status and future perspectives. Endocr Rev 2003;24:102–32.

13. Nam-Goong IS, Kim HY, Gong G, et al. Ultrasonography-guided fine-needle aspiration of thyroid incidentaloma: correlation with pathological findings. Clin Endocrinol 2004;60:21–8.

14. Thyroid cancer (n.d.). Steer Statistic American Cancer Society. Thyroid, cancer, key statistics. Available at: www.cancer.org/cancer/thyroid. Accessed May 21, 2013.

15. Davies L, Welch HG. Increasing incidence of thyroid cancer in the United States, 1973-2002. JAMA 2006; 295:2164–7.

16. Morris LG, Sikora AG, Tosteson TD, et al. The increasing incidence of thyroid cancer: the influence of access to care. Thyroid 2013;23:885–91.

17. Chen AY, Jemal A, Ward EM. Increasing incidence of differentiated thyroid cancer in the United States, 1988-2005. Cancer 2009;115:3801–7.

18. Grebe SK, Hay ID. Follicular cell-derived thyroid carcinoma. In: Arnold A, editor. Cancer treatment and research. Endocrine neoplasms, vol. 18. Norwell (MA): Kluwer Academic; 1997. p. 91–140.

19. Lam KY, Lo CY. Metastatic tumors of the thyroid gland: a study of 79 cases in Chinese patients. Arch Pathol Lab Med 1998;122:37–41.

20. Black BM, Kirk TA, Woolner LB. Multicentricity of papillary adenocarcinoma of the thyroid; influence on treatment. J Clin Endocrinol Metab 1960;20:130–5.

21. Kim EK, Park CS, Chung WY, et al. New sonographic criteria for recommending fine-needle aspiration biopsy of nonpalpable solid nodules of the thyroid. AJR Am J Roentgenol 2002;178:687–91.

22. Sillery JC, Reading CC, Charboneau JW, et al. Thyroid follicular carcinoma: sonographic features of 50 cases. AJR Am J Roentgenol 2010;194:44–54.

23. Pitt SC, Moley JF. Medullary, anaplastic, and metastatic cancers of the thyroid. Semin Oncol 2010;37:567–79.

24. Lee S, Shin JH, Han BK, et al. Medullary thyroid carcinoma: comparison with papillary thyroid carcinoma and application of current sonographic criteria. AJR Am J Roentgenol 2010;194:1090–4.

25. Widder S, Pasieka JL. Primary thyroid lymphomas. Curr Treat Options Oncol 2004;5:307–13.

26. Reading CC, Charboneau JW, Hay ID, et al. Sonography of thyroid nodules: a classic pattern diagnostic approach. Ultrasound Q 2005;21:157–65.

27. Hoang JK, Lee WK, Lee M, et al. US features of thyroid malignancy: pearls and pitfalls. Radiographics 2007;27:847–65.

28. Kim MJ, Kim EK, Park SI, et al. US-guided fine-needle aspiration of thyroid nodules: indications, techniques, results. Radiographics 2008;28:1869–89.

29. Gharib H, Papini E, Paschke R, et al. AACE/AME/ETA thyroid nodule guidelines. Endocr Pract 2010;16(Supp1):1–43.

30. Cooper DS, Doherty G, Haugen BR, et al. Revised American Thyroid Association management guideline for patients with thyroid nodules and differentiated thyroid cancer. Thyroid 2009;19:1167–214.

31. Moon WJ, Baek JH, Jung SL, et al. Ultrasonography and the ultrasound and ultrasound based management of thyroid nodules: consensus statement and recommendations. Korean J Radiol 2011;12:1–14.

32. Hamberger B, Gharib H, Melton LJ, et al. Fine needle aspiration biopsy of thyroid nodules; impact on thyroid practice and cost of care. Am J Med 1982;73:381–4.

33. Kwak JY, Han KH, Yoon JH, et al. Thyroid imaging reporting and data system for US features of nodules: a step in establishing better stratification of cancer risk. Radiology 2011;260:892–9.

34. Tollin SR, Mery GM, Jelveh N, et al. The use of fine-needle aspiration biopsy under ultrasound guidance to assess the risk of malignancy in patients with a multinodular goiter. Thyroid 2000;10:235–41.

35. Frates MC, Bendon CB, Doubilet PM, et al. Prevalence and distribution of carcinoma in patients with solitary and multiple thyroid nodules on sonography. J Clin Endocrinol Metab 2006;91:3411–7.

36. Cibas ES, Ali SZ. The Bethesda System for reporting thyroid cytopathology. Thyroid 2009;19:1159–65.

37. Baloch ZW, Livolsi VA, Asa SL, et al. Diagnostic terminology and morphologic criteria for cytologic diagnosis of thyroid lesions: a synopsis of the National Cancer Institute Thyroid Fine-Needle Aspiration State of the Science Conference. Diagn Cytopathol 2008;36:425–37.

38. Papanicolaou Society of Cytopathology Task Force on Standards of Practice. Guidelines for Papanicolaou Society of Cytopathology for fine-needle aspiration procedure reporting. Diagn Cytopathol 1997;17:239–47.

39. Baloch ZW, LiVolsi VA. Post fine-needle aspiration histologic alterations of thyroid revisited. Am J Clin Pathol 1999;112:311–6.

40. LiVolsi VA, Merino MJ. Worrisome histologic alterations following fine-needle aspiration of the thyroid (WHAFFT). Pathol Annu 1994;29:99–120.

41. Singh RS, Wang HH. Timing of repeat thyroid fine-needle aspiration on the management of thyroid nodules. Acta Cytol 2011;55:544–8.

42. Anderson L, Middleton WD, Teefey SA, et al. Hashimoto thyroiditis: part 1, sonographic analysis of the nodular form of Hashimoto thyroiditis. AJR Am J Roentgenol 2010;195:208–15.

Parathyroid Sonography

Vincent M. Mellnick, MD*, William D. Middleton, MD

KEYWORDS

- Parathyroid adenoma • Hyperparathyroidism • Parathyroid hormone

KEY POINTS

- Ultrasonography plays a crucial role in preoperative localization of abnormal parathyroid glands to facilitate minimally invasive surgical techniques.
- The accuracy of ultrasonography in characterizing parathyroid disease is augmented by correlation with scintigraphy, although neither technique excels in multigland disease or after failed surgical resection.
- Cystic degeneration of parathyroid adenomas, parathyroid cysts, lipoadenomas, and parathyroid carcinoma are uncommon entities but could be encountered on sonography.
- Normal structures and other diseases may simulate parathyroid disease on sonography, including thyroid nodules and septa, cervical lymph nodes, and blood vessels.
- Fine-needle aspiration of parathyroid lesions for parathyroid hormone levels can be a useful adjunct to identify abnormal glands. Cytologic analysis of parathyroid lesions cannot consistently differentiate them from thyroid tissue.

DISCUSSION OF PROBLEM/CLINICAL PRESENTATION

Physiology

The parathyroid glands regulate calcium homeostasis by secretion of parathyroid hormone (PTH) from chief cells, which in turn increases renal reabsorption of calcium, decreases renal phosphate excretion, and stimulates osteoclasts. Hyperparathyroidism is classically categorized into primary, secondary, and tertiary subtypes. Although they may be asymptomatic, patients with hyperparathyroidism commonly present with symptoms of hypercalcemia, namely urinary tract stones, hypertension and abdominal and bone pain, as well as psychiatric symptoms, most commonly depression.

Primary Hyperparathyroidism

- Increased serum PTH and calcium levels
- Caused by parathyroid adenomas (90%), double adenomas (5%), hyperplasia (5%), and carcinomas (<1%)
- Treatment usually surgical excision
- Preoperative imaging commonly used

Primary hyperparathyroidism is caused by hyperfunctioning of the parathyroid glands themselves and manifests biochemically with abnormally increased serum levels of both PTH and calcium. Causes include adenomas, hyperplasia, and carcinoma of the parathyroid gland. This condition is most commonly caused by a single adenoma (approximately 90% of cases). Less commonly, it may occur in the setting of multigland disease, defined as either 2 adenomas (5%), or 4-gland hyperplasia (5%).[1,2] Parathyroid carcinoma accounts for less than 1% of cases of primary hyperparathyroidism and tends to produce worse laboratory abnormalities and more severe clinical symptoms.[2] Patients with multiple endocrine neoplasia (MEN) syndromes and other inherited causes of hyperparathyroidism comprise a small subset of primary hyperparathyroidism cases, occurring more commonly with type I MEN than in MEN IIA. Primary hyperparathyroidism is most

Disclosures: None.
Mallinckrodt Institute of Radiology, Washington University School of Medicine, 510 South Kingshighway Boulevard, St Louis, MO 63110, USA
* Corresponding author. Mallinckrodt Institute of Radiology, Washington University School of Medicine, 510 South Kingshighway Boulevard, Box 8131, St Louis, MO 63110.
E-mail address: mellnickv@mir.wustl.edu

Ultrasound Clin 9 (2014) 339–349
http://dx.doi.org/10.1016/j.cult.2014.02.001
1556-858X/14/$ –

often treated with surgical resection of the hypersecreting gland or glands.

Secondary Hyperparathyroidism

- Increased serum PTH and decreased serum calcium levels
- Caused by glandular hyperplasia as a result of end-stage renal disease (ESRD), vitamin D deficiency
- Treatment usually medical
- Imaging use controversial

Secondary hyperparathyroidism is PTH oversecretion occurring in response to hypocalcemia, most commonly caused by chronic renal insufficiency and vitamin D deficiency. This condition typically manifests with multiglandular hyperplasia and biochemically with high serum PTH and low calcium levels. Medical management is the mainstay of treatment of secondary hyperparathyroidism, with only approximately 5% of ESRD requiring surgery after failed pharmacologic therapy.[3] Preoperative localization of parathyroid glands using ultrasonography or scintigraphy can be performed in select cases, such as with persistent hyperparathyroidism after subtotal resection, but its use before primary parathyroidectomy remains controversial because of the high likelihood of multigland disease and a wide range of accuracy in the literature.[4–8]

Tertiary Hyperparathyroidism

- Increased serum PTH and calcium levels
- Caused by persistent glandular hyperplasia after correction of causative disease
- Treatment commonly surgical
- Imaging use controversial

Tertiary hyperparathyroidism occurs when longstanding secondary hyperparathyroidism results in parathyroid hyperplasia that secretes PTH autonomously regardless of serum calcium level, usually in the setting of ESRD. This disorder remains despite correction of the underlying cause, classically seen as persistent hyperparathyroidism after renal transplantation. Biochemically, these patients have increased serum calcium and PTH levels, frequently accompanied by hyperphosphatemia. Total or subtotal parathyroidectomy is usually the treatment of choice for tertiary hyperparathyroidism. Similar to secondary hyperparathyroidism, preoperative imaging can be used in some cases, but it is not commonly used, because of the frequent need for bilateral neck exploration and the varying reported sensitivity in this setting.[4–8]

Surgical approach

Depending on the subtype of hyperparathyroidism that a patient has and the number of glands affected, bilateral neck exploration (in patients with multigland disease) or unilateral minimally invasive surgery may be performed. Minimally invasive parathyroidectomy with either radioguidance or serum PTH monitoring has decreased morbidity and shorter hospital stays than those observed with more radical dissections of the neck.[9,10] However, this approach relies on preoperative imaging, with precise localization of the abnormal gland. In patients with secondary or tertiary hyperparathyroidism, a subtotal parathyroidectomy may be performed to avoid hypoparathyroidism, in some cases with autologous transplantation of parathyroid tissue into the patient's forearm.

ANATOMY

- Normal parathyroid glands rarely seen by imaging
- Most patients have 4 glands (2 superior, 2 inferior)
- Inferior glands less predictable in location than superior glands and may be seen in the cervical thymus (26%) or mediastinum (2%)

The normal parathyroid glands are small and are rarely seen by imaging. The typical average size of the individual glands is approximately $5 \times 3 \times 1$ mm and 40 to 50 mg.[11] Most patients have 4 glands (2 superior and 2 inferior), although approximately 3% to 5% of patients have a fifth gland.[12] The presence of fewer than 4 glands is rare, documented in less than 3% of patients.[13]

The superior parathyroid glands are closely associated with the thyroid gland, with a fairly predictable location posterior to the midthyroid (>90%). The superior glands may uncommonly be found more inferior than the midthyroid gland (4%), or above the superior margin of the thyroid (3%). Even less commonly, the superior parathyroid glands may be seen in retropharyngeal (1%), retroesophageal, or intrathyroidal locations (**Figs. 1** and **2**).[12–15]

The inferior glands are associated with the thymus, with a more variable location spanning from posterior to the midthyroid to the upper anterior and middle mediastinum. The inferior parathyroids are most commonly seen inferior, posterior, or lateral to the lower thyroid pole (69%). However, they are often seen in the cervical portion of the thymus (26%), mediastinum (2%), or rarely in the carotid sheath (see **Fig. 1**; **Fig. 3**).[12–15]

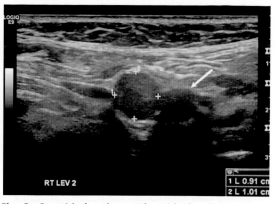

Fig. 3. Carotid sheath parathyroid gland. Transverse view of the high right neck shows a nodule (*cursors*) lateral to the common carotid artery (*arrow*), near the level of the bifurcation. This nodule was removed and shown to be an ectopic parathyroid adenoma.

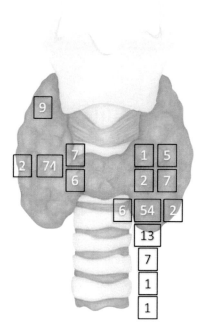

Fig. 1. Normal parathyroid gland location. Percentage of superior (*left-hand side of image*) and inferior (*right-hand side of image*) parathyroid glands found at various locations relative to the thyroid gland. (*Data from* Gilmour JR. The gross anatomy of the parathyroid glands. J Pathol Bacteriol 1938;46(1):133–49. *Courtesy of* Shanna Mellnick, BS, St. Louis, MO.)

IMAGING PROTOCOLS
Ultrasonography

- High frequency linear transducer
- Patient neck hyperextended for better visualization
- Scan from hyoid bone to thoracic inlet
- Curved array may help with deep glands and glands in the low neck and mediastinum
- Sensitivity high for adenomas, but lower in multigland, postoperative cases

The chief advantage of sonography lies in precise anatomic localization of the parathyroid glands when pathologically enlarged. Generally, sonographic evaluation for parathyroid adenomas begins with use of a high frequency (12–15 MHz) linear transducer. The patient should ideally be scanned supine, with a pillow beneath the shoulders to hyperextend the neck. Images should be obtained from approximately the hyoid bone to the thoracic inlet. In some instances, use of a high frequency curved array (such as those used for pediatric head or transvaginal sonography) may be helpful, particularly to find deeply located adenomas such as in the upper mediastinum (**Fig. 4**). Color or power Doppler may be a useful adjunct to further characterize suspected adenomas by their internal vascularity. Ultrasonography has a sensitivity of 72% to 89% for detecting parathyroid adenomas, but this is substantially lower after previous failed surgery.[16] Sensitivity of ultrasonography is also low in the setting of multigland disease, ranging from 26% to 69% in the literature.[2,17–19]

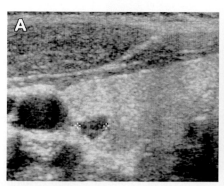

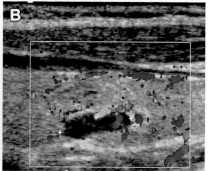

Fig. 2. Intrathyroidal parathyroid gland. Transverse grayscale (*A*) and longitudinal color Doppler (*B*) ultrasonography images show a hypoechoic, solid lesion (*cursors*) in the posterior aspect of thyroid gland with increased internal vascularity. This finding was operatively confirmed to be an ectopic intrathyroidal parathyroid adenoma.

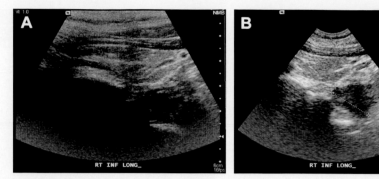

Fig. 4. Value of curved array. Ultrasonography with a linear array (*A*) shows a poorly characterized hypoechoic nodule. This parathyroid adenoma is better seen in (*B*) (*cursors*), obtained with a curved array, which enabled better penetration.

Parathyroid Scintigraphy

- Technetium 99m sestamibi
- Two-hour delayed images show retained parathyroid uptake
- Single-photon emission computed tomography (SPECT) may offer better anatomic localization
- High sensitivity in primary hyperparathyroidism, but lower in multigland disease

Scintigraphy provides functional imaging of the parathyroid glands. Technetium 99m sestamibi is most commonly used in parathyroid scintigraphy. There is normal, physiologic uptake of the tracer by both the thyroid and the parathyroid glands. However, parathyroid adenomas take up more tracer and retain it longer than these adjacent normal tissues, allowing for identification of adenomas on 2-hour delayed images. Planar images are the mainstay of parathyroid scintigraphy, but SPECT images, including when paired with anatomic computed tomography (CT) images, are being used with increasing frequency (**Fig. 5**).[20,21] In the setting of primary

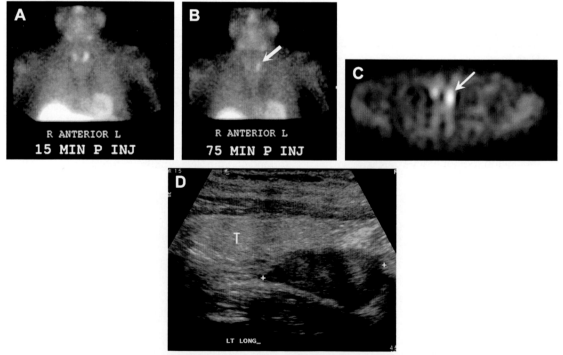

Fig. 5. Parathyroid adenoma on sestamibi and ultrasonography. Planar 15-minute (*A*) and 75-minute (*B*) images from sestamibi show persistent increased uptake at the inferior left aspect of the thyroid (*B, arrow*), better seen separate from the thyroid on axial SPECT (*C, arrow*). A parathyroid lesion (*cursors*) was confirmed immediately posterior to the thyroid (T) on sonography (*D*).

hyperparathyroidism, sestamibi scan has a sensitivity of 88% in 1 metanalysis.[2] However, similar to sonography, the accuracy of scintigraphy in multigland disease is substantially lower, ranging from 30% to 44%.[1,2]

Combined approach

A combined approach using both ultrasonography and scintigraphy is used at many centers, with improved accuracy compared with using either modality alone. Ultrasonography provides better anatomic localization of enlarged parathyroid glands relative to the thyroid, whereas scintigraphy can confirm the hyperfunctionality of a gland and also identify glands that may be invisible by ultrasonography, such as deep in the mediastinum. When ultrasonography and sestamibi are combined, their additive sensitivity is 73% to 95%.[17,22] In cases in which a sestamibi scan shows ambivalent or negative results, positive ultrasonography had an accuracy of 92% and 76%, respectively, in 1 study.[23] One shortcoming that is not overcome with the combined approach is decreased accuracy in the setting of multigland disease, the sensitivity for which ranges from 30% to 60% (**Fig. 6**).[18,24]

DIAGNOSTIC CRITERIA
Parathyroid Adenoma

- Solid, hypoechoic lesion
- Oval, with long axis oriented craniocaudally
- Variable vascularity, may have feeding vessel
- Echogenic interface with thyroid gland
- Cystic degeneration, parathyroid cysts, lipoadenomas are uncommon variants

The typical appearance of a parathyroid adenoma on sonography is of a solid, homogeneously

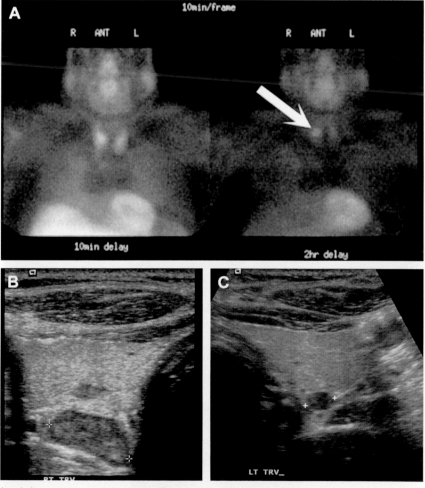

Fig. 6. Multigland disease. Sestamibi scan performed initially shows increased uptake in the right aspect of the thyroid on the 2-hour delayed images (*A, arrow*). A parathyroid adenoma (*cursors*) was confirmed in this location on sonography (*B*). However, an additional lesion (*cursors*) was found on the left side on ultrasonography (*C*). Both sonographically detected lesions were proved to be adenomas at surgery.

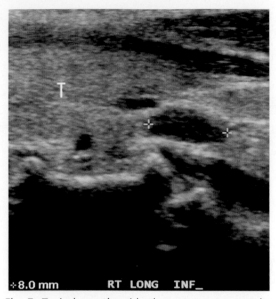

Fig. 7. Typical parathyroid adenoma on sonography. Grayscale longitudinal image shows an oval, hypoechoic lesion (*cursors*), with its long axis in the craniocaudal direction and located inferior to the right thyroid lobe (T). These are classic sonographic findings of a parathyroid adenoma.

hypoechoic nodule that is oval, with the long axis in the craniocaudal direction (**Fig. 7**). Although many parathyroid adenomas show increased internal vascularity (particularly peripherally) relative to the adjacent thyroid gland, this is variable (**Fig. 8**). Doppler may also show an extrathyroidal feeding vessel.[14] A tissue clear plane between the lesion and the thyroid gland, manifest as an echogenic interface, helps differentiate parathyroid adenomas from exophytic thyroid nodules (**Fig. 9**).

Cystic degeneration of parathyroid adenomas is uncommon, representing approximately 4% of all abnormal parathyroid glands and occurring in 1% to 2% of patients with primary hyperparathyroidism.[25–27] This appearance may occur in the setting of true parathyroid cysts or with hemorrhage and cystic degeneration of a solid parathyroid adenoma (**Fig. 10**). These adenomas may be functional or nonfunctional and tend to be larger than homogeneously solid parathyroid adenomas.[25] Another rare variant of adenoma, parathyroid lipoadenoma, is most commonly seen in patients beyond the fourth decade of life and is composed of glandular and adipose elements. These lesions have a clinical presentation similar to typical parathyroid adenomas but may have

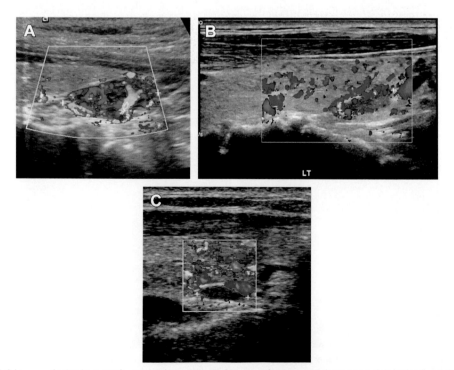

Fig. 8. Variable vascularity in parathyroid adenomas. Color Doppler images show parathyroid adenomas (*cursors*) with hypervascularity (*A*), isovascularity (*B*), and hypovascularity (*C*) relative to the thyroid gland, showing the range of blood flow that can be seen in these lesions.

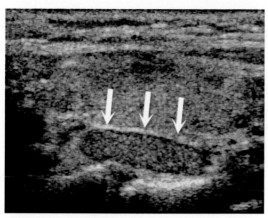

Fig. 9. Echogenic interface between thyroid and parathyroid adenoma. Grayscale ultrasonography shows a parathyroid adenoma with an echogenic interface (*arrows*) with the overlying thyroid gland, a feature that helps distinguish a parathyroid adenoma from a posteriorly located thyroid nodule.

lower uptake on sestamibi scans, because of internal fat tissue.[28,29]

Parathyroid Carcinoma

- Rare
- Severe laboratory abnormalities
- Lobulated, irregular borders
- Calcification and radial vascularity also possible

Parathyroid carcinoma comprises a small subset of solid parathyroid lesions, appearing in approximately 0.5% to 3% of all patients with primary hyperparathyroidism.[30–33] Clinically, parathyroid carcinomas present with higher serum PTH and calcium levels than do parathyroid adenomas.[30,32] On sonography, parathyroid carcinomas are larger than adenomas, showing a median measurement of 38.5 mm and 23.3 mm, respectively, in 1 study

(**Fig. 11**).[30] Other ultrasonographic findings that may suggest parathyroid carcinoma include irregular shape with a rounded rather than oval appearance, invasive or lobulated borders, radially oriented vascularity, and calcification.[30]

Diagnostic Pitfalls

- Thyroid nodules and septa
- Cervical lymph nodes
- Vascular structures

Many structures in or abutting the thyroid gland may be confused for a parathyroid adenoma. Awareness of these structures and their specific sonographic features can help avoid these pitfalls when encountered. Correlation with scintigraphy is also imperative when ultrasonographic findings are ambivalent.

Thyroid septum
A septum within the thyroid gland may mimic an extrathyroidal lesion, but careful observation of isoechogenicity with the thyroid gland and contiguity of the lesion with the remainder of the gland may help differentiate these cases from adenomas, although this may be difficult in the setting of a heterogeneous gland or multinodular goiter (**Fig. 12**).

Lymph nodes
Central lymph nodes abutting the thyroid gland may also present a diagnostic dilemma because of their hypoechogenicity relative to the thyroid gland as well as their location in places that parathyroid adenomas are commonly observed. These nodes may be seen with increased frequency in patients with neck inflammation, including those with Hashimoto thyroiditis (**Fig. 13**). A characteristic fatty hilum with associated hilar vessel is a key feature to help distinguish lymph nodes from parathyroid adenomas.

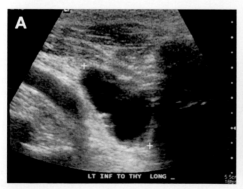
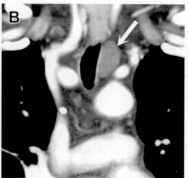

Fig. 10. Parathyroid cyst. Sonography shows an anechoic structure (*cursors*) inferior to the left thyroid (*A*), which was low attenuation on CT (*B, arrow*). This cyst was acellular when aspirated, but had increased PTH assay levels, confirming a parathyroid origin.

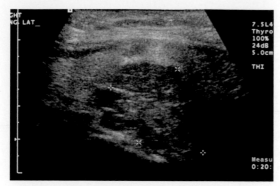

Fig. 11. Parathyroid carcinoma. Longitudinal view of the right neck shows a solid, lobulated, hypoechoic mass (*cursors*) posterior to the thyroid.

Blood vessels

Hypoechoic blood vessels, particularly dilated veins, may be situated posterior to the thyroid gland and simulate a solid lesion. Doppler ultrasonography should differentiate these cases from parathyroid lesions, showing uniform flow within

the lumen and an appropriate vascular waveform (**Fig. 14**). For deep locations such as the upper mediastinum, this modality may require using a lower frequency to optimize penetration.

PATHOLOGY

Although the imaging findings on ultrasonography and scintigraphy are the major determinants of operative planning, ultrasound-guided aspiration of a parathyroid lesion may be useful in equivocal cases, such as in the case of discrepancy between ultrasonography and scintigraphy or to confirm multigland disease.

Cytology

- Fine-needle aspiration may be performed in cases of equivocal preoperative diagnosis
- Cytology is of controversial use because of overlap with thyroid histologically
- Aspiration of cystic lesions is typically acellular

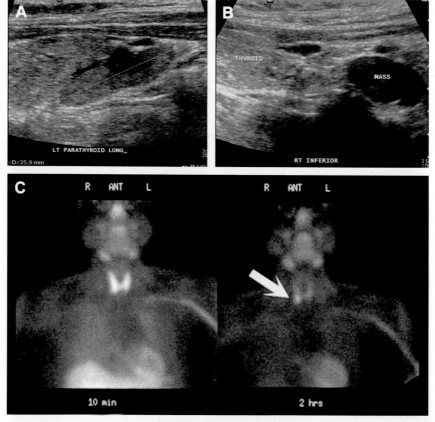

Fig. 12. Thyroid septum mimicking a parathyroid lesion. Initial sonography (*A*) shows an apparent oval mass at the inferior left thyroid (*cursors*). However, careful inspection showed isoechogenicity with the thyroid tissue and that this appearance was caused by a thyroid septum. Further evaluation (*B*) showed an unusually low parathyroid adenoma (MASS) inferior to the right thyroid (RT). Follow-up scintigraphy (*C*) confirmed persistent uptake only at the right inferior aspect of the thyroid gland (*arrow*). ANT, anterior; L, left; R, right.

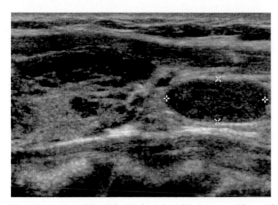

Fig. 13. Cervical lymph node mimicking a parathyroid lesion. Sonography shows an oval, hypoechoic lesion (*cursors*) inferior to the thyroid gland. The thyroid is heterogeneous in appearance because of underlying Hashimoto thyroiditis. Further ultrasonography showed several other similar appearing nodules, which represented mildly enlarged lymph nodes caused by chronic inflammation.

Because of the small size of most parathyroid adenomas, those that are biopsied are typically investigated with fine-needle aspiration. Although positive staining for PTH as well as cytologic characteristics such as cohesive cellular tissue fragments admixed with single naked nuclei showing stippled chromatin (among other features) are typical of parathyroid lesions, much of the literature has historically shown that fine-needle aspiration cannot reliably differentiate between thyroid and parathyroid lesions.[34–38] Compounding this problem is that many aspirates must pass through the thyroid gland to reach the parathyroid lesion, resulting in cellular contamination. Aspiration of cystic parathyroid lesions typically yields an acellular specimen.[34]

PTH Assay

- Aspiration with suction using a 25-gauge needle
- At least 3 passes, rinsed in 1 mL saline
- Specimen on ice, delivered promptly to laboratory
- Parathyroid tissue level higher than serum, greater than 1000 pg/mL

The low sensitivity and aforementioned limitations of cytology for diagnosing parathyroid lesions have led many to advocate for performing a PTH assay on parathyroid lesion aspirates.[39,40] This procedure is typically performed with a 25-gauge needle using suction, usually requiring at least 3 separate passes. The needle and tubing should be rinsed in 1 mL of saline in a test tube. The tube should then be placed in ice and immediately delivered to the laboratory to preserve the specimen. Aspirates from hypersecreting parathyroid glands, including cystic parathyroid lesions, should yield higher PTH assay values than those from serum. Diagnostic cutoff values for PTH levels in parathyroid lesions in the literature vary depending on dilution of the specimen, but greater than 1000 pg/mL has been suggested.[41,42]

WHAT THE REFERRING PHYSICIAN NEEDS TO KNOW

Referring surgeons and endocrinologists rely on radiologists to localize enlarged parathyroid glands under sonography and, in many instances, to correlate those results with parathyroid scintigraphy. Although diagnosing multigland disease remains a challenge for both modalities, communicating its presence when observed is of paramount importance, because of the potential need

A   **B**

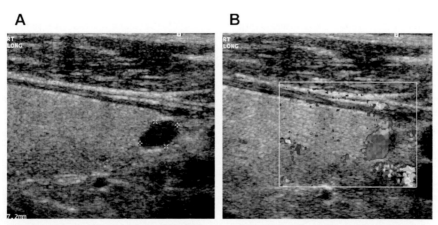

Fig. 14. Cervical vein mimicking a parathyroid lesion. (*A*) Sonography shows an oval, hypoechoic lesion (*cursors*) inferior to the thyroid gland, suggesting a possible parathyroid lesion. However, color Doppler (*B*) shows uniform flow within the lesion, characteristic of a blood vessel rather than an adenoma.

for a bilateral neck exploration as opposed to minimally invasive techniques. Atypical features, particularly those that suggest parathyroid carcinoma, should also be communicated with the referring physician, because this also has implications for surgical planning. The radiologist may also play an important diagnostic role in select cases by offering ultrasound-guided fine-needle aspiration for tissue PTH levels.

SUMMARY

Hyperparathyroidism can lead to symptoms related to hypercalcemia and warrant treatment, which is often surgical. Evaluation of the parathyroid glands with sonography requires knowledge of the classic and variant appearances of parathyroid lesions as well as the range of anatomic locations in which they may occur. The accuracy of ultrasonography in characterizing parathyroid disease is augmented by correlation with scintigraphy; although neither sonography nor scintigraphy excels in detecting multigland disease or after failed resection, they are still used in those settings, with varying sensitivities reported in the literature. Because of the increasing use of minimally invasive techniques, ultrasonography, and when appropriate, ultrasound-guided fine-needle aspiration, play a crucial role in preoperative characterization of abnormal parathyroid glands.

REFERENCES

1. Fraker DL, Harsono H, Lewis R. Minimally invasive parathyroidectomy: benefits and requirements of localization, diagnosis, and intraoperative PTH monitoring. Long-term results. World J Surg 2009; 33(11):2256–65.
2. Ruda JM, Hollenbeak CS, Stack BC Jr. A systematic review of the diagnosis and treatment of primary hyperparathyroidism from 1995 to 2003. Otolaryngol Head Neck Surg 2005;132(3):359–72.
3. Gasparri G, Camandona M, Abbona GC, et al. Secondary and tertiary hyperparathyroidism: causes of recurrent disease after 446 parathyroidectomies. Ann Surg 2001;233(1):65–9.
4. Lai EC, Ching AS, Leong HT. Secondary and tertiary hyperparathyroidism: role of preoperative localization. ANZ J Surg 2007;77(10):880–2.
5. Fuster D, Ybarra J, Ortin J, et al. Role of preoperative imaging using 99mTc-MIBI and neck ultrasound in patients with secondary hyperparathyroidism who are candidates for subtotal parathyroidectomy. Eur J Nucl Med Mol Imaging 2006;33(4): 467–73.
6. Pons F, Torregrosa JV, Vidal-Sicart S, et al. Preoperative parathyroid gland localization with technetium-

99m sestamibi in secondary hyperparathyroidism. Eur J Nucl Med 1997;24(12):1494–8.
7. Perie S, Fessi H, Tassart M, et al. Usefulness of combination of high-resolution ultrasonography and dual-phase dual-isotope iodine 123/technetium Tc 99m sestamibi scintigraphy for the preoperative localization of hyperplastic parathyroid glands in renal hyperparathyroidism. Am J Kidney Dis 2005; 45(2):344–52.
8. Low RA, Katz AD. Parathyroidectomy via bilateral cervical exploration: a retrospective review of 866 cases. Head Neck 1998;20(7):583–7.
9. Fuhrman GM, Bolton JS. Minimally invasive parathyroid surgery. Ochsner J 2000;2(3):168–71.
10. Said SM, Cassivi SD, Allen MS, et al. Minimally invasive resection for mediastinal ectopic parathyroid glands. Ann Thorac Surg 2013;96(4):1229–33.
11. Grimelius L, Bondeson L. Histopathological diagnosis of parathyroid diseases. Pathol Res Pract 1995;191(4):353–65.
12. Akerstrom G, Malmaeus J, Bergstrom R. Surgical anatomy of human parathyroid glands. Surgery 1984;95(1):14–21.
13. Wang C. The anatomic basis of parathyroid surgery. Ann Surg 1976;183(3):271–5.
14. Johnson NA, Tublin ME, Ogilvie JB. Parathyroid imaging: technique and role in the preoperative evaluation of primary hyperparathyroidism. AJR Am J Roentgenol 2007;188(6):1706–15.
15. Gilmour JR. The gross anatomy of the parathyroid glands. J Pathol Bacteriol 1938;46(1):133–49.
16. Rotstein L, Irish J, Gullane P, et al. Reoperative parathyroidectomy in the era of localization technology. Head Neck 1998;20(6):535–9.
17. Siperstein A, Berber E, Mackey R, et al. Prospective evaluation of sestamibi scan, ultrasonography, and rapid PTH to predict the success of limited exploration for sporadic primary hyperparathyroidism. Surgery 2004;136(4):872–80.
18. Sugg SL, Krzywda EA, Demeure MJ, et al. Detection of multiple gland primary hyperparathyroidism in the era of minimally invasive parathyroidectomy. Surgery 2004;136(6):1303–9.
19. Milas M, Stephen A, Berber E, et al. Ultrasonography for the endocrine surgeon: a valuable clinical tool that enhances diagnostic and therapeutic outcomes. Surgery 2005;138(6):1193–200 [discussion: 1200–1].
20. Papathanassiou D, Flament JB, Pochart JM, et al. SPECT/CT in localization of parathyroid adenoma or hyperplasia in patients with previous neck surgery. Clin Nucl Med 2008;33(6):394–7.
21. Civelek AC, Ozalp E, Donovan P, et al. Prospective evaluation of delayed technetium-99m sestamibi SPECT scintigraphy for preoperative localization of primary hyperparathyroidism. Surgery 2002;131(2): 149–57.

22. Lumachi F, Zucchetta P, Marzola MC, et al. Advantages of combined technetium-99m-sestamibi scintigraphy and high-resolution ultrasonography in parathyroid localization: comparative study in 91 patients with primary hyperparathyroidism. Eur J Endocrinol 2000;143(6):755–60.

23. Davis ML, Quayle FJ, Middleton WD, et al. Ultrasound facilitates minimally invasive parathyroidectomy in patients lacking definitive localization from preoperative sestamibi scan. Am J Surg 2007; 194(6):785–90 [discussion: 790–1].

24. Haciyanli M, Lal G, Morita E, et al. Accuracy of preoperative localization studies and intraoperative parathyroid hormone assay in patients with primary hyperparathyroidism and double adenoma. J Am Coll Surg 2003;197(5):739–46.

25. Johnson NA, Yip L, Tublin ME. Cystic parathyroid adenoma: sonographic features and correlation with 99mTc-sestamibi SPECT findings. AJR Am J Roentgenol 2010;195(6):1385–90.

26. Randel SB, Gooding GA, Clark OH, et al. Parathyroid variants: US evaluation. Radiology 1987; 165(1):191–4.

27. Clark OH. Parathyroid cysts. Am J Surg 1978; 135(3):395–402.

28. Turner WJ, Baergen RN, Pellitteri PK, et al. Parathyroid lipoadenoma: case report and review of the literature. Otolaryngol Head Neck Surg 1996;114(2): 313–6.

29. Nguyen BD. Parathyroid imaging with Tc-99m sestamibi planar and SPECT scintigraphy. Radiographics 1999;19(3):601–14 [discussion: 615–6].

30. Sidhu PS, Talat N, Patel P, et al. Ultrasound features of malignancy in the preoperative diagnosis of parathyroid cancer: a retrospective analysis of parathyroid tumours larger than 15 mm. Eur Radiol 2011; 21(9):1865–73.

31. Koea JB, Shaw JH. Parathyroid cancer: biology and management. Surg Oncol 1999;8(3):155–65.

32. Robert JH, Trombetti A, Garcia A, et al. Primary hyperparathyroidism: can parathyroid carcinoma be anticipated on clinical and biochemical grounds? Report of nine cases and review of the literature. Ann Surg Oncol 2005;12(7):526–32.

33. Sheehan JJ, Hill AD, Walsh MF, et al. Parathyroid carcinoma: diagnosis and management. Eur J Surg Oncol 2001;27(3):321–4.

34. Absher KJ, Truong LD, Khurana KK, et al. Parathyroid cytology: avoiding diagnostic pitfalls. Head Neck 2002;24(2):157–64.

35. Gooding GA, Clark OH, Stark DD, et al. Parathyroid aspiration biopsy under ultrasound guidance in the postoperative hyperparathyroid patient. Radiology 1985;155(1):193–6.

36. Abati A, Skarulis MC, Shawker T, et al. Ultrasound-guided fine-needle aspiration of parathyroid lesions: a morphological and immunocytochemical approach. Hum Pathol 1995;26(3):338–43.

37. Bergenfelz A, Forsberg L, Hederstrom E, et al. Preoperative localization of enlarged parathyroid glands with ultrasonically guided fine needle aspiration for parathyroid hormone assay. Acta Radiol 1991;32(5):403–5.

38. Dimashkieh H, Krishnamurthy S. Ultrasound guided fine needle aspiration biopsy of parathyroid gland and lesions. Cytojournal 2006;3:6.

39. Owens CL, Rekhtman N, Sokoll L, et al. Parathyroid hormone assay in fine-needle aspirate is useful in differentiating inadvertently sampled parathyroid tissue from thyroid lesions. Diagn Cytopathol 2008; 36(4):227–31.

40. Agarwal AM, Bentz JS, Hungerford R, et al. Parathyroid fine-needle aspiration cytology in the evaluation of parathyroid adenoma: cytologic findings from 53 patients. Diagn Cytopathol 2009;37(6): 407–10.

41. Kiblut NK, Cussac JF, Soudan B, et al. Fine needle aspiration and intraparathyroid intact parathyroid hormone measurement for reoperative parathyroid surgery. World J Surg 2004;28(11):1143–7.

42. Maser C, Donovan P, Santos F, et al. Sonographically guided fine needle aspiration with rapid parathyroid hormone assay. Ann Surg Oncol 2006; 13(12):1690–5.

Ultrasonography in the Assessment of Lymph Node Disease

Hans-Peter Weskott, MD[a],*, Sanshan Yin, MD[b]

KEYWORDS

- Reactive lymph nodes • Metastatic lymph nodes • Lymphoma • Ultrasonography • Color Doppler
- B-Flow • Contrast agent

KEY POINTS

- The lymphatic system consists of a network of interconnected lymphatic channels collecting lymph fluid from the interstitium. The lymph may contain antigens entering a lymph node (LN) while LNs take up and filter the lymph on its way through the lymph node meshwork.
- Ultrasonography has become the first imaging modality in patients with inflammatory or malignant diseases to evaluate both peripheral and abdominal LN status. Several sonographic imaging modes including B-mode, elastography, color and pulsed-wave Doppler techniques, B-flow, and contrast-enhanced ultrasonography (CEUS) can be applied to characterize LNs.
- The sensitivity for detecting regional LN metastases on B-mode depends on the primary tumor, size, and echogenicity, but is limited by the minuscule size of tumor infiltrations. Besides gray-scale patterns, evaluating the vascularity and perfusion add great value in characterizing LNs and distinguishing normal from suspicious LNs.
- A typical reactive LN has an oval shape with an even thickness of its preserved cortex and regular vessel architecture.
- LN metastases are mostly round shaped and hypoechoic to cystic; an echogenic hilum is missed and its vessel architecture is chaotic.
- The presence of a dominantly peripheral vascularity in LNs is highly suspicious of malignancy.
- At present, no single gray-scale or color Doppler criterion exists that can reliably differentiate between reactive LN enlargement and involvement of a non-Hodgkin lymphoma.
- There are considerable overlaps of sonographic features, especially between inflammatory and non-Hodgkin lymphomas.
- Ultrasound-guided biopsies are in most cases successful in defining the characteristics of LNs.
- The use of contrast agents is most advantageous in the detection of tissue perfusion, thus confirming the effect of chemotherapy or radiation therapy.

 Videos of color Doppler and B-flow examinations accompany this article at http://www.ultrasound.theclinics.com/

THE LYMPHATIC SYSTEM

The lymphatic system consists of a network of interconnected lymphatic channels collecting lymph fluid from the interstitium by blind-ending lymphatic capillaries to carry it to the next regional lymph nodes (LNs). It is estimated that about 2 L of lymph fluid is produced within 24 hours. The

The authors have nothing to disclose.
[a] Central Ultrasound Department, Klinikum Siloah, KRH, Hannover, Germany; [b] Department of Ultrasound, Key Laboratory of Carcinogenesis and Translational Research, Peking University Cancer Hospital & Institute, Beijing 100142, People's Republic of China
* Corresponding author.
E-mail address: weskotthp@t-online.de

Ultrasound Clin 9 (2014) 351–371
http://dx.doi.org/10.1016/j.cult.2014.03.008

size of these tiny tubes allows only small molecules and particles (including antigens) to pass this network. The lymphatic vessels have a valve system that allows the lymph to flow only in one direction, preventing intraluminal fluid to flow backward.

Depending on the size of an LN, the lymph enters an LN by 1 or several afferent lymph vessels and runs through a reticular meshwork to be filtered and analyzed on its way through the LN. The cleared lymph is drained by the efferent lymphatic vessels and enters the systemic circulation via the thoracic duct into the left and right subclavian vein. The efferent lymph vessels may also function as an afferent lymphatic vessel when it again enters the next LN for clearance. Some lymphatic vessels may bypass the first (sentinel LN) or secondary LN and enter the next, or one of the next, LNs (Fig. 1).[1]

Lymph nodes have a capsule of dense connective tissue. Each LN is composed of 3 parts. The subcapsular cortex consists of the primary and secondary follicles, which are surrounded and separated by the interfollicular cortex. The secondary follicles develop when they encounter antigens. The lymph may contain antigens entering an LN via the afferent lymphatic vessels, whereas most lymphocytes enter the LN via blood vessels. B lymphocytes home to follicles in the superficial cortex where they interact with follicular dendritic cells. The paracortex consists of the deep cortical units where T lymphocytes home to the deep cortical unit (DCU) and interact with dendritic cells (Fig. 2). When coming in contact with antigens via specialized venules, namely high endothelial venules (HEV), the palisades of the HEV open to allow lymphocytes to migrate to the interstitium to encounter specific antigens. HEVs are specialized postcapillary venous swellings characterized by plump endothelial cells as opposed to the usual thinner endothelial cells found in regular venules. HEVs enable naïve lymphocytes to move in and out of the LNs from the circulatory system. In contrast to the endothelial cells from other vessels, the endothelial cells of HEV have a plump appearance different from the flat morphology of endothelial cells that line other vessels, and are therefore called high endothelial cells by reference to their thickness. Lymphocytes that are not involved in this process leave the LN via the efferent lymphatic vessels. The medulla with the medullary cords is located in the center of the LN. The LNs take up and filter the lymph on its way through the LN meshwork. This meshwork provides lymphocytes, antigen-presenting cells, and macrophages to interact with immunocompetent cells.[2] The feeding and draining blood vessels enter the LN from the hilum and branch arbitrarily up to the follicles (Fig. 3). Some LNs are supplied by accessory arteries and veins entering the LN extrahilarly.

In contrast to LNs, lymphatic nodules have no capsule; they are also known as mucosa-associated lymphatic tissue (MALT) and can be found most often in the upper gastrointestinal (GI) tract. Part of the MALT is made up of Peyer plaques of the terminal ileum. The GI tract is the most frequent extranodal site of non-Hodgkin lymphomas (NHLs), but accounts for only about 5% of all NHLs.

ULTRASONOGRAPHY EXAMINATION MODES

Sonographic assessment of LNs includes number and size of LN, shape, echotexture (including microcalcifications and cystic changes), B-mode architecture, margin, stiffness, vascular patterns, and evaluating the tenderness of enlarged LNs. To evaluate these different morphologic and perfusion features, several sonographic imaging modes are available. Besides B-mode, stain and shear-wave based elastography, color and pulsed-wave (PW) Doppler techniques, B-flow, contrast-enhanced ultrasonography (CEUS), and ultrasound-guided biopsies have become valuable tools in the diagnostic workup of LN. B-Mode is the basic

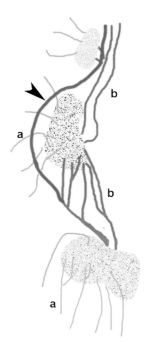

Fig. 1. Scheme of lymph node (LN) chains (a, afferent vessels; b, efferent vessels). *Arrowhead* indicates a bypassing efferent lymphatic vessel draining fluid into a secondary LN.

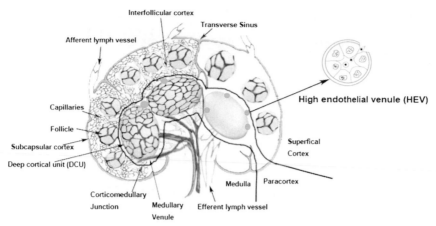

Fig. 2. The lymphoid lobules, the functional unit of an LN. The outer zone consists of the follicles, followed by the paracortex and the medulla. The lymph runs through a reticular meshwork where immune competent cells interact with antigens. High endothelial venules are postcapillary venules with cuboidal endothelial cells that enable lymphocytes to migrate into the lymph node parenchyma from the blood-supplying vessels.

ultrasonographic examination technique for detection, characterization, and sizing, and locating LNs. Whenever possible, high-frequency linear probes should be applied. For imaging intranodal vessels, the most sensitive technique with the lowest chance of artifacts must be chosen. Color Doppler and PW Doppler techniques are used to demonstrate the LN vasculature, adding PW Doppler velocities and velocity ratios such as resistive index (RI) and pulsatility index (PI) numbers, which can easily be calculated. B-Flow is a non-Doppler subtraction technique that is capable of imaging vessels with almost no blooming artifact, is far less angle dependent, and does not need a "color box," as flow information is generated over the whole image.[3]

B-Flow is therefore the best imaging modality for architecture, although it is limited because flow direction is only indicated when Doppler information is added (**Fig. 4**). In addition, a 3-dimensional imaging technique might help to better visualize the tissue adjacent LNs or evaluate scars after LN dissection.

In the manner of finger palpation attempting to evaluate the stiffness of subcutaneous tumors (and their tenderness), elastography is used to demonstrate the stiffness of LNs and to differentiate between hard and soft areas of an LN.[4–6] Two different technical solutions are offered. Strain elastography uses the external pressure of the transducer to compress tissue and image the displacement of scatterers on a color map between different shades of red and blue (**Fig. 5**). Shear-wave elastography uses short, high-intensity pulses to depict tissue deformation perpendicular to the direction of sound-wave propagation.

Contrast agents are most sensitive in detecting LN perfusion with a high spatial resolution, but dedicated software is needed. Evaluation of contrast kinetics and direction of enhancement are important criteria in characterizing LNs.[7] Because in rare cases adverse reactions may occur, the indication for using contrast agents has to be considered carefully (contrast agents for LN examinations are available for off-label use only).

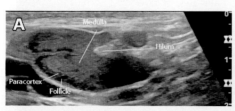 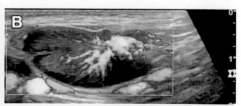

Fig. 3. (A, B) Reactive LN in the groin of a patient with atopic dermatitis. (A) B-mode shows the echo-poor cortical follicles surrounded by the paracortex, the central medulla, and the echogenic hilum. It is suspected that LNs in these patients may show a plasma cellular lymphadenitis. (B) Bidirectional color power Doppler confirms its rich vasculature running straight through the medulla. ([A] Data from Müller KM. Plasma cellular lymphadenitis in neurodermitis. Path Res Pract 1983;178:88–90.)

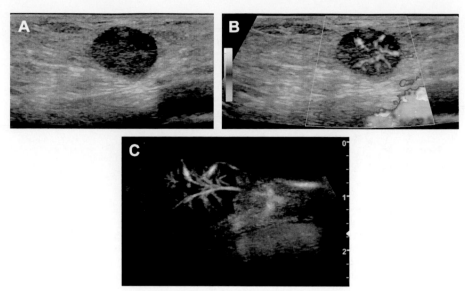

Fig. 4. (*A–C*). Reactive LN in the right groin (mononucleosis). (*A*) B-mode image. (*B*) Power Doppler image. (*C*) B-Flow image. On color Doppler a central vascular supply with regular branching arteries is shown, and intranodal veins are missed. B-Flow shows additional tiny peripheral vessels.

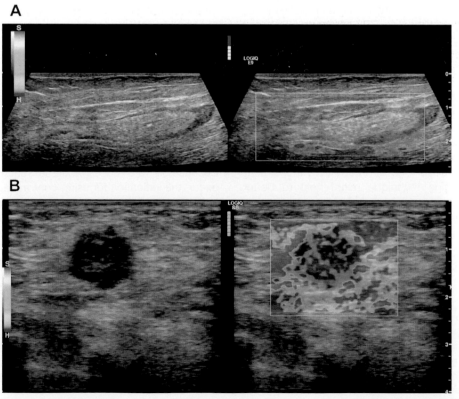

Fig. 5. (*A*) Strain elastography of a reactive LN demonstrating that the cortex is harder than the hilum. (*B*) LN metastasis in the left axilla (melanoma). Hard tissue is displayed in blue, soft tissue in red.

LYMPH NODE DETECTION

It is accepted that ultrasonography is superior to palpation in detecting and characterizing subcutaneous LNs. In the evaluation of peripheral LN status, ultrasonography has become the first-line imaging modality in patients with inflammatory or malignant diseases. Detection rate and characterization of abdominal LNs depend on the scanning conditions, equipment, and, last but not least, the operator's skills and knowledge.

It is estimated that at least 1000 LNs exist in humans. Tiny LNs smaller than 2 mm do not differ from surrounding tissue in their acoustic properties, and therefore cannot be detected. Ultrasonography examinations aim at the detection and characterization of all diseased (benign and malignant) LNs. In patients with known disease, the goals of imaging are staging, evaluation of response to therapy, and identification of new or recurrent disease or of complications of therapy. Lymphatic vessels and nodes follow the course of vessels; their location can be defined in different compartments such as the neck, axilla, groin, or abdomen. When using high-frequency linear probes, superficial LNs down to 2 to 3 mm can be identified when surrounded by fatty tissue. LN metastases between 0.2 and 2 mm are regarded as micrometastases and those below 0.2 mm as submicrometastases, and are mostly found in sentinel LNs by the pathologist.[8] These tiny metastases cannot be detected by any sonographic mode.

For anatomic regions in which transcutaneous ultrasonography examination is not possible, such as the mediastinum or perihilar region of the lung, endoscopic ultrasonography should be considered, but computed tomography (CT) is often the imaging modality of choice. The same is true in patients with unfavorable abdominal scanning conditions. Depending on the location, endosonography is a highly reliable examination tool for detecting and characterizing mediastinal and paraesophageal LNs or LNs in the liver hilum or the parapancreatic space.[9–12] Its ability to perform fine-needle aspiration punctures is another important advantage.

Lymphatic vessels and their nodes follow the course of the vessels. In the neck the location of LNs can be classified into 8 regions (Fig. 6), separated by muscles, trachea, and bones.

Breast cancer metastases spread in the main to the axillary LNs, infrasupraclavicular region, and internal mammary region (see Fig. 6B). The axilla may be challenging because of unfavorable scanning conditions, as in thin patients or after LN dissection.

A review study on thyroid cancer by Mulla and colleagues[13] reported on poor sensitivity for the detection of LN metastases, as low as 27% for ultrasonography and CT in comparison with histologic workup after LN dissection.

In the groin, superficial LNs can be found supramedially, and lateral and inferior to the inguinal ligament. Medial of the inguinal vessels, deep LNs are found (see Fig. 6C). The highest LN of

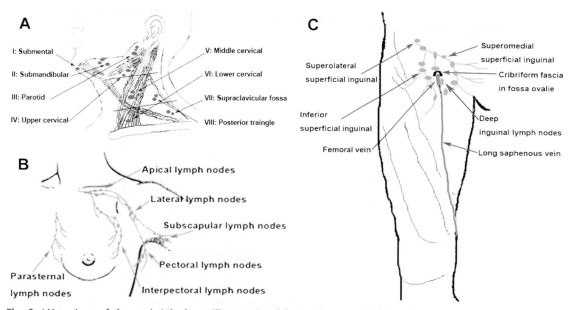

A

I: Submental
II: Submandibular
III: Parotid
IV: Upper cervical
V: Middle cervical
VI: Lower cervical
VII: Supraclavicular fossa
VIII: Posterior traingle

B

Apical lymph nodes
Lateral lymph nodes
Subscapular lymph nodes
Pectoral lymph nodes
Parasternal lymph nodes
Interpectoral lymph nodes

C

Superolateral superficial inguinal
Inferior superficial inguinal
Femoral vein
Superomedial superficial inguinal
Cribriform fascia in fossa ovalie
Deep inguinal lymph nodes
Long saphenous vein

Fig. 6. LN regions of the neck (*A*), the axillary region (*B*), and the groin (*C*).

the leg is located within the proximal femoral canal close to the inguinal ligament and medial to the femoral vein, or may be the first node in the pelvis (the Cloquet node). This region must also be looked for very carefully.[14] If this LN is enlarged it can sometimes be mistaken for a femoral hernia.

It is not only important to detect LN but also to depict focal changes in the LN cortex (**Fig. 7**). Therefore, detection is already part of the LN characterization.

Distinguishing normal from malignant LNs is critical for accurate staging, prognosis, and determination of optimal therapeutic options. Besides gray-scale patterns, vascularity and perfusion add great value in characterizing LNs and distinguishing normal from malignant LNs.

LYMPH NODE VASCULATURE AND PERFUSION

Vessel leakiness is a hallmark of inflammation and cancer. In inflammation, plasma extravasation occurs in a coordinated manner to enable the immune response but also to maintain tissue perfusion. In tumors similar mechanisms operate, but are not well regulated (**Fig. 8**). Therefore, blood perfusion in tumors is nonuniform, and global or focal leakage interacts with the LN perfusion.[15] Acute inflammation is characterized by vasodilatation, increased permeability, and increased blood flow, which are induced by various endogenous mediators. Malignant tumors have a higher vessel density that can comprise up to 10% of a tumor volume. In most cancerous tumors the native vasculature is destroyed and, within a network of imperfect tumor vessels with a chaotic architecture, the vessel branching patterns are abnormal. Tumor vessels often have atrioventricular shunts. Pericytes are missed or loosely associated with the tumor endothelium.[16] The diameter of tumor arteries may vary or be split. The vessel density may therefore differ within a tumor or malignant LN (see **Fig. 8B**).

For characterizing LNs, it is thus mandatory to image their vasculature by applying Doppler techniques, B-flow, or, if needed, ultrasonography contrast agents (see **Fig. 8**) (the latter still being off-label).

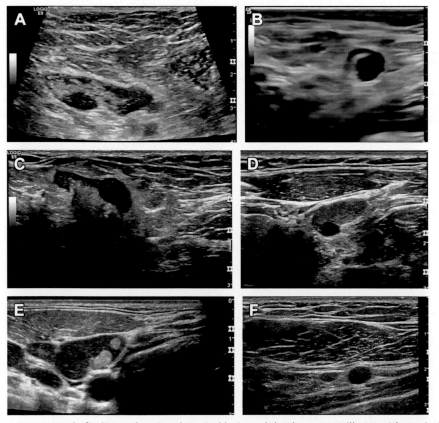

Fig. 7. (*A–F*) Various B-mode findings of regional cortical lesions. (*A*) Echo-poor axilla LN with cortical thickening in a sarcoidosis patient. (*B*) Melanoma metastasis in an inguinal LN. (*C*) Hodgkin disease of an inguinal LN. (*D*) Focal LN inflammation of the neck. (*E*) Focal fatty infiltration in a lymphoma LN of the neck. (*F*) Infraclavicular metastases of 3 mm and 5 mm in melanoma. All diagnoses were confirmed by LN dissection or biopsy.

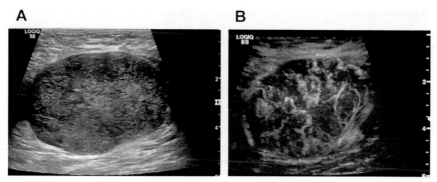

Fig. 8. B-Mode (*A*) and B-flow (*B*) images of intranodal vessel density distribution and architecture of an LN metastasis (melanoma).

Tumor vessels have no muscle layer; their wall is characterized by pores of different sizes. Within one tumor a pore size ranging from 200 nm to 1.2 μm has been described.[17] Depending on the size of these pores, fluid will leak into the interstitium, thus increasing the intratumoral pressure and leading to an ischemia, which itself stimulates neoangiogenesis. At the same time there is an intravascular increase of the hematocrit, which also contributes to hypoxia and necrosis formation of the tumor center.[18] When intranodular pressure is rising, the RI number will increase as well. Small venous vessels are compressed and can no longer be detected by means of color Doppler techniques. Only in the LN periphery can bigger draining veins be seen. At this stage an intratumoral ischemia starts to develop. With a further increase in pressure, the smaller and, later, larger intratumoral arteries will be missed. Ahuja and colleagues[19–22] already pointed out that peripheral vascularity is not found in normal or reactive nodes, and the presence of peripheral vascularity, regardless of sole peripheral or mixed vascularity, is highly suspicious of malignancy. As long as the organ has an intact capsule, the pressure will increase. When the capsule is invaded by tumor and destroyed, the intratumoral pressure will in most cases drop again, as the interstitial fluid of the LN pours into the adjacent fatty tissue (**Fig. 9**). CEUS is capable of demonstrating tumor infiltration in the tissue adjacent to the LN if a neovascularization has been built up (**Fig. 10**).

The RI number will then decrease again, and color Doppler will then demonstrate a lower intranodular vasculature. Thus a primary tumor with several LN metastases may all show different vascular patterns. This variation can be explained not only because of the number of shunts and the number of larger neovessels; it can also be assumed that differences in the intranodular pressure are responsible for the different intratumoral perfusion patterns. It is well known that compared with reactive nodes, metastatic nodes have higher RI and PI numbers.[19,20,23–25]

Perfusion patterns are less variable in inflammatory LNs where, owing to local edema, ischemia develops, which may lead to abscess and necrosis.

The controversy about the value of RI and PI measurements for differentiating benign from malignant nodes can probably be solved by the influence of the intranodular pressure on the resistance values that may change even within a single malignant LN.

A reduced or even partly missed vasculature may also be caused by a high local density of small tumor cells, as can be seen, for example, in lymphomas. Owing to these densely packed tumor cells, intranodal vessels will be mechanically compressed.

Color Doppler or B-flow can depict the changes of vascularity during systole and diastole, especially in metastatic LNs (**Fig. 11**, Video 1). B-Flow can additionally characterize the intranodal tumor vessels (Video 2).

REACTIVE LYMPH NODES

Enlarged LNs may be caused by inflammatory, autoimmune, or malignant disease. Bacterial and viral diseases such as mononucleosis, herpes, hepatitis, infections of the intestine, or nasopharyngeal space are the most common reasons of reactive lymphadenitis. Mononucleosis often exists together with an enlarged spleen. In acute and chronic active hepatitis, enlarged LNs in the liver hilum are apparent (**Fig. 12**).

Reactive LNs are detected and characterized by their typical B-mode appearance: The echo-poor cortex can be easily depicted within the surrounding echogenic fatty tissue, and will enlarge with the acuity and severity of inflammation. When using

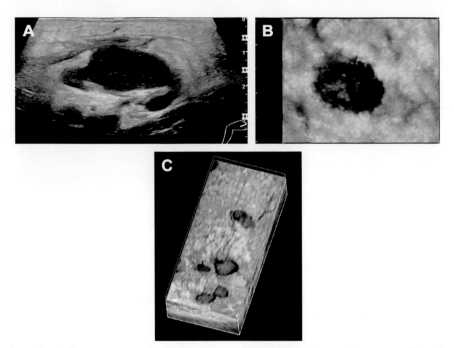

Fig. 9. (*A*) Absceding inflammatory LN. (*B*) Tumor destroyed the LN capsule causing surrounding edema (c-plane image). (*C*) Five LN metastases with edema imaged in a c-plane mode, both metastases from a melanoma.

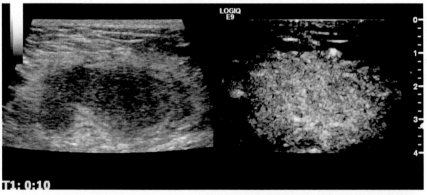

Fig. 10. Tumor invasion of the perinodal fat. On contrast-enhanced ultrasonography (CEUS), the neovasculature shows the tumor-supplying vessels, making the size of the LN bigger than on B-mode.

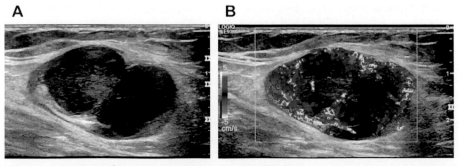

Fig. 11. (*A*, *B*) Two metastases of a melanoma in one LN. See cine loop.

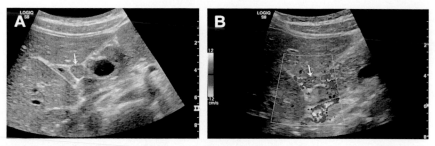

Fig. 12. (*A*) Lymph nodes of a patient with chronic hepatitis in the liver hilum (*arrow*). (*B*) Color Doppler depicts the central supplying artery.

high-frequency curved or linear transducers, echo-poor to cystic follicles within the cortex can sometimes be seen.

Reactive lymphadenopathy is a nonneoplastic enlargement in response to antigenic stimuli. Clinically reactive LNs are mostly tender and mobile. Depending on the cellular response, 3 histologic types can be differentiated. A follicular hyperplasia is most common (differential diagnoses: rheumatoid arthritis, Sjögren syndrome, and toxoplasmosis). Second, a paracortical hyperplasia with a preferred stimulation of T cells can histologically be diagnosed (as in infectious mononucleosis or other viral infections). Third least common is sinus hyperplasia, as seen in hemophagocytosis and sinus histiocytosis.

It must be noted that infectious material can cause a focal cortical thickening. In most cases a local infectious focus can be detected clinically or by ultrasonography. This focus is characterized by a regular segmental vascularization (**Fig. 13**). As focal cortical thickening is also suspicious for tumor invasion, a biopsy should be considered.

A typical reactive LN has an oval shape with an even thickness of its cortex. A hilum where the supplying vessels enter can be seen in all early cases. In bigger LNs the vessels can already be identified even on gray-scale images. Color Doppler demonstrates direction and pulsatility of blood flow. The vessels branch tree-like from the hilum to the cortex.

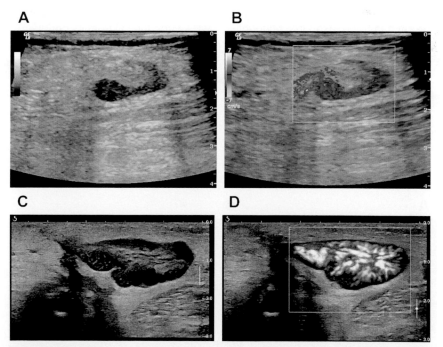

Fig. 13. (*A*) Segmental thickening of an axillary LN. (*B*) color Doppler shows segmental hypervascularization. Biopsy and follow-up confirmed an inflammatory cortical reaction. (*C*, *D*) Acute inflammatory LN with an uneven thickening of the cortex after bypass surgery of the superficial femoral artery (infected skin ulcerations of the calf).

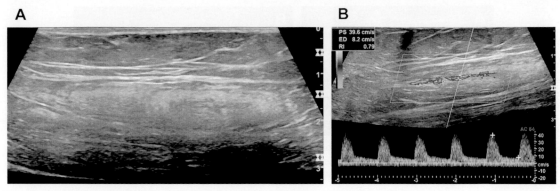

Fig. 14. (*A, B*) Fatty involution of an oval-shaped LN, resistive index 0.76.

Besides acute inflammatory LNs, fatty involution of LNs are often found, especially in the axilla and groin, and can be mistaken for subcutaneous lipoma, as the thin cortex may sometimes be difficult to image (**Fig. 14**).

The RI number in inflammatory LNs reflects its intranodal pressure, and may therefore be of great variability, but in most cases will be less than 0.70.

Regular branching vessels arising from the hilum are not specific for reactive LNs or lymphomas. In a few cases cancerous LN transformation still shows an increased but regular flow (**Figs. 15 and 16**).

As a consequence, no single criterion allows a reliable diagnosis of LN enlargement. In addition to morphologic and hemodynamic criteria, the clinical background has to be taken into account.

Tables 1 and **2** list the criteria that help to distinguish between reactive and metastatic LN and lymphoma.

CANCEROUS LYMPH NODES

Ultrasonography is mainly regarded as the first-line imaging modality in the management of metastatic disease or lymphomas, especially in superficial regions. LNs are the most frequent site of metastatic spread. The sensitivity for detecting regional LN metastases on B-mode depends on the primary tumor, size, cortical thickness and echogenic hilum, and echogenicity (see **Fig. 7A–F**). LN metastases are mostly round shaped and hypoechoic to cystic, and an echogenic hilum is missed. The sensitivity for detecting LN vascularity and perfusion depends on the sonographic technique applied. Color Doppler and B-flow can only depict the major vessels supplying an LN. In cases of early lymphatic tumor, seeding the central vessels may still be recognized while the tumor nodule is building up its own vasculature. Besides the regular central vessels, tumor vessels will invade the LN from its periphery. As the tumor vessels are to a certain extent leaky, the intratumoral pressure will differ between different primaries. It is also known that neoangiogenesis is not only building up blood but also lymphatic vessels (lymphangiogenesis by vascular endothelial growth factor C[26]). It is assumed that lymphangionenesis in a sentinel LN promotes tumor spread to distant sites.[27] Whether

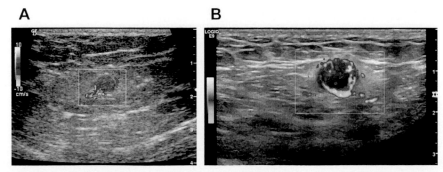

Fig. 15. (*A, B*) Two tiny, round-shaped LNs. (*A*) Reactive LN with regular branching central vessels under interferon therapy. (*B*) LN metastasis with vessels in the LN periphery.

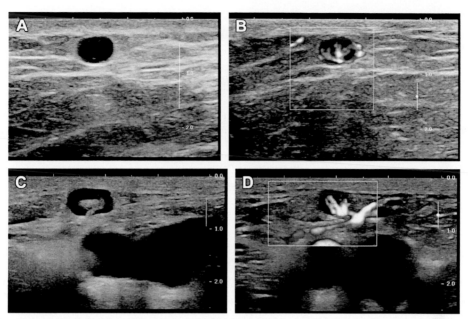

Fig. 16. (*A*, *B*) Round-shaped LN with regularly branching central vessels and vessels at its capsule (melanoma metastasis). (*C*, *D*) Reactive, tender LN with echo-poor thickened cortex, echogenic hilum, and a Solbiati index lower than 2.

Table 1
Lymph node characteristics on B-mode imaging

Criterion	Reactive LN	Lymphomas	LN Metastases
Size	Measurement of the biggest LN in relevant regional lymph locations in 2 scan planes (follow up!)		
Shape	Oval (length: width >2)	Oval to round	Mostly round
Number	Single to a few	A few to many LNs in different LN stations	A few to multiple locoregional LNs
Location	Mostly 1 or a few LNs of the first draining LN station	Mostly LN in 1 or multiple LN stations	Mostly 1 or multiple regional LN stations, not all LN stations
Spatial arrangement	Size and number increases toward inflammatory focus	Unsystematic or chain-like to packet-like	Along the draining LN station
Echogenicity	Echo-poor cortex	Echo-poor to cystic appearance	Echo-poor
Architecture	Preserved (except: abscess, TB, sarcoidosis)	Preserved to destroyed	Totally to partial destroyed
Cortex	Thickened, concentric, or eccentric	Thickened, concentric, or eccentric	Infiltrated, mostly in nodules
Hilus	Echogenic	Thin or absent	Compressed, often absent
Margin	Sharp, undefined in abscess	Sharp	Sharp; undefined with surrounding edema
Abdominal involvement	Lymphotropic viruses such as mononucleosis, sarcoidosis, tuberculosis (liver, spleen)	Most common in NHL, infiltration of all organs possible (liver, spleen, kidneys, glands). Not so often in Hodgkin disease	Possible, mostly liver and abdominal LN

Abbreviations: LN, lymph node; NHL, non-Hodgkin lymphoma; TB, tuberculosis.

Table 2
Lymph node characteristics on vascular/perfusion patterns

Ultrasound Mode	Criterion	
	Malignant Lymphomas/Reactive LN	Metastatic
Color-coded duplex ultrasonography/ B-flow	Poor to rich vasculature	Mostly poor vasculature except when primary tumor is hypervascularized
	Preserved vessel architecture. Tree-like vessel branching, often seen up to the capsule. "Hilus amputation" in high tumor cell density or inflammatory edema	Mostly chaotic vessel architecture. Seldom axillary LNs in breast cancer; vessel architecture may be preserved
	Central hilar vessels	Often peripheral vessels
	Arterial and venous flow	Mostly only arterial flow or even no flow (in the LN center)
Contrast-enhanced ultrasonography	Centrifugal	Mostly centripetal
	Completely or only central vascularized	Intranodal ischemia/necrosis may be seen
	Enhancement only within the LN, except local abscess	Enhancement may exceed the LN margin when tumor penetrates capsule

lymphangiogenesis contributes to the tumor's drainage and thus reduces intranodal pressure is not yet clear.

The diagnostic confidence in abdominal staging is lower than that of CT and magnetic resonance imaging, especially in the thorax.

Regional LN stations are found along the course of the major vessels and organ-supplying vessels. In the case of a lymphatic spread, tumor cells enter an LN via the afferent lymphatic vessels and start to grow where they enter the cortex; thus, neovascularization starts within the cortex (**Fig. 17**).

When staging tumor patients, knowledge of the lymphatic pathways of the primary tumor is mandatory. Transport through the lymphatic system is the most common pathway for the initial dissemination of carcinomas. The initial route of tumor cells in most patients with melanoma or breast cancer is via the lymph vessels to the regional nodes. Especially in melanoma, tumor cells may stay within a lymph vessel and start to grow (transit metastasis, **Fig. 18**).

The site of cancerous LN infiltration in breast cancer depends on the quadrant location of the tumor. Tumors of the upper outer quadrant spread to LN of the axilla in 75%. Other sites of metastatic spread in early disease are supraclavicular and infraclavicular LN, and interpectoral LN (Rotter LN).

Applying these B-mode features, the negative predictive value is low in detecting LN metastases in breast cancer.[28] Comparing sentinel node biopsy with dissection in patients with breast cancer, a sensitivity of 71% to 100% has been reported.[29] Fine-needle aspiration of suspicious axillary LN in breast cancer has sensitivity of only 42%. Reasons for the unsatisfactory results have been explained by lymphovascular invasion and the sampling technique of fine-needle puncture.[30] Therefore, negative sonographic results do not exclude axillary LN metastases. A negative Solbiati index, preserved B-mode, and intranodal vessel architecture are reasons for not recognizing tumor-infiltrate axillary LN on basic ultrasonography examination. **Fig. 19** exemplifies that a single ultrasonographic criterion is often of little diagnostic value, and that it is important to decide on which LN to biopsy.

In patients with melanoma or other skin tumors such as Merkel cell carcinomas, regional LNs must be examined carefully; tumors distal of the elbow or the knee, the bend of the elbow, or the hollow of the knee should also be examined. Malignant LN metastases of the neck are most often found in head and neck cancers, lung cancer, melanoma, breast cancer, and lymphoma. Melanoma preferentially spreads via the lymphatics, making the first regional nodal basin the most important area of investigation. Cystic or calcified changes will increase the likelihood of cancerous LN. Tiny calcifications or cystic changes on LNs in the neck are suspicious for thyroid cancer metastases, but not specific (**Figs. 20 and 21**).

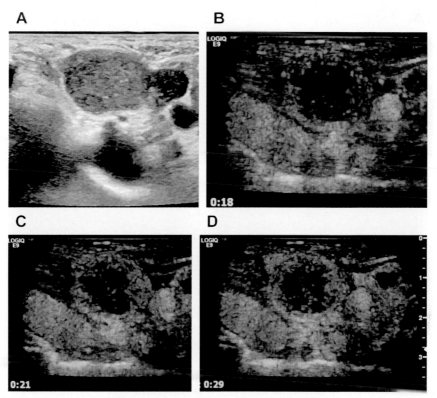

Fig. 17. (A–D) Lymph node metastasis from a squamous lung cancer. Contrast follows a centripetal enhancement pattern, being typical for malignant transformation of an LN.

A negative LN on ultrasonography is not sensitive enough to stage patients in small cancerous part tumors, and LN dissection for staging is still recommended. Ultrasonography is more helpful during follow-up, with regard to the size of metastases with the aforementioned technical and individual scanning limitations.

Highly differentiated tumors may also be characterized by rich intratumoral vasculature, and often mirror the vascularity of the primary tumor. Hypervascularized LNs can therefore be found in patients with thyroid, ovarian, breast, and renal cell cancer, and others in whom the primary tumor is also hypervascularized (see **Tables 1** and **2**).

A leakage of fluid into the surrounding fatty tissue causes a constant flow of tumor cells into the neighboring soft tissue. If a surgical intervention is planned this finding has to be taken into account, as the resected amount of tissue has to include the edema around the cancerous LN.

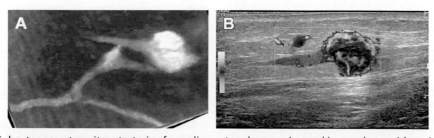

Fig. 18. (A) Subcutaneous transit metastasis of a malignant melanoma imaged in a c-plane with an inverted gray-scale map. The efferent lymphatic vessel is tumor-infiltrated by the transit metastasis. Subcutaneous veins can be seen close to the tumor. (B) Hypervascularization of the transit metastases.

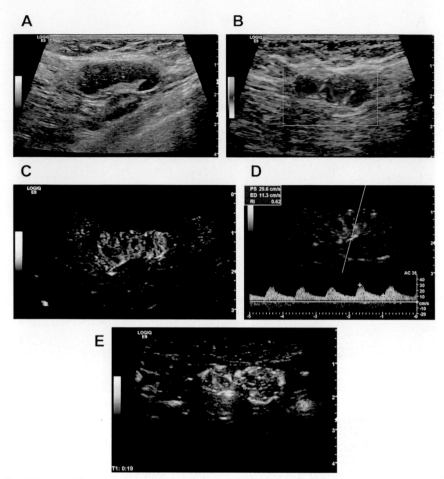

Fig. 19. (*A–E*) A 55-year-old woman with an incidental finding of an enlarged axillary LN. Although oval shaped (*A*), with a regular branching of the intranodal vessels on color Doppler and B-flow (*B, C*) plus a low resistive index of 0.62 (*D*), the LN has a thickened cortex, which was the indication for core biopsy. On B-flow–CEUS enlarged peripheral veins could be detected (*E*). Immune histology confirmed an LN metastasis of a ductal adenocarcinoma of the breast.

LYMPHOMAS

Two types of lymphoma can be differentiated, Hodgkin lymphoma and NHL. Four histologic subtypes of Hodgkin disease have been described: lymphocytic predominance, mixed cellularity, lymphocytic depletion, and nodular sclerosis (**Figs. 22 and 23**). Nodular sclerosis is the most common subtype, accounting for about 70%, whereas the lymphocytic depletion subtype is rare.[31]

NHLs arise from B cells (90%), T cells (~10%), and natural killer cells (~1%). NHLs are also described by how quickly the cancer is growing: indolent or aggressive. Indolent and aggressive NHLs are equally common in adults. In children, aggressive NHL is more common.

Histology is needed for a final specific diagnosis in patients with suspected lymphoma. Some investigators prefer as a first diagnostic step a core biopsy with sensitivity of 89% and specificity of 97%,[32] others a primary LN dissection. **Fig. 24** shows a case of a cutaneous T-cell lymphoma with an axillary tumor-infiltrated LN.

Extranodal involvement is more common in NHL than in Hodgkin disease, ranging between 20% and 40% versus 4% and 5% of cases.[23,33,34] Extranodal involvement is more common in patients with recurrent disease[35] or immunodeficiency-related disease[35–39] than in patients with an initial manifestation. As lymphomas can involve almost any organ and tissue, the possible differential diagnoses are great.

In most cases the LNs are echo-poor or even cystic; they may be lined up in chains and in most cases the swollen LNs do not hurt (**Fig. 25**C, D). Some LNs may have lost their

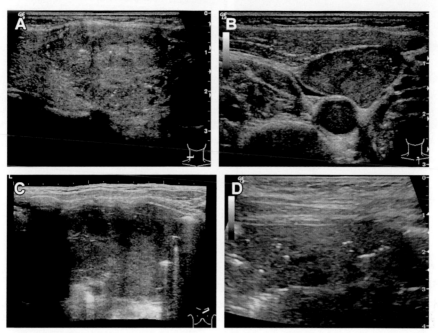

Fig. 20. (*A*) Papillary thyroid cancer with tiny calcifications. (*B*) LN metastasis of the same patient showing similar microcalcifications. (*C, D*) Infraclavicular masses of another patient with tiny calcifications. Histology confirmed Hodgkin lymphoma.

architecture while in others the cortex and hilum can still be differentiated. In B-mode, only minor changes of the cortex may be present.

In other cases multiple-cystic appearing LNs around the aorta may mimic an abdominal aortic aneurysm or Ormond disease (see **Fig. 25**A, B). Abdominal lymphoma can be seen intraperitoneally and retroperitoneally, and have the same characteristics as the peripheral LNs except that they mostly have to be examined with lower frequencies.

A lymphomatous LN may look like a reactive one; only a rich vasculature in the absence of an infectious focus can support the idea of a lymphatic disease. A focal infiltration may cause an echopoor, hypervascularized cortical thickening (see **Tables 1** and **2**).

No gray-scale or color Doppler criterion thus exists that can reliably differentiate between reactive LN enlargement and NHL involvement. As in other malignancies, lymphomas are also characterized by a high microvessel density (MVD); especially aggressive lymphomas have a high MVD. As in cancerous tumors, a high MVD is associated with a poor prognosis.[32,40–42] However, even CEUS cannot always detect a high microvessel density, as an elevated interstitial pressure may prevent its detection. To date there have been no reports on whether CEUS can contribute to the differentiation of different subtypes of NHL.

In most cases, color-flow imaging demonstrates a rich vasculature of lymphomas with clearly visible arteries and veins. The normal architecture is preserved, especially in NHL with low

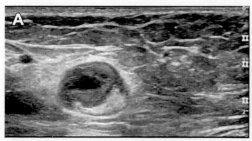
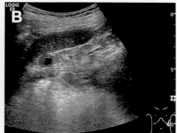

Fig. 21. (*A*) Central necrosis in a cortical LN metastasis in the groin (melanoma), cystic area in LN at the splenic hilum. (*B*) Central necrotic area of an LN metastasis of a colon cancer at the splenic hilum.

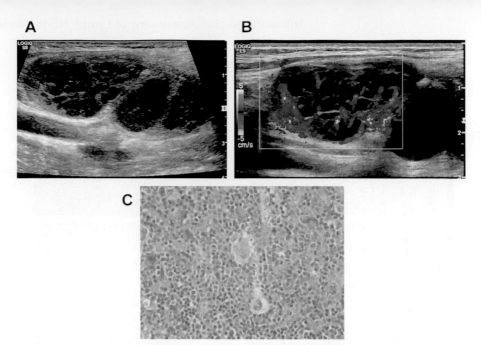

Fig. 22. (*A*) Hodgkin lymphoma of the neck (nodular sclerosis). (*B*) Color Doppler shows a rich vasculature. (*C*) On ultrasound-guided core biopsy, Reed-Sternberg cells were identified (HE stain). (*Courtesy of* L. Wilkens, MD, Hannover, Germany.)

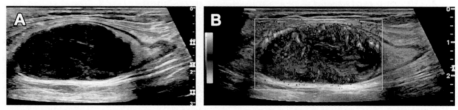

Fig. 23. (*A*, *B*) Large Hodgkin infiltration of an inguinal LN. Tumor vessels show a regular branching from the LN supplying central vessels.

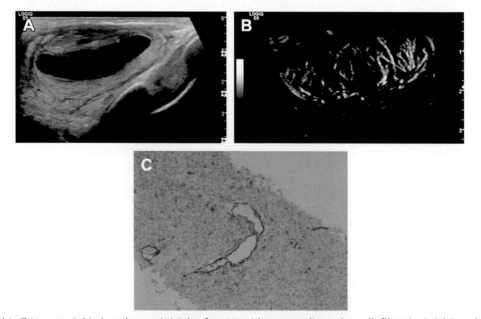

Fig. 24. (*A–C*) Non-Hodgkin lymphoma. (*A*) Echo-free LN with surrounding edema (infiltration). (*B*) Regular vessel branching imaged with B-flow. (*C*) CD31 stain demonstrated the larger vessels and the tiny tumor cell infiltration. (*Courtesy of* L. Wilkens, MD, Hannover, Germany.)

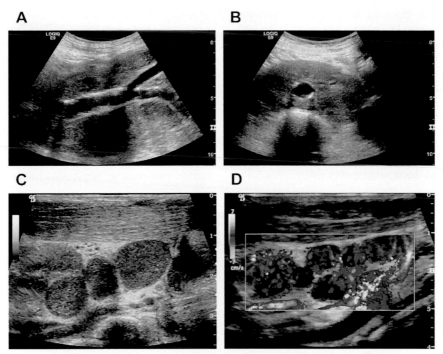

Fig. 25. (*A*, *B*) Para-aortic Infiltration of a non-Hodgkin lymphoma. (*C*, *D*) Multiple NHL nodes of the neck; color Doppler shows its rich vasculature.

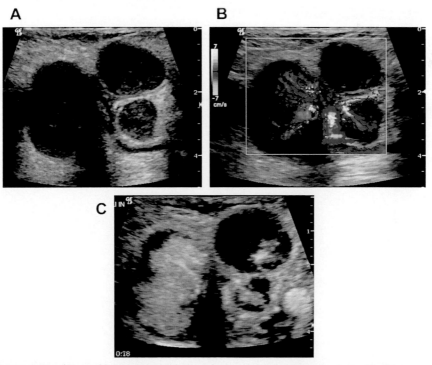

Fig. 26. (*A*) Inguinal LN infiltrated by non-Hodgkin lymphoma. (*B*) Color Doppler shows the bigger central vessels, and no peripheral vessels can be seen (hilar amputation). (*C*) CEUS shows more tiny vessels, but still no peripheral, subcapsular vessels can be seen.

malignancy.[7] In contrast to cancerous nodules, however, the native vessels are not destroyed, nor does neovascularization substitute native vessels. Color Doppler and CEUS may also show a distorted vascular branching and vessel amputation (**Fig. 26**).

Although most NHL transformed LNs have a typical gray-scale appearance, some show an echo-poor perinodular infiltration, as has been seen in inflammatory edema of soft tissue.

Sonographically detected enlarged LNs in patients with no history of malignancy present a challenge. There are considerable overlaps, especially between inflammatory and NHL LNs. A combination of several features, including the patient's clinical presentation, is helpful in the diagnosis.

FOLLOW-UP

Number, size, echogenicity, and vascularity of formally recognized malignant LNs are the most important criteria in the early follow-up. Local tumor recurrence, especially after surgery, is

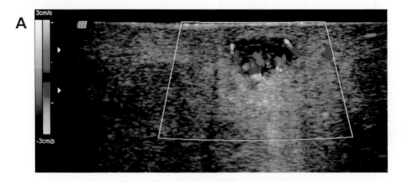

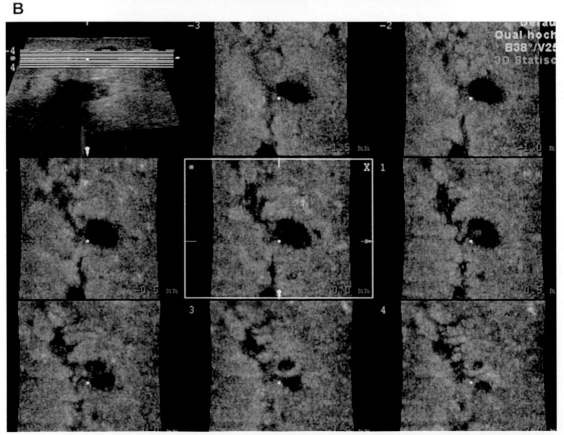

Fig. 27. Local tumor recurrence 2 months after LN dissection of an LN metastasis melanoma. (*A*) Subcutaneous hypervascularized metastasis (4 mm). (*B*) The c-plane image shows the metastasis adjacent to the scar.

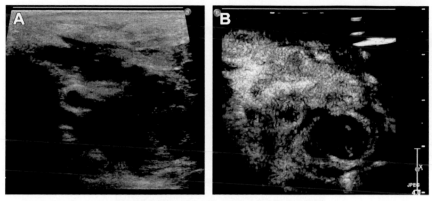

Fig. 28. (*A, B*) A 35-year-old man after axillary LN dissection (melanoma). (*A*) Suspected local hematoma. (*B*) Marked diffuse hyperenhancement without clinical signs of inflammation. Core biopsy confirmed diffuse tumor cell infiltration.

another challenge for ultrasonography. After surgery a scarred tissue, local edema, seroma, hemorrhage, or infection will be a challenge for most of the sonographic techniques applied. After LN dissection the scar has to be examined carefully. Owing to local spread of tumor cells probably caused by pressure on the node during intraoperative manipulation, tumor cells might either spread diffusely into the surrounding fatty tissue or start to grow locally (**Figs. 27** and **28**). Especially during follow-up, contrast agents are helpful in demonstrating local tumor tissue vascularization, and confirming the effect of chemotherapy (**Fig. 29**) and radiation therapy. During follow-up after radiation therapy CEUS will show a hyperemia of the irradiation field, and the tumor should be without enhancement (**Fig. 30**).

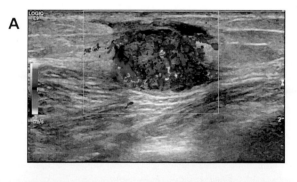

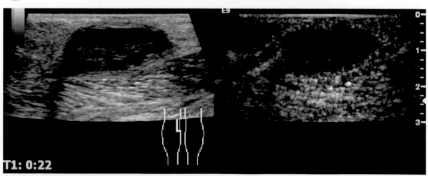

Fig. 29. (*A*) Transit metastasis (melanoma) shows rich chaotic vasculature before regional perfusion therapy. (*B*) CEUS shows the avascular mass 2 weeks after therapy.

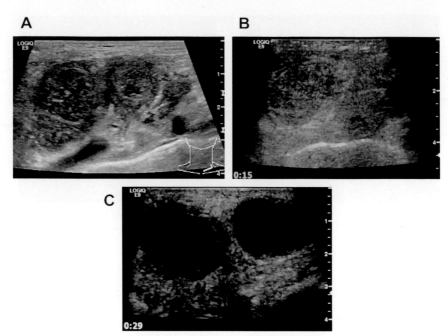

Fig. 30. (A) B-mode and (B) CEUS examination (hybrid mode) images of non-Hodgkin lymphoma in the axilla before radiation therapy. (C) Follow-up with CEUS 2 weeks after radiation therapy. Hyperemia of the tissue is adjacent to the nonenhanced LN.

SUPPLEMENTARY DATA

Videos related to this article can be found online at http://dx.doi.org/10.1016/j.cult.2014.03.008.

REFERENCES

1. Kubik S, Wirth W. In: Viamonte M, Rüttimann A, editors. Atlas of lymphography. Thieme Publ; 1980.
2. Willard-Mack CL. Normal structure, function, and histology of lymph nodes. Toxicol Pathol 2006; 34(5):409–24.
3. Weskott HP. B-flow—a new method for detecting blood flow. Ultraschall Med 2000;21(2):59–65.
4. Bhatia KS, Lee YY, Yuen EH, et al. Ultrasound elastography in the head and neck. Part I. Basic principles and practical aspects. Cancer Imaging 2013; 13(2):253–9.
5. Bhatia KS, Lee YY, Yuen EH, et al. Ultrasound elastography in the head and neck. Part II. Accuracy for malignancy. Cancer Imaging 2013;13(2):260–76.
6. Choi YJ, Lee JH, Lim HK, et al. Quantitative shear wave elastography in the evaluation of metastatic cervical lymph nodes. Ultrasound Med Biol 2013; 39(6):935–40.
7. Weskott HP. Ultrasound in the diagnostic management of malignant lymphomas. Radiologe 2012; 52(4):347–59 [in German].
8. van Rijk MC, Peterse JL, Nieweg OE, et al. Additional axillary metastases and stage migration in breast cancer patients with micrometastases or submicrometastases in sentinel lymph nodes. Cancer 2006;107:467–71.
9. Pech O, May A, Günter E, et al. The impact of endoscopic ultrasound and computed tomography on the TNM staging of early cancer in Barrett's esophagus. Am J Gastroenterol 2006;101(10):2223–9.
10. Tangoku A, Yamamoto Y, Furukita Y, et al. The new era of staging as a key for an appropriate treatment for esophageal cancer. Ann Thorac Cardiovasc Surg 2012;18(3):190–9.
11. Zhang R, Ying K, Shi L, et al. Combined endobronchial and endoscopic ultrasound-guided fine needle aspiration for mediastinal lymph node staging of lung cancer: a meta-analysis. Eur J Cancer 2013; 49(8):1860–7.
12. Lee TH, Cho JY, Bok GH, et al. Intra-abdominal tuberculous lymphadenitis diagnosed using an endoscopic ultrasonography-guided ProCore Needle Biopsy. Clin Endosc 2013;46(1):77–80.
13. Mulla MG, Knoefel WT, Gilbert J, et al. Lateral cervical lymph node metastases in papillary thyroid cancer: a systematic review of imaging-guided and prophylactic removal of the lateral compartment. Clin Endocrinol (Oxf) 2012;77(1):126–31.
14. Love TP, Delman KA. Management of regional lymph node basins in melanoma. Ochsner J 2010;10(2): 99–107.
15. Sun C, Jain RK, Munn LL. Ann non-uniform plasma leakage affects local hematocrit and blood

flow: implications for inflammation and tumor perfusion. Biomed Eng 2007;35(12):2121–9.

16. Jain RK, Booth MF. What brings pericytes to tumor vessels? J Clin Invest 2003;112(8):1134–6.

17. Goldberg BB, Merton DA, Liu JB, et al. Contrast-enhanced ultrasound imaging of sentinel lymph nodes after peritumoral administration of Sonazoid in a melanoma tumor animal model. J Ultrasound Med 2011;30(4):441–53.

18. Wu J, Long Q, Xu S, et al. Study of tumor blood perfusion and its variation due to vascular normalization by anti-angiogenic therapy based on 3D angiogenic microvasculature. J Biomech 2009; 42(6):712–21.

19. Ahuja A, Ying M. Sonographic evaluation of cervical lymph nodes. AJR Am J Roentgenol 2005;184(5): 1691–9.

20. Ahuja A, Ying M, Yuen YH, et al. Power Doppler sonography to differentiate tuberculous cervical lymphadenopathy from nasopharyngeal carcinoma. AJNR Am J Neuroradiol 2001;22:735–40.

21. Hobbs SK, Monsky WL, Yuan F, et al. Regulation of transport pathways in tumor vessels: role of tumor type and microenvironment. Proc Natl Acad Sci U S A 1998;95(8):4607–12.

22. Ahuja A, Ying M. Sonographic evaluation of cervical lymphadenopathy: is power Doppler sonography routinely indicated? Ultrasound Med Biol 2003;29: 353–9.

23. Doolabh N, Anthony T, Simmang C, et al. Primary colonic lymphoma. J Surg Oncol 2000;74:257–62.

24. Chang DB, Yuan A, Yu CJ, et al. Differentiation of benign and malignant cervical lymph nodes with color Doppler sonography. Am J Roentgenol 1994;162: 965–8.

25. Ying M, Ahuja A, Brook F. Repeatability of power Doppler sonography of cervical lymph nodes. Ultrasound Med Biol 2002;28:737–44.

26. Wu QW, She HQ, Liang J, et al. Expression and clinical significance of extracellular matrix protein 1 and vascular endothelial growth factor-C in lymphatic metastasis of human breast cancer. BMC Cancer 2012;12: 47. http://dx.doi.org/10.1186/1471-2407-12-47.

27. Hirakawa S, Brown LF, Kodama S, et al. VEGF-C–induced lymphangiogenesis in sentinel lymph nodes promotes tumor metastasis to distant sites. Blood 2007;109(3):1010–7.

28. Lee B, Lim AK, Krell J, et al. The efficacy of axillary ultrasound in the detection of nodal metastasis in breast cancer. Am J Roentgenol 2013;200(3): W314–20.

29. Lyman GH, Giuliano AE, Somerfield MR, et al. American Society of Clinical Oncology guideline recommendations for sentinel lymph node biopsy in early-stage breast cancer. J Clin Oncol 2005; 23(30):7703–20.

30. Park SH, Kim EK, Park BW, et al. False negative results in axillary lymph nodes by ultrasonography and ultrasonography-guided fine-needle aspiration in patients with invasive ductal carcinoma. Ultraschall Med 2013;34(6):559–67.

31. Ioma P, Granata C, Rossi A, et al. Multimodality imaging of Hodgkin Disease and non-Hodgkin lymphomas in children. Radiographics 2007;27: 1335–54.

32. Demharter J, Müller P, Wagner T, et al. Percutaneous core-needle biopsy of enlarged lymph nodes in the diagnosis and subclassification of malignant lymphomas. Eur Radiol 2001;11(2):276–83.

33. Charnsangavej C. Lymphoma of the genitourinary tract. Radiol Clin North Am 1990;28:865–77.

34. Metser U, Goor O, Lerman H, et al. PET-CT of extranodal lymphoma. Am J Roentgenol 2004;182: 1579–86.

35. Urban BA, Fishman EK. Renal lymphoma: CT patterns with emphasis on helical CT. Radiographics 2000;20:197–212.

36. Honda H, Barloon TJ, Franken EA Jr, et al. Clinical and radiologic features of malignant neoplasms in organ transplant recipients: cyclosporine-treated vs untreated patients. Am J Roentgenol 1990;154: 271–4.

37. Gassel AM, Westphal E, Hansmann ML, et al. Malignant lymphoma of donor origin after renal transplantation: a case report. Hum Pathol 1991;22:1291–3.

38. Miller FH, Parikh S, Gore RM, et al. Renal manifestations of AIDS. Radiographics 1993;13:587–96.

39. Tsang K, Kneafsey P, Gill MJ. Primary lymphoma of the kidney in the acquired immunodeficiency syndrome. Arch Pathol Lab Med 1993;117:541–3.

40. Tzankov A, Heiss S, Ebner S, et al. Angiogenesis in nodal B cell lymphomas: a high throughput study. J Clin Pathol 2007;60(5):476–82.

41. Farinha P, Kyle AH, Minchinton AI, et al. Vascularization predicts overall survival and risk of transformation in follicular lymphoma. Haematologica 2010; 95(12):2157–60.

42. Cardesa-Salzmann TM, Colomo L, Gutierrez G, et al. High microvessel density determines a poor outcome in patients with diffuse large B cell lymphoma treated with rituximab plus chemotherapy. Haematologica 2011;96(7):996–1001.

Ultrasonography of Lumps and Bumps

Jason M. Wagner, MD*, Bradley K. Lamprich, MD

KEYWORDS

• Sonography • Soft tissue • Superficial • Subcutaneous • Mass • Lipoma

KEY POINTS

- A superficial lump or bump may be caused by a large number of nonneoplastic conditions or by soft tissue neoplasms, most of which are benign.
- Sonography of superficial lumps begins with a focused history and physical examination and requires careful attention to technical detail.
- The diagnosis of soft tissue hematoma should be approached with caution, because hematomas and sarcomas can have similar sonographic features.
- Lipomas have variable echogenicity, but have characteristic sonographic features including wavy echogenic lines, smooth borders, wider-than-tall shape, and minimal or no internal Doppler signal.
- Soft tissue masses that are intramuscular or greater than 5 cm generally require additional evaluation with magnetic resonance.

 Videos of muscle hernia involving the tibialis anterior and dynamic compression of an abscess accompany this article at http://www.ultrasound.theclinics.com/

INTRODUCTION

A palpable lump or bump is a common reason for patients to seek medical care. The incidence of soft tissue tumors is estimated at 3 per 1000 people per year, with about 99% of these tumors having a benign histology.[1] In addition to tumors, patients also frequently present with nonneoplastic causes of a palpable lump, such as epidermal inclusion cysts, ganglion cysts, hematomas, and foreign bodies.[2,3] The diagnostic challenge posed by soft tissue masses is that a small number of these lesions are malignant and potentially life threatening. For instance, in the United States, it is estimated that 300,000 patients present each year with a benign lipoma, but 10,000 patients present with a soft tissue sarcoma and approximately 4000 patients die each year because of soft tissue sarcoma.[4]

The goal of managing patients presenting with a palpable lump is therefore to identify potentially aggressive neoplasms while minimizing the burden of excessive imaging and invasive procedures on patients with benign disease. We do not advocate imaging for all lumps and we recognize that experienced clinicians often effectively diagnose and manage some superficial lumps such as lipomas and cysts based on history and physical examination. However, clinical evaluation can be difficult because of the nonspecific signs and symptoms of soft tissue tumors, necessitating further evaluation with imaging.[4,5]

Ultrasonography is an attractive imaging modality for palpable lumps because of its low cost, lack of ionizing radiation, high spatial resolution in superficial structures, and ability to easily correlate imaging findings with palpation.[1,6,7] In addition, ultrasonography can assess blood flow in a lesion

Department of Radiological Sciences, University of Oklahoma Health Sciences Center, College of Medicine, P.O. Box 2690, Garrison Tower, Suite 4G4250, Oklahoma City, OK 73126, USA
* Corresponding author.
E-mail address: jason-wagner@ouhsc.edu

Ultrasound Clin 9 (2014) 373–390
http://dx.doi.org/10.1016/j.cult.2014.02.004
1556-858X/14/$ – see front matter © 2014 Elsevier Inc. All rights reserved.

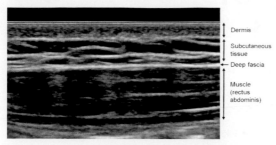

Fig. 1. Parasagittal longitudinal view of the anterior abdominal wall showing the major tissue layers.

without the need for contrast administration.[6] We recommend ultrasonography as the initial imaging evaluation of palpable masses that are clinically thought to be less than 5 cm in size and superficial. For lesions that are clinically thought to be large or deep, ultrasonography evaluation may be limited, and we recommend beginning with magnetic resonance (MR) for extremity lesions and computed tomography (CT) or MR for lesions of the neck and trunk. This article explores the sonographic evaluation of superficial lumps. Although much of this article is applicable to the evaluation of superficial lumps in older children, certain topics such as superficial vascular lesions in young children are not addressed in this article.

ANATOMY

The primary anatomic concern for evaluation of superficial lesions is identification of tissue layers (Fig. 1). Accurate localization of lesions into the correct tissue layer (Fig. 2) aids in determining differential diagnosis and appropriate management.

SONOGRAPHIC TECHNIQUE

Sonographic evaluation of a palpable lump should begin with a focused history and physical examination. Relevant history includes multiplicity of lesions, duration of the lump, rate of growth (or decrease in size), pain or other local symptom, signs or symptoms of infection, prior trauma or procedure, administration of anticoagulation, and history of major systemic illness or malignancy. Relevant findings on physical examination include size, firmness, mobility, and tenderness of the mass as well as inflammatory changes or discoloration of the overlying skin. Inspection of the skin for evidence of primary skin malignancy is important because these lesions may be difficult to detect with conventional ultrasonography. Palpation of the lump allows correlation of the palpable findings with the sonographic findings (Fig. 3), which is particularly important with small mobile masses in redundant tissues.

Sonography of a superficial lump is generally performed with a high-frequency linear transducer using a mound of coupling gel. Extended field of view imaging is helpful to show larger lesions (Fig. 4). Lower frequency transducers should be used to evaluate for deep lesions, particularly in the thigh (see Fig. 4). Color Doppler, or power Doppler, should be used on all lesions, with pulsed Doppler used when appropriate. With most superficial lesions, it is necessary to optimize the color Doppler settings for low flow by decreasing the

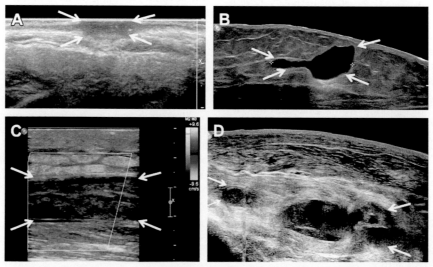

Fig. 2. Lesion localization. (A) Intradermal squamous cell carcinoma (arrows). (B) Subcutaneous postprocedure seroma (arrows). (C) Intrafascial abscess caused by methicillin-resistant Staphylococcus aureus (arrows). (D) Extensive hematoma in the gluteus medius muscle following bone marrow biopsy (arrows).

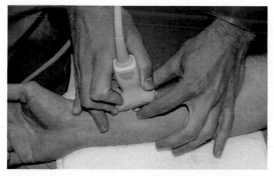

Fig. 3. Correlate physical examination findings with sonography by trapping the lesion between the index finger and thumb to immobilize the lesion, then place the transducer directly over the lesion. This maneuver is repeated in orthogonal planes.

color scale (pulse repetition frequency) and increasing the gain (Fig. 5). We train our sonographers to increase the gain until there is abundant Doppler flash artifact and then slowly decrease the gain to evaluate for slow flow. A light touch with the transducer is necessary, because too much pressure can decrease or eliminate flow in superficial structures (Fig. 6).

DIAGNOSTIC ALGORITHM

We use a diagnostic algorithm for evaluating palpable lumps with ultrasonography (Fig. 7). The initial sonographic evaluation of a lump yields 3 possible outcomes: no sonographic abnormality, a specific nonneoplastic diagnosis, or a possible neoplasm. When no sonographic abnormality can be found in the area of patient concern, we use the history and physical examination findings to guide further management. In most cases, we suggest clinical follow-up with repeat imaging if there is a concerning change. If we find the patient's history or physical examination concerning, or we think that we may be missing lesions because of anatomic or technical limitations, then we recommend further imaging with MR or CT.

FOREIGN BODY

Ultrasonography is sensitive and specific in the diagnosis of foreign bodies.[8,9] Glass and metal foreign bodies (Fig. 8) are generally echogenic and may produce comet tail artifact.[10] Metal foreign bodies may also produce acoustic shadowing. Wooden foreign bodies (Fig. 9) are

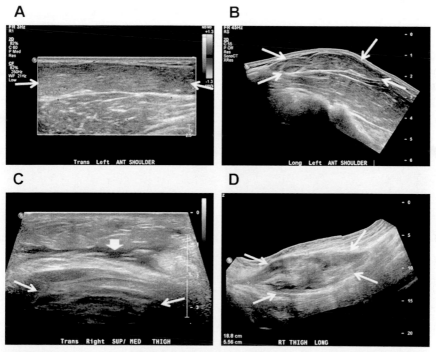

Fig. 4. The importance of using extended field of view and sufficient depth. Initial imaging of a palpable shoulder mass (A) shows apparently homogeneous subcutaneous adipose tissue (thin arrows). Further imaging with extended field of view (B) shows a large lipoma (thin arrows). Initial evaluation of the proximal thigh with a high-frequency linear transducer (C) shows subcutaneous edema (thick arrow), but only provides a hint of more extensive deep disorder (thin arrows). Evaluation of the thigh with a lower frequency curved transducer (D) using extended field of view imaging shows a large intramuscular mass (thin arrows), which proved to be a hematoma in this hospitalized patient with excessive anticoagulation.

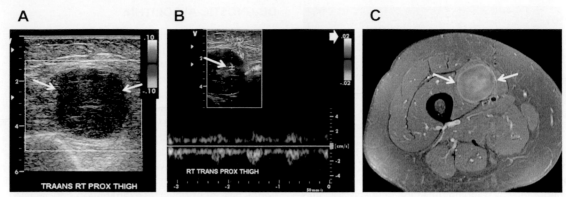

Fig. 5. The importance of color Doppler optimization. A 56-year-old woman who presented with a firm, painless thigh mass noticed after minor trauma. Initial sonographic evaluation (*A*), showed a hypoechoic intramuscular mass (*arrows*) without blood flow by color Doppler imaging, which was initially thought to be a hematoma. Further imaging with optimized color Doppler parameters (*B*) shows internal blood flow with an arterial waveform (*thin arrow*). Note the lower color scale (*thick arrow*). The patient was referred for MR imaging (*C*), which showed an enhancing mass (*arrows*). This was a benign myxoma at excision.

echogenic with acoustic shadowing and may have surrounding hypoechoic tissue if they are sub-acute.[10] The shadowing from a linear foreign body is often best appreciated when scanning perpendicular to the long axis of the structure.

SHADOWING STRUCTURES

There are multiple causes of superficial lumps with acoustic shadowing other than foreign bodies, such as bones and soft tissue calcifications. In our experience, a radiograph is often helpful in clarifying or confirming the diagnosis when a shadowing structure is detected with ultrasonography

(**Fig. 10**). Specifically, we use ultrasonography to guide placement of a metallic marker and then obtain radiographs, including a view that is at a tangent to the marker.

FAT NECROSIS

Fat necrosis is a benign process associated with aseptic saponification of adipose tissue, usually in the breast or subcutaneous tissue.[11] Fat necrosis can present as a palpable, possibly painful, nodule, with a variable history of trauma.[12] Fat necrosis can have a variable sonographic appearance, including a well-defined isoechoic mass

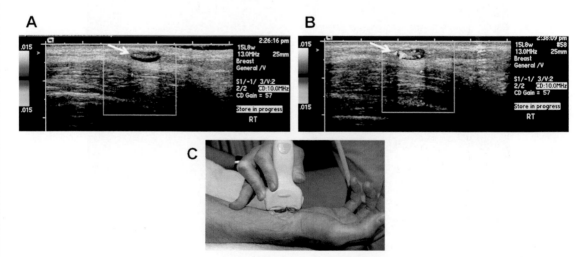

Fig. 6. The importance of a light touch. Both images are of a superficial benign-appearing lymph node at the axillary margin of the breast in a young woman and are taken with identical color Doppler settings. (*A*) Blood flow in the node (*arrow*) is only minimally detected because of excessive pressure from the transducer. (*B*) More robust blood flow (*arrow*) and was obtained by supporting the weight of the transducer and allowing only minimal contact with skin, but no pressure, which is accomplished by resting the ring and small finger on the patient (*C*) and lifting the transducer to eliminate pressure on the imaged tissues.

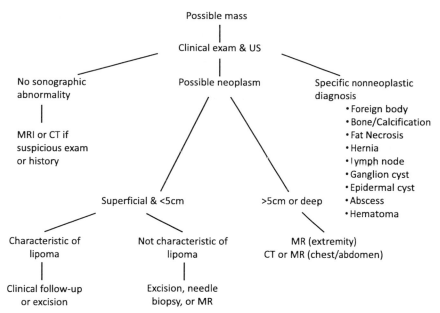

Fig. 7. Diagnostic algorithm for the sonographic evaluation of a soft tissue lump. US, ultrasonography.

with a hypoechoic halo and a poorly defined hyperechoic region in the subcutaneous fat.[12] Fat necrosis may have partial acoustic shadowing, possibly caused by calcification (**Fig. 11**). Although fat necrosis in the breast has a classic appearance on mammography, this appearance is uncommonly seen on radiographs of other parts of the body (**Fig. 12**). Because of its variable sonographic

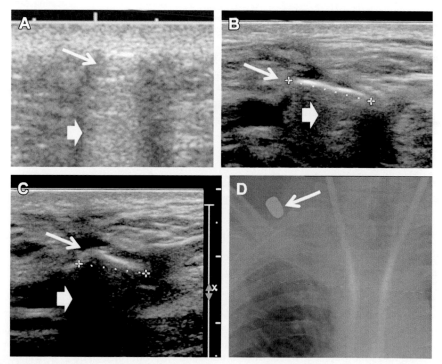

Fig. 8. Foreign bodies. (*A*) Glass foreign body (*thin arrow*) producing comet tail artifact (*thick arrow*). (*B, C*) Metal foreign body (*thin arrow*) that showed echogenic comet tail artifact (*thick arrow*) on a longitudinal image (*B*) and acoustic shadowing (*thick arrow*) on a transverse image (*C*). (*D*) Corresponding chest radiograph shows this metal foreign body to be a bullet in the supraclavicular fossa.

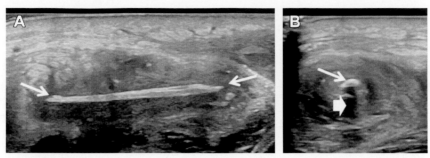

Fig. 9. Wooden foreign body (*thin arrows*) in the antecubital fossa. The image oriented with the long axis of the structure (*A*) allows measurement of the length of the structure but does not show clear acoustic shadowing. The image oriented perpendicular to the axis of the foreign body (*B*) shows deep acoustic shadowing (*thick arrow*).

appearance and symptomatic presentation, fat necrosis may require MR imaging or biopsy (see **Fig. 11**).

HERNIA AND LYMPH NODE

Both hernias and lymph nodes may be the cause of a palpable lump in an appropriate body site.

Both of these topics are discussed elsewhere in this issue.

A muscle hernia is a less commonly recognized cause of a lower extremity lump, potentially presenting as a painful mass present only with exercise. The most common location for a muscle hernia is the tibialis anterior (Video 1).[13] Ultrasonography is well suited for the evaluation of

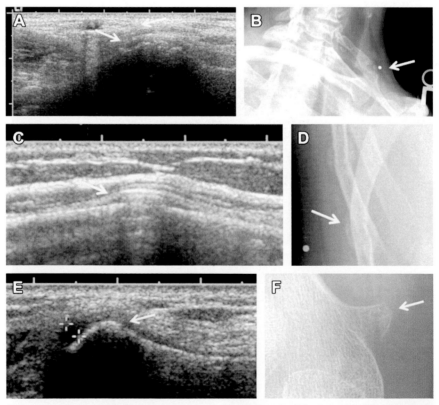

Fig. 10. Benefit of radiograph correlation for shadowing structures found on sonography. (*A*) A 52-year-old man who presented with a hard neck mass (*arrow*) and a history of a recent 23-kg (50-lb) intentional weight loss. The shadowing structure had sonographic characteristics of bone and was confirmed to be a cervical rib (*arrow in B*). (*C, D*) A 42-year-old man with a painful right upper quadrant mass that was found to be a healing rib fracture (*arrows*). (*E, F*) A 19-year-old man with a tender hard mass (*arrows*) at the lateral aspect of the knee that had a sonographic bone signature and was continuous with the adjacent femur. This mass was confirmed to be an osteochondroma. The calipers (*E*) measure the cartilaginous cap (*arrow*).

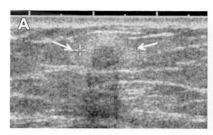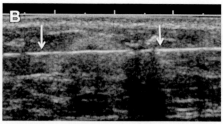

Fig. 11. Fat necrosis, proved by biopsy. A 61-year-old woman with a mildly tender, firm lump in the subcutaneous tissues of the chest wall. The mass was near the margin of the breast, but not within the breast. The mass (A) was centrally hypoechoic with surrounding hyperechogenicity and subtle acoustic shadowing (arrows). The patient could not recall trauma to the area. The patient had a history of treated ovarian cancer and strongly desired a biopsy (B, arrows indicate the needle).

a muscle hernia because of its ability to image the affected area immediately after vigorous exertion, which may be necessary if no abnormality can be found at rest.

GANGLION CYST

Ganglion cysts are common and account for 60% of wrist and hand masses (Fig. 13).[14] Ganglion cysts are found less commonly near other joints of the upper and lower extremities (Fig. 14). The diagnosis of a ganglion cyst is often made clinically, although ultrasonography imaging is useful in cases with atypical features or for preoperative planning.[14] Ganglion cysts are typically anechoic

with enhanced acoustic transmission. Thin septations and internal debris may be present. A stalk attaching the cyst to an adjacent joint may be observed in some cases with careful interrogation. Like all superficial masses, Doppler interrogation is needed to exclude a vascular lesion or a solid mass (Fig. 15).

EPIDERMAL CYSTS

An epidermal inclusion cyst is a common dermal or subcutaneous lesion that commonly occurs on the hair-bearing portions of the body, including the scalp, face, neck, and trunk.[15,16] Epidermal inclusion cysts contain keratin debris surrounded by

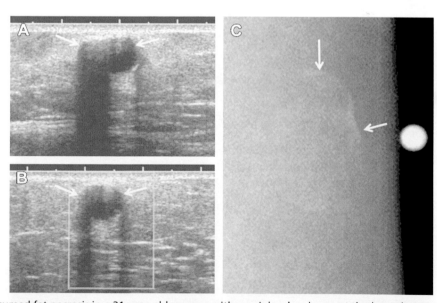

Fig. 12. Presumed fat necrosis in a 21-year-old woman with a painless hard mass at the lateral aspect of the knee. Longitudinal (A) and transverse (B) ultrasonography images of the mass show a hypoechoic partially shadowing mass (arrows) with no internal color Doppler signal. The mass could not be visualized on conventional radiographs of the knee, but an oblique view performed at a tangent to the mass with soft tissue technique revealed thin, smooth, partial rim calcification (arrows in C). The patient had a history of trauma 6 months earlier and was diagnosed with posttraumatic fat necrosis based on these studies. The patient was followed for 3 years with no clinical change.

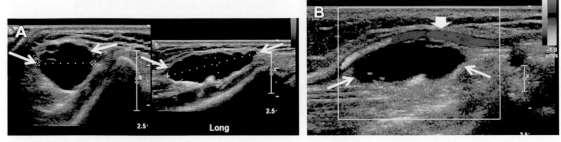

Fig. 13. (*A*) Transverse and longitudinal images of a ganglion cyst (*thin arrows*) immediately proximal to the wrist. (*B*) Color Doppler evaluation shows no flow within the cyst (*thin arrows*), which is immediately adjacent to the radial artery (*thick arrow*).

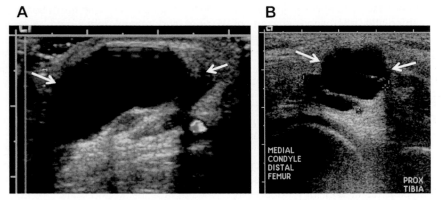

Fig. 14. (*A*) Cyst at the anterior aspect of the ankle (*thin arrows*), related to the tibiotalar joint. (*B*) Parameniscal cyst (*thin arrows*) at the medial aspect of the knee.

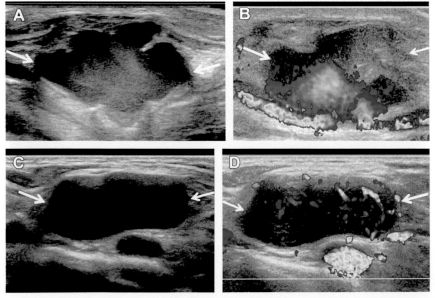

Fig. 15. Importance of color Doppler evaluation of possible cysts. (*A*) Lobulated lesion (*arrows*) in the forearm could be confused with a debris-containing cystic structure or abscess on grayscale imaging. (*B*) Color Doppler imaging showed this to be a pseudoaneurysm of the radial artery (*arrows*). (*C*) A lesion in the supraclavicular fossa (*arrows*) appears cystic on grayscale imaging. (*D*) Color Doppler shows abundant internal blood flow (*arrows*). Biopsy of this lesion showed follicular lymphoma.

a wall of stratified squamous epithelium, probably caused by traumatic implantation of epidermis into the deeper tissues.[16] Subcutaneous epidermal inclusion cysts are typically well-circumscribed, oval, mildly echogenic masses with increased acoustic through-transmission, a hypoechoic rim, and no internal Doppler signal.[17] The internal echogenicity of epidermal inclusion cysts has been described as a pseudotestis pattern.[15] Scattered internal echogenic and hypoechoic linear structures can often be seen. Epidermal inclusion cysts commonly have a dermal attachment, manifested as a focal extension into the dermis (Fig. 16).

Ruptured epidermal inclusion cysts may present as painful superficial lesions with surrounding erythema and swelling.[18] Ruptured epidermal cysts often have a lobulated shape, a poorly defined border, and increased vascularity by color Doppler imaging.[16,18] Because of these sonographic features and the presence of symptoms, ruptured epidermal cysts can be confused on clinical examination and imaging for more aggressive lesions (Fig. 17). Ruptured epidermal cysts are frequently excised because they can be complicated by abscess formation and may recur after antibiotic therapy.[18]

ABSCESS

Ultrasonography is the ideal modality for evaluating symptomatic patients for superficial abscess.[19,20] The differential diagnosis is often uncomplicated cellulitis (Fig. 18) versus abscess within an area of cellulitis. This distinction can be difficult by physical examination alone, but is important for instituting the correct therapy.[20] Abscesses often are irregularly shaped collections occurring within edematous, hyperechoic tissue with surrounding increased vascularity. The contents of an abscess can range from hypoechoic to hyperechoic (Fig. 19). Real-time sonography during dynamic compression is helpful in diagnosis of abscess, particularly when the contents are hyperechoic (Video 2).[19,20] When an abscess is identified, ultrasonography can be used to aspirate the collection (Fig. 20).

HEMATOMA

Hematomas present as an avascular collection that may be hyperechoic acutely, but generally is hypoechoic once established.[21,22] A variable degree of internal linear echoes may be seen within a hematoma (Fig. 21). A hematoma may be deformable with dynamic compression, but, in our experience, the contents of a hematoma show less motion with compression compared with abscess contents.

Although hematomas are common, the diagnosis must be approached with caution. The sonographic appearance of soft tissue neoplasm and hematoma can be similar (Fig. 22). When ultrasonography has been implicated in the delayed

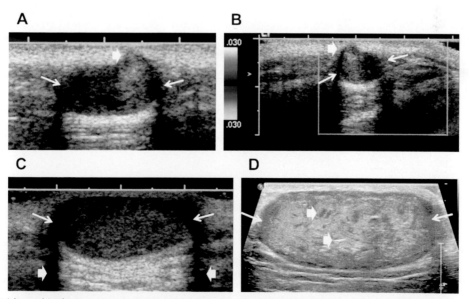

Fig. 16. Epidermal inclusion cysts. Longitudinal (A) and transverse (B) images through an epidermal inclusion cyst (*thin arrows*) showing no internal color Doppler (B) signal and a dermal attachment (*thick arrows*). (C) Epidermal inclusion cyst (*thin arrows*) that shows the pseudotestis pattern of internal echogenicity, increased acoustic through-transmission, and refractive edge shadowing (*thick arrows*). (D) Larger epidermal inclusion cyst (*thin arrows*) with internal echogenic and hypoechoic linear structures (*thick arrows*).

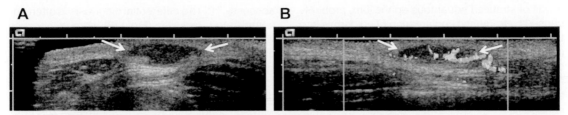

Fig. 17. (*A*, *B*) Ruptured epidermal inclusion cyst involving the deep dermis and superficial subcutaneous tissues with an irregular, lobulated border and prominent blood flow with color Doppler.

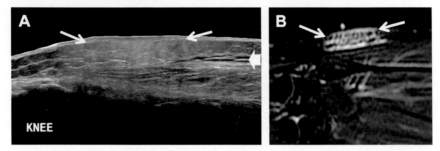

Fig. 18. Cellulitis. (*A*) Longitudinal sonographic image of the lateral aspect of the knee shows focal thickening and increased echogenicity of the subcutaneous tissues (*thin arrows*) and adjacent edema near the deep fascia (*thick arrow*). (*B*) Fat-saturated T2-weighted MR image of the same knee rotated into the same orientation as the ultrasonography image shows a corresponding area of increased subcutaneous signal (*arrows*).

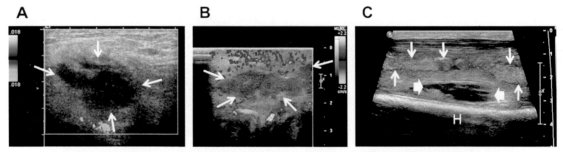

Fig. 19. Abscesses. (*A*) Axillary abscess with hypoechoic content (*arrows*). (*B*) Perineal abscess with intermediate echogenicity contents and surrounding hypervascularity (*arrows*). (*C*) Intramuscular abscesses in the upper extremity. The more superficial collection is hyperechoic (*thin arrows*) and the deeper collection (*thick arrows*) has near-anechoic contents. The deeper collection abuts the humerus (H).

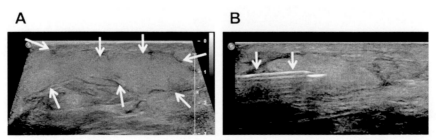

Fig. 20. (*A*) Extensive abscess (*arrows*) in the superficial aspect of the thigh with hyperechoic contents that are nearly isoechoic with the adjacent inflamed subcutaneous fat. The collection is difficult to see on a still image, but is easily shown with dynamic compression (see Video 2). (*B*) Ultrasonography-guided diagnostic aspiration (*arrows*).

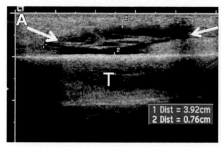
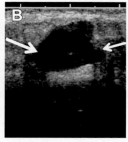
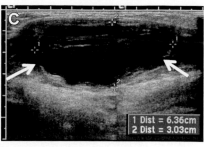

Fig. 21. Superficial hematomas. (A) Hematoma (arrows) anterior to the midshaft of the tibia (T) in a 21-year-old man who dropped a 20-kg (45-lb) weight on his shin. (B) Anterior abdominal hematoma (arrows) associated with an injection site of low-molecular-weight heparin. (C) Hematoma (arrows) in the antecubital fossa of an elderly woman with excessive anticoagulation (International Normalized Ratio >8) and a history of minor trauma.

diagnosis of a soft tissue sarcoma, hematoma is the most common incorrect sonographic diagnosis.[23–25] Sarcomas can also have internal hemorrhage and present as intramuscular hematomas, which can be a difficult diagnosis with both ultrasonography and MR.[26,27]

Therefore, a good explanation is required for bleeding, such as major trauma, surgery, or excessive anticoagulation, before seriously considering the diagnosis of soft tissue hematoma. Spontaneous intramuscular hematoma is rare and must be approached with a high degree of clinical suspicion.[28] In addition, many patients associate the onset of a soft tissue mass with minor trauma.[4] We generally recommend that soft tissue hematomas be followed clinically or with imaging and, if there is doubt of the diagnosis of hematoma, we recommend consultation with an orthopedic oncologist.

CAN ULTRASONOGRAPHY CHARACTERIZE SOFT TISSUE NEOPLASMS?

Although 99% of soft tissue neoplasms are benign, 1% are malignant and can be life threatening. The goal of imaging characterization is therefore to identify all potentially aggressive lesions and direct these patients to appropriate management. The role of ultrasonography in the characterization of soft tissue neoplasms is controversial, with several studies indicating poor diagnostic performance of ultrasonography.[29,30] Inampudi and colleagues[29] reported the results of sonography of 39 masses with known pathology (1 malignancy) and found a 64% accuracy of the sonographic diagnosis. Wu and colleagues[30] reported a series of 397 masses with known pathology (4 malignancies) and found a 58% accuracy of the sonographic diagnosis. Other studies have found ultrasonography to be effective in the diagnosis of superficial lesions.[2,7,31]

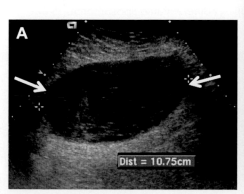
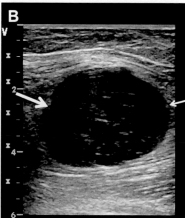

Fig. 22. The similar sonographic appearance of hematoma and neoplasm. (A) Postoperative hematoma of the abdominal wall (arrows). (B) Intramuscular myxoma (arrow; the same lesion as shown in Fig. 5). Both lesions are well defined and hypoechoic with predominantly linear internal echogenic structures.

For instance, Wagner and colleagues[2] reported a series of 72 masses with known pathology (1 malignancy) and found a 93% concordance between the initial diagnosis and the final pathology, as well as 96% accuracy for the diagnosis of lipoma.

Lakkaraju and colleagues[32] reported a prospective study in which ultrasonography was used to triage 358 consecutive patients referred during a 6-month period to a tertiary care center for evaluation of a palpable mass. Ultrasonography was used to categorize 284 patients into one of 5 benign categories, which included lipomas less than 5 cm with no worrisome clinical or imaging features. All of these patients were referred back to their primary care physician for clinical follow-up of the mass. At 24 to 30 months' follow-up, none of these patients had developed malignancy. In this study, all lesions greater than 5 cm, deep to the fascia, clinically painful, or enlarging were referred for additional imaging with MR. In addition, superficial lipomas less than 5 cm with internal heterogenicity and superficial lesions that could not be characterized as benign were referred for MR. Of the patients referred for MR, 6 were diagnosed with sarcoma.

A limitation of the study by Lakkaraju and colleagues[32] is that the ultrasonography examinations were all performed by experienced musculoskeletal radiologists and their results might not be replicated by all practitioners. Nevertheless, we think that well performed sonography can effectively triage patients into those with a high likelihood of benign disease versus those who need additional evaluation for possible malignancy. This opinion is reflected in our diagnostic algorithm (see **Fig. 7**). When a possible neoplasm is identified by ultrasonography, the next step is to determine whether the lesion is greater than 5 cm or deep to the fascia. If a lesion has either of these features, then we recommend further evaluation with MR for extremity lesions and CT or MR for lesion of the neck, chest, abdomen, and pelvis (**Fig. 23**).

Although more expensive than ultrasonography and generally requiring intravenous contrast, MR is well established in the diagnosis of soft tissue masses,[33,34] including fatty masses[35,36] and superficial sarcomas.[37]

If a possible neoplasm is superficial, less than 5 cm, and meets criteria for a lipoma with no concerning imaging or clinical features, then we diagnose the lesion as being compatible with lipoma and recommend clinical follow-up with repeat imaging or biopsy if there is a concerning clinical change. Simple excision of these lesions may be considered if the lesion is causing a cosmetic problem or physical symptoms because of its location, such as near the beltline. Superficial lesions that are possible neoplasms and do not meet strict criteria for lipoma should be considered for MR imaging or tissue sampling.

WILL ULTRASONOGRAPHY MISDIAGNOSE SUPERFICIAL SARCOMA AS LIPOMA?

Will following this algorithm with only clinical follow-up of subcutaneous lesions smaller than 5 cm that have clinical and imaging features of lipoma lead to an adverse patient outcome because of delayed diagnosis of sarcoma? We think that an adverse outcome caused by following our proposed diagnostic algorithm is unlikely, although the literature is not definitive on this topic. Furthermore, we doubt that a prospective study containing large numbers of both benign and malignant superficial lesions is feasible because of the rarity of superficial malignant lesions and the resulting need for a large number of patients. To further explore this question, based on the available literature, the incidence and natural history of superficial sarcoma must first be addressed. This article focuses on superficial liposarcoma because we think that the most likely type of sarcoma to potentially be misdiagnosed as a lipoma is well-differentiated liposarcoma.

A   **B**

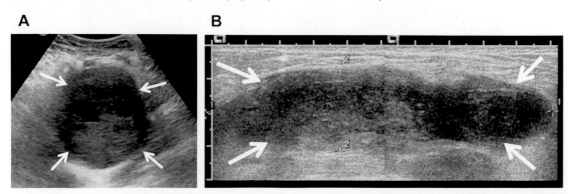

Fig. 23. Large malignant masses. (*A*) Intramuscular sarcoma in the proximal thigh (*arrows*). (*B*) Extensive solid groin mass (*arrows*) extending into the superficial soft tissues, found to be non-Hodgkin lymphoma.

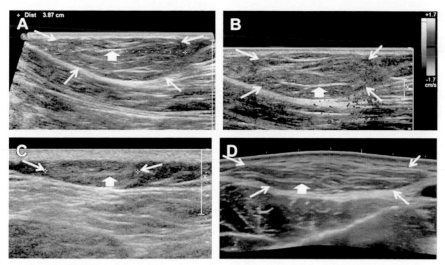

Fig. 24. (*A, B*) Subcutaneous lipoma (*thin arrows*) of the thigh of a 65-year-old woman, with no internal color Doppler signal despite sensitive settings. Subcutaneous lipomas (*thin arrows*) of the lower back (*C*) in a 64-year-old woman and the upper back (*D*) in a 31-year-old man. Note the gently curved linear echogenic structures (*thick arrows*) with the lipomas.

Although 99% of soft tissue tumors are benign and 99% of the benign tumors are superficial, 19% to 33% of extremity and trunk wall sarcomas are superficial.[38,39] In addition, 95% of benign soft tissue tumors are less than 5 cm at presentation,[38] but only 10% of malignant soft tissue tumors are less than 5 cm at presentation.[39] These statistics confirm the need to carefully evaluate all lesions greater than 5 cm and lesions located deep to the fascia but they also indicate that only a small minority of superficial lesions less than 5 cm are malignant.

In the large series reported by Datir and colleagues,[39] the most common types of malignant soft tissue tumors presenting at less than 5 cm were synovial sarcoma, spindle cell sarcoma, and leiomyosarcoma. In a series of 74 superficial malignancies, Calleja and colleagues[37] found

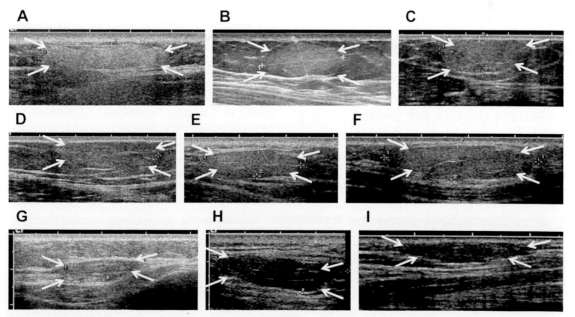

Fig. 25. (*A–I*) Nine different pathology-proven lipomas (*thin arrows*) showing a range of echogenicities, from hyperechoic (*A–C*) to hypoechoic (*H–I*) compared with the adjacent subcutaneous fat.

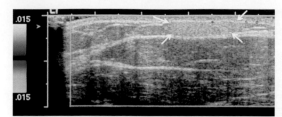

Fig. 26. Subcutaneous angiolipoma (*arrows*) in the upper extremity of a 38-year-old man. The mass is solid, homogeneously hyperechoic, and shows only a minimal amount of peripheral color Doppler signal.

> **Box 1**
> **Sonographic features of lipomas**
>
> - Hyperechoic to hypoechoic
> - Smooth borders (better appreciated on real-time imaging)
> - No refractive or edge shadowing
> - No deep shadowing
> - May have deep acoustic enhancement
> - Minimal or no color Doppler signal
> - Wavy echogenic internal lines; otherwise uniform echogenicity
> - Wider than tall (height<60% of width)
> - Subcutaneous (not intradermal)
> - Oval or gently lobulated
> - Clinical: soft or rubbery, mobile, slowly growing

only 8 (11%) to be liposarcoma. In a large series of 367 superficial malignancies with a median size of 3 cm, Salas and colleagues[40] found 12 (3.3%) well-differentiated liposarcomas, 9 (2.5%) myxoid liposarcoma, and 1 (0.3%) dedifferentiated liposarcoma. Subcutaneous and cutaneous pleomorphic liposarcoma has also been reported.[41] Subcutaneous and dermal liposarcoma seems to have a less aggressive clinical course than deep-seated liposarcoma, with reports of local recurrences but not distant metastasis.[41–44]

Therefore, superficial sarcomas less than 5 cm do rarely occur, although massively outnumbered by small superficial benign lesions, particularly lipomas. A small proportion of superficial malignancies are liposarcoma, although they seem to have an indolent clinical course. Can ultrasonography successfully separate these rare subcutaneous liposarcomas from the larger group of benign lipomas? Based on the prospective study by Lakkaraju and colleagues,[32] the answer may be yes, because no sarcoma was missed with ultrasonography and one of the detected malignancies was liposarcoma. In addition, Chiou and colleagues[7] reported different sonographic features of liposarcoma compared with lipoma.

DIAGNOSTIC CRITERIA FOR LIPOMA

Lipoma is the most common benign soft tissue tumor.[1] Lipomas are most common between the ages of 40 and 60 years, are more frequent in obese individuals, and are rare in children.[45]

Although we have encountered pathologically proven lipomas in older teenagers, we view the diagnosis of lipoma in a child with suspicion. Approximately 5% of patients with a lipoma have multiple lipomas.[45]

On clinical examination, lipomas are usually soft or rubbery, mobile, and nontender, with no overlying skin changes. Angiolipoma, a common benign pathologic variant of lipoma, is frequently tender to palpation, is most common in young men, and has predilection to occur in the forearm or the trunk.[38,46,47] In our experience, lipomas in some locations, such as the beltline, may be tender because of irritation from clothing or other causes of repetitive trauma.

By sonography, subcutaneous lipomas are solid masses with smooth, well-defined borders, which are often more easily appreciated on real-time scanning (**Fig. 24**). In a series of 66 lipomas reported by Chiou and colleagues,[7] 63 (96%) had well-defined borders, whereas 13 of 14 (93%) liposarcomas had infiltrated margins. Lipomas have variable echogenicity (**Fig. 25**). Wagner and colleagues[2] reported a series of 39 pathology-proven lipomas, in which 26% were hyperechoic,

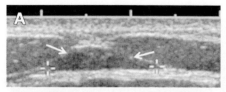
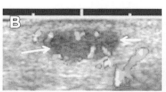
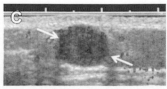

Fig. 27. Benign superficial masses. (*A*) Neurofibroma (*arrows*) involving the chest wall of a 29-year-old man. (*B*) Pilomatricoma (*arrows*) involving the hand of a 10-year-old girl. (*C*) Fibrohistiocytic proliferation (*arrows*) with benign features involving the back of a 9-year-old girl.

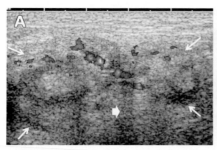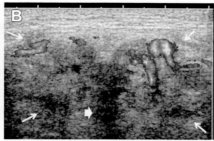

Fig. 28. (*A, B*) Soft tissue hemangioma (*thin arrows*) in the buttock of a 27-year-old woman. The mass has ill-defined borders, mixed echogenicity, moderate signal on power Doppler, and areas of acoustic shadowing (*thick arrows*).

59% were isoechoic, and 15% were hypoechoic with respect to the adjacent subcutaneous fat. Angiolipomas are generally hyperechoic (**Fig. 26**).[46]

Lipomas may have deep acoustic enhancement, but should not have acoustic shadowing or refractive edge shadowing. Lipomas generally have an oval or gently lobulated shape and are usually significantly wider than tall, particularly when greater than 2 cm. In our experience, a subcutaneous mass with a spherical shape is not a lipoma.

Gently curved (wavy) echogenic lines are commonly seen within lipomas (see **Fig. 23**). Wagner and colleagues[2] reported these lines in 29 of 39 (74%) lipomas. The 10 lipomas that did not contain these lines were mostly subcentimeter and hyperechoic. In this series, wavy echogenic lines were also observed in 3 fat-containing hernias, but in no other lesions. Chiou and colleagues[7] report echogenic lines in 59 of 66 (89%) lipomas and found these lines in no other lesions, including liposarcoma.

With color Doppler imaging, lipomas (including angiolipomas) should have no more than minimal Doppler signal.[2] A lesion with more than minimal color Doppler signal should not be diagnosed as a lipoma. In the series reported by Chiou and

colleagues,[7] 8 of 14 (57%) liposarcomas had moderate or greater color Doppler signal. A summary of the sonographic features of lipoma is given in **Box 1**.

SUPERFICIAL NEOPLASMS OTHER THAN LIPOMA

There are a wide variety of superficial tumors encountered less frequently than lipomas, including fibrohistiocytic, fibrous, vascular, and nerve sheath tumors.[38] Although there may be some hints to a specific diagnosis, such as continuity with a nerve seen in nerve sheath tumors, characteristic location in giant cell tumor of the tendon sheath, and characteristic symptoms in abdominal wall endometriosis, we generally regard superficial tumors other than lipoma as nonspecific (**Fig. 27**). Most of these lesions require excision or some other form of tissue sampling, although correlation with patient history and presentation is needed. Hemangiomas in the soft tissues have a characteristic appearance with a high vessel density and shadowing caused by phleboliths (**Fig. 28**).[48] However, the vascular patterns of soft tissue hemangiomas and sarcomas can be similar.[1]

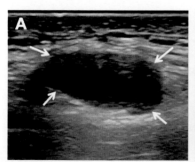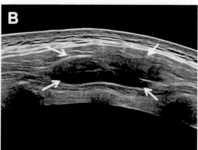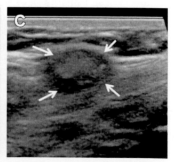

Fig. 29. (*A*) Metastatic melanoma (*arrows*) involving the back of a 21-year-old man. (*B*) Metastatic germ cell tumor (*arrows*) involving the muscle of the posterior chest wall in a 22-year-old man. (*C*) Metastatic papillary ovarian cancer (*arrows*) involving the anterior abdominal wall of a 46-year-old woman.

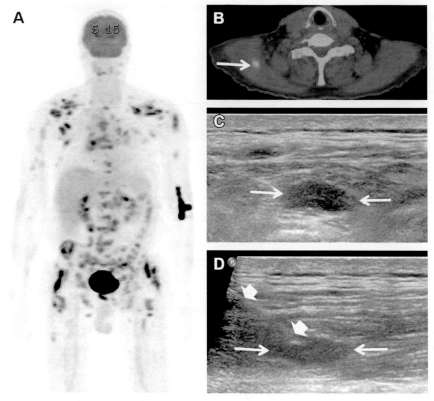

Fig. 30. Diffuse metastatic disease including intramuscular lesions. A 54-year-old man who presented with evidence of diffuse metastatic disease, as shown on a maximum intensity projection image (*A*) from positron emission tomography (PET)/CT. (*B*) Axial fused image from the PET/CT shows a focus of hypermetabolism (*thin arrow*) in the right trapezius. (*C, D*) This mass (*thin arrows*) was localized for the purpose of biopsy (*thick arrows* indicates biopsy needle). The diagnosis was widely metastatic esophageal cancer.

In studies evaluating patients referred to tertiary sarcoma services, the most commonly observed malignant soft tissue masses are sarcomas.[32,39] In our more general clinical experience and in the case series reported by Chiou and colleagues,[7] metastasis is the most common malignant diagnosis. In our experience, soft tissue metastatic lesions are solid hypoechoic masses with variable internal Doppler signal, although we have encountered hyperechoic metastatic ovarian adenocarcinoma (**Fig. 29**). Patients occasionally present with diffuse metastatic disease including superficial lesions. In these cases, ultrasonography-guided biopsy of a superficial lesion may be the easiest and safest method to establish a tissue diagnosis (**Fig. 30**).

SUMMARY

Ultrasonography should be the first-line imaging modality for evaluation of superficial lumps and bumps and can often establish a specific diagnosis. Careful attention to technique is necessary, particularly optimization of color Doppler. This article presents a diagnostic algorithm that can effectively triage patients who have a high likelihood of benign disease versus those who need additional imaging or tissue sampling.

SUPPLEMENTARY DATA

Videos related to this article can be found online at http://dx.doi.org/10.1016/j.cult.2014.02.004.

REFERENCES

1. Widmann G, Riedl A, Schoepf D, et al. State-of-the-art HR-US imaging findings of the most frequent musculoskeletal soft-tissue tumors. Skeletal Radiol 2009;38(7):637–49.
2. Wagner JM, Lee KS, Rosas H, et al. Accuracy of sonographic diagnosis of superficial masses. J Ultrasound Med 2013;32(8):1443–50.
3. Crundwell N, O'Donnell P, Saifuddin A. Non-neoplastic conditions presenting as soft-tissue tumours. Clin Radiol 2007;62(1):18–27.
4. Balach T, Stacy GS, Haydon RC. The clinical evaluation of soft tissue tumors. Radiol Clin North Am 2011;49(6):1185–96, vi.

5. Ahuja AT, King AD, Kew J, et al. Head and neck lipomas: sonographic appearance. AJNR Am J Neuroradiol 1998;19:505–8.

6. Bodner G, Schocke MF, Rachbauer F, et al. Differentiation of malignant and benign musculoskeletal tumors: combined color and power Doppler US and spectral wave analysis. Radiology 2002;223:410–6.

7. Chiou HJ, Chou YH, Chiu SY, et al. Differentiation of benign and malignant superficial soft-tissue masses using grayscale and color Doppler ultrasonography. J Chin Med Assoc 2009;72(6):307–15.

8. Jacobson JA, Powell A, Craig JG, et al. Wooden foreign bodies in soft tissues: detection at US. Radiology 1998;206:45–8.

9. Bray PW, Mahoney JL, Campbell JP. Sensitivity and specificity of ultrasound in the diagnosis of foreign bodies in the hand. J Hand Surg Am 1995;20(4):661–6.

10. Teefey SA, Middleton WD, Boyer MI. Sonography of the hand and wrist. Semin Ultrasound CT MR 2000; 21(3):192–204.

11. Robinson P, Farrant JM, Bourke G, et al. Ultrasound and MRI findings in appendicular and truncal fat necrosis. Skeletal Radiol 2008;37(3):217–24.

12. Walsh M, Jacobson JA, Kim SM, et al. Sonography of fat necrosis involving the extremity and torso with magnetic resonance imaging and histologic correlation. J Ultrasound Med 2008;27:1751–7.

13. Kramer DE, Pace JL, Jarrett DY, et al. Diagnosis and management of symptomatic muscle herniation of the extremities: a retrospective review. Am J Sports Med 2013;41(9):2174–80.

14. Freire V, Guerini H, Campagna R, et al. Imaging of hand and wrist cysts: a clinical approach. AJR Am J Roentgenol 2012;199(5):W618–28.

15. Huang CC, Ko SF, Huang HY, et al. Epidermal cysts in the superficial soft tissue: sonographic features with an emphasis on the pseudotestis pattern. J Ultrasound Med 2011;30:11–7.

16. Jin W, Ryu KN, Kim GY, et al. Sonographic findings of ruptured epidermal inclusion cysts in superficial soft tissue. J Ultrasound Med 2008;27:171–6.

17. Kim HK, Kim SM, Lee SH, et al. Subcutaneous epidermal inclusion cysts: ultrasound (US) and MR imaging findings. Skeletal Radiol 2011;40(11):1415–9.

18. Yuan WH, Hsu HC, Lai YC, et al. Differences in sonographic features of ruptured and unruptured epidermal cysts. J Ultrasound Med 2012;31:265–72.

19. Bureau NJ, Chhem RK, Cardinal E. Musculoskeletal infections: US manifestations. Radiographics 1999; 19:1585–92.

20. Adhikari S, Blavias M. Sonography first for subcutaneous abscess and cellulitis evaluation. J Ultrasound Med 2012;31:1509–12.

21. vanSonnenberg E, Simeone JF, Mueller PR, et al. Sonographic appearance of hematoma in liver, spleen and kidney: a clinical, pathologic, and animal study. Radiology 1983;147:507–10.

22. Jain N, Goyal N, Mukherjee K, et al. Ultrasound of the abdominal wall: what lies beneath? Clin Radiol 2013;68:85–93.

23. Doyle AJ, Miller MV, French JG. Ultrasound of soft-tissue masses: pitfalls in interpretation. Australas Radiol 2000;44:275–80.

24. Brouns F, Stas M, De Wever I. Delay in diagnosis of soft tissue sarcomas. Eur J Surg Oncol 2003;29(5): 440–5.

25. Coates M. Ultrasound and soft-tissue mass lesions – a note of caution. N Z Med J 2003;116(1187):1–2.

26. Ward WG Sr, Rougraff B, Quinn R, et al. Tumors masquerading as hematomas. Clin Orthop Relat Res 2007;465:232–40.

27. Kontogeorgakos VA, Martinez S, Dodd L, et al. Extremity soft tissue sarcomas presented as hematomas. Arch Orthop Trauma Surg 2010;130(10): 1209–14.

28. Taieb S, Penel N, Vanseymortier L, et al. Soft tissue sarcomas or intramuscular haematomas? Eur J Radiol 2009;72(1):44–9.

29. Inampudi P, Jacobson JA, Fessell DP, et al. Soft-tissue lipomas: accuracy of sonography in diagnosis with pathologic correlation. Radiology 2004;233(3): 763–7.

30. Wu S, Tu R, Liu GL, et al. Role of ultrasound in the diagnosis of common soft tissue lesions of the limbs. Ultrasound Q 2013;29(1):67–71.

31. Kuwano Y, Ishizaki K, Watanabe R, et al. Efficacy of diagnostic ultrasonography of lipomas, epidermal cysts and ganglions. Arch Dermatol 2009;145(7): 761–4.

32. Lakkaraju A, Sinha R, Garikipati R, et al. Ultrasound for initial evaluation and triage of clinically suspicious soft-tissue masses. Clin Radiol 2009;64(6): 615–21.

33. Berquist TH, Ehman RL, King BF, et al. Value of MR imaging in differentiating benign from malignant soft-tissue masses: study of 95 lesions. AJR Am J Roentgenol 1990;155:1251–5.

34. Moulton JS, Blebea JS, Dunco DM, et al. MR imaging of soft-tissue masses: diagnostic efficacy and value of distinguishing between benign and malignant lesions. AJR Am J Roentgenol 1995;164: 1191–9.

35. Gaskin CM, Helms CA. Lipomas, lipoma variants, and well-differentiated liposarcomas (atypical lipomas): results of MRI evaluations of 126 consecutive fatty masses. AJR Am J Roentgenol 2004;182:733–9.

36. Kransdorf MJ, Bancroft LW, Peterson JJ, et al. Imaging of fatty tumors: distinction of lipoma and well-differentiated liposarcoma. Radiology 2002; 224:99–104.

37. Calleja M, Dimigen M, Saifuddin A. MRI of superficial soft tissue masses: analysis of features useful in distinguishing between benign and malignant lesions. Skeletal Radiol 2012;41(12):1517–24.

38. Fletcher CD, Rydolm A, Singer S, et al. Soft tissue tumours: epidemiology, clinical features, histopathological typing and grading. In: Fletcher CDM, Unni KK, Mertens F, editors. World Health Organization classification of tumours: pathology and genetics of tumours of soft tissue and bone. Lyon (France): International Agency for Research on Cancer; 2002. p. 12–8.

39. Datir A, James SL, Ali K, et al. MRI of soft-tissue masses: the relationship between lesion size, depth, and diagnosis. Clin Radiol 2008;63(4):373–8 [discussion: 379–80].

40. Salas S, Stoeckle E, Collin F, et al. Superficial soft tissue sarcomas (S-STS): a study of 367 patients from the French Sarcoma Group (FSG) database. Eur J Cancer 2009;45(12):2091–102.

41. Gardner JM, Dandekar M, Thomas D, et al. Cutaneous and subcutaneous pleomorphic liposarcoma: a clinicopathologic study of 29 cases with evaluation of MDM2 gene amplification in 26. Am J Surg Pathol 2012;36:1047–51.

42. Allen PW, Strungs I, MacCormac LB. Atypical subcutaneous fatty tumors: a review of 37 referred cases. Pathology 1998;30:123–35.

43. Dei Tos A, Mentzel T, Fletcher CD. Primary liposarcoma of the skin: a rare neoplasm with unusual high grade features. Am J Dermatopathol 1998; 20(4):332–8.

44. Guillen DR, Coccerell CJ. Cutaneous and subcutaneous sarcomas. Clin Dermatol 2001;19:262–8.

45. Nielsen GP, Mandahl N. Lipoma. In: Fletcher CD, Unni KK, Mertens F, editors. World Health Organization classification of tumours: pathology and genetics of tumours of soft tissue and bone. Lyon (France): International Agency for Research on Cancer; 2002. p. 20–2.

46. Bang M, Kang BS, Hwang JC, et al. Ultrasonographic analysis of subcutaneous angiolipoma. Skeletal Radiol 2012;41(9):1055–9.

47. Choong K. Sonographic appearance of subcutaneous angiolipomas. J Ultrasound Med 2004;23: 715–7.

48. Lin J, Jacobson JA, Fessell DP, et al. An illustrated tutorial of musculoskeletal sonography: part 4, musculoskeletal masses, sonographically guided interventions, and miscellaneous topics. AJR Am J Roentgenol 2000;175:1711–9.

Ultrasonography of the Breast

Boris Brkljačić, MD, PhD*, Gordana Ivanac, MD, PhD

KEYWORDS

• Ultrasonography • Breast • Benign changes • Malignant lesions

KEY POINTS

• Ultrasonography (US) is extensively used for the diagnosis of breast diseases; it is convenient for the patient and enables high-resolution visualization of breast lesions without exposure of patients to radiation.
• As a real-time, dynamic modality, US is ideal for tissue sampling guidance.
• Sonographic features of irregular margins, hypoechogenicity, vertical orientation, and others speak in favor of invasive cancers, but a considerable overlap between benign and malignant US features exists, which requires correlation with mammography, magnetic resonance imaging, and often, image-guided biopsy.

INTRODUCTION

Continuous advances in ultrasonography (US) technology enable visualization of the breast with high resolution and greatly expand the use of sonography for the diagnosis of breast diseases.[1] US examination is well tolerated and convenient for the patient; it does not expose breast to radiation or other harmful effects and may be repeated whenever indicated. As a real-time, dynamic modality, US is ideal for tissue sampling guidance, because it enables monitoring of the accurate placement of the needle within the breast lesion during the biopsy. It is also used for preoperative lesion marcation and clip placement, or guidance of minimally invasive treatment, such as radiofrequency ablation.[2,3] Color and power Doppler are routinely used to evaluate vascularization of lesions, and three-dimensional (3D) US and sonoelastography are established in clinical practice.[4] Automated US is being investigated extensively, especially for screening. For optimal US examination, the proper equipment and transducer should be selected, the proper imaging technique should be used, and knowledge of the normal sonographic anatomy of the breast as well as of the sonographic features of benign and malignant lesions is needed. US findings need to be correlated with mammography and magnetic resonance (MR) imaging findings.[2]

EQUIPMENT FOR BREAST US AND EXAMINATION TECHNIQUE

Scanners with linear transducers are used in the high-frequency range of 10 to 15 MHz. The selection of imaging frequencies for particular parts of the breasts and particular lesions should be tailored individually, according to the breast volume, its structure, and the location/depth of the lesion within the breast. Higher frequencies improve resolution, but sound beam penetration decreases, which may be a disadvantage in larger breasts. Transducer apertures should allow a scanning width of 4.5 to 6.5 cm, and some manufacturers produce transducers with longer apertures.[4]

Disclosure statement: the authors have nothing to disclose.
Breast Unit, Department of Diagnostic and Interventional Radiology, University Hospital "Dubrava", University of Zagreb School of Medicine, Avenija G.Šuška 6, Zagreb 10000, Croatia
* Corresponding author.
E-mail address: boris.brkljacic@zg.htnet.hr

Ultrasound Clin 9 (2014) 391–427
http://dx.doi.org/10.1016/j.cult.2014.03.003
1556-858X/14/$ – see front matter © 2014 Elsevier Inc. All rights reserved.

B-mode, grayscale imaging features are the most important in the evaluation of lesions. Most high-end US systems have compound imaging, harmonic imaging, color and power Doppler, and elastography. Compound imaging uses electronic beam steering, and a composite image is obtained by averaging frames from multiple images obtained from different angles within the plane of imaging. Harmonic imaging can further improve spatial and contrast resolution; harmonic echo frequencies are used to generate the image while the original, fundamental tissue echo frequencies are suppressed by phase inversion between 2 consecutive transmit pulses. An extended field of view is less useful for the breast than for the muscles and other superficial structures, but may be used to show multifocal lesions within the breast lobe.[4–6]

Strain or shear-wave sonoelastography is used to measure the stiffness of breast lesions. In both forms, elastographically determined stiffness of a lesion is coded in different colors superimposed on the grayscale image. Strain elastography is more operator dependent because it requires manual compression with a transducer. It provides mostly qualitative information, with stiff tissues coded blue or dark, whereas elastic tissues are coded in bright-reddish colors.[7,8] Shear-wave elastography is less operator dependent, does not require compression, but only light transducer pressure, and ultrafast imaging is used to capture the velocity of the shear waves, which travel faster in hard tissues than in soft tissues. Shear-wave elastography provides quantitative information, because the elasticity of the different tissues can be measured and expressed in kilopascals, and elasticity ratios can be measured between the breast lesions and normal tissue or fat. In shear-wave elastography, stiff lesions are coded in reddish or bright colors, and elastic tissues in dark colors, opposite to strain elastography.[9–12]

3D US is available for use in breast sonography, with both automated and handheld 3D transducers. Automated supine breast 3D US is advertised for screening, and 3D US may have a role in assessing the response of cancer to neoadjuvant chemotherapy.[13]

Transducers with color and power Doppler use high Doppler frequencies ($\geq$7 MHz), which enable good visualization of lesion vessels. A malignant vascular pattern is described as hypervascular, with vessels arising along the edge of the tumor, extending into the center, often branching and very irregular, with low resistance index.[14,15] Vessels in benign lesions are supposed to be smooth and aligned parallel with the surface of the lesion. However, these general rules do not always apply in clinical circumstances, and there is often an overlap of many Doppler features in malignant and benign breast lesions; grayscale features are crucial in differentiating benign and malignant lesions and selecting lesions for biopsy.[16,17]

US is operator dependent, and meticulous technique is needed to optimize the examination and to scan all of the breast tissue so that no area is missed.[1–4] The medial quadrants are usually examined in the supine position; when outer quadrants are examined, the patient should be placed in the contralateral posterior oblique position, with the arm extended over the head. This position flattens the breast tissue over the chest wall and decreases the thickness of the tissue to be examined. The breast parenchyma should be carefully followed through in every direction until it is substituted with peripheral fat tissue. After the breast, the axilla should be examined for enlarged lymph nodes. If a breast lesion is palpated only when the patient is in the upright position, the examination may be performed with the patient in the sitting position.[2,18–20]

Scanning can be performed in parallel parasagittal planes, from top to the bottom, and with continuous transverse increments (from lateral to medial and back). The alternative radial technique requires centripetal imaging in the radial and antiradial planes, centering at the nipple and stretching outwards, corresponding to the normal pattern of lobar beast anatomy.[2–5] Whatever the technique, it is mandatory to visualize lesions in at least 2 orthogonal planes. To avoid absorption and scattering artifacts, uniformly controlled tissue compression by the transducer and perpendicular insonation (characterized by strong reflectivity of the fascia pectoralis) is needed. Optimal imaging of a particular lesion requires focusing the sound beam at the depth at which the lesion is localized. All lesions should be dynamically examined regarding elasticity, mobility, and delineation against the neighboring tissue. The sound beam striking a diagonal interface (Cooper ligaments) can be reflected away from the transducer, causing acoustic shadowing. Most echoes in glandular and fatty tissue are scatter echoes, which occur at tissue interfaces with irregular surfaces. The size of these interfaces is similar to or smaller than the sound beam wavelength, so the sound wave is scattered in various directions, and the intensity of the echo that returns to the transducer is weak. To maintain equal brightness and intensity of the image at different depths, time-gain compensation is used. The optimum gain settings should be adjusted according to the echogenicity of the fatty tissue. It should not appear too dark in the image to allow distinguishing between hypoechoic lesions such as carcinomas and cysts.[2,18–20]

NORMAL BREAST ANATOMY AND SONOGRAPHIC ANATOMY

The mature breast is composed of parenchyma (lobules), milk ducts, fat, and connective tissue. On average, there are 15 to 20 lobes in each breast, arranged centripetally around the nipple. There is a preponderance of glandular tissue in the upper outer portion of the breast, where approximately half of all cancers originate. Each lobe organizes around a lactiferous duct, and ducts converge into 6 to 10 larger collecting ducts, which open in the nipple. The lobule with its terminal branches forms the terminal duct-lobular unit. The parenchyma is imbedded in fatty tissue and supported by connective tissue, mainly Cooper ligaments, which arise from the stoma tissue and insert into the prefectural fascia and the skin. Axillary lymph nodes are the main drainage site of the lymph, but lower inner quadrants mainly drain into the internal mammary lymph node chain. Breast cancer can develop anywhere within the ductal epithelium, including the accessory mammary tissue, which should be carefully examined on US. During puberty, the ducts increase in length, and terminal alveoli increase in number. The immature glandular tissue is initially hypoechoic, like surrounding fat. With maturity, the echogenicity of the glandular tissue increases, sometimes not uniformly over the whole tissue volume, producing alternating hypoechoic and hyperechoic areas. In mature breast, the glandular tissue sonographically appears hyperechoic. Surrounding fatty tissue and interspersed fat lobules appear hypoechoic. Cooper ligaments appear as fine linear hyperechoic structures traversing the fat. They sometimes reflect the sound beam away, producing acoustic shadows, which can be eliminated by compression and changing the position of the transducer. The skin appears as a hyperechoic double-contour line; the thickness does not exceed 3 mm. The retroareolar ducts run almost parallel to the direction of the sound beam penetration and reflect sound echoes away from the probe, so an acoustic shadow behind the nipple is produced, which often impairs visualization of the retroareolar region.[2,18]

The role of US is particularly important in glandular, mammographically dense breasts, in which small cystic and solid lesions are hidden on mammography by the surrounding dense parenchyma. On US, these lesions can be visualized because of the different echogenicity between the lesions and surrounding parenchyma.[21,22]

With involution, parenchyma becomes atrophic, and fatty and fibrous tissues predominate. Fatty breast appears hypoechoic, with only scarce moderately echogenic patches of parenchymal tissue. The connective tissue remains hyperechoic. During pregnancy, lobular hyperplasia, hyperemia, and fluid retention in breast tissue occur. Sonographically, the echogenicity of the tissue decreases with increased water content.[2,18,23,24] In late pregnancy, the distended ducts can be recognized as tubular hypoechoic/anechoic structures. Hormone replacement therapy (HRT) causes proliferation of the breast parenchyma. The glandular tissue under HRT stimulation generally appears homogeneous and hyperechoic, but variations are possible (**Figs. 1–4**).[2,25]

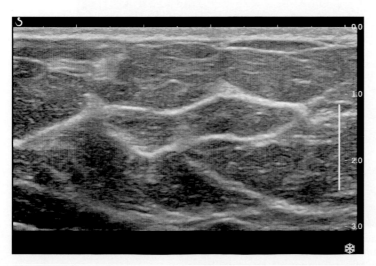

Fig. 1. Normal B-mode US image of the involutive breast. Sixty-year-old patient with fatty breasts, with completely atrophic parenchyma. Fat is hypoechoic, and connective tissue (Cooper ligaments) is hyperechoic. Superficially, skin is seen as a hyperechoic double-contour line. Examination was performed with a 15-MHz linear transducer.

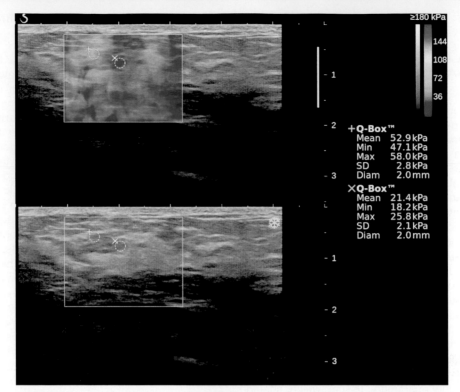

Fig. 2. Normal B-mode US and shear-wave elastography image of the dominantly glandular (mammographically dense) breast. Glandular parenchyma is echogenic, and fat is hypoechoic. On the upper part of the image, shear-wave sonoelastography is performed with colors related to stiffness superimposed on the grayscale image. Maximum elasticity value of parenchyma is 58 kPa and of fatty tissue 25.8 kPa. Diam, diameter; Max, maximum; Min, minimum; SD, standard deviation.

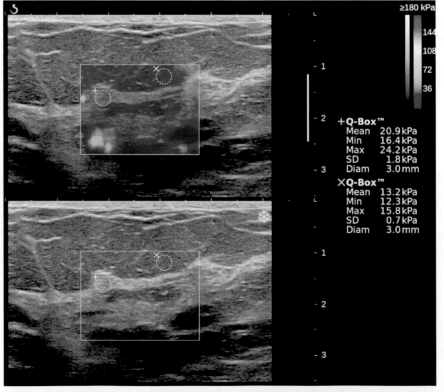

Fig. 3. Normal B-mode US and shear-wave elastography image of the moderately dense breast, with echogenic parenchyma with elastographic maximum elasticity value (Emax) of 24 kPa, and hypoechoic fat with Emax of 16 kPa. Diam, diameter; Max, maximum; Min, minimum; SD, standard deviation.

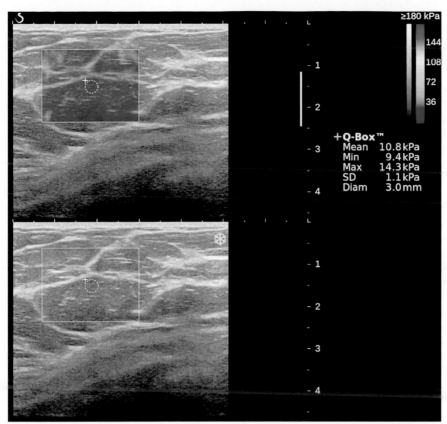

Fig. 4. Normal B-mode US and shear-wave elastography image of the involutive breast, with only fatty tissue visible and glandular parenchyma completely atrophic. Maximum elasticity value of fat is 14 kPa. Diam, diameter; Max, maximum; Min, minimum; SD, standard deviation.

TYPES OF BREAST LESIONS, SONOGRAPHIC FEATURES, AND THE BREAST IMAGING-REPORTING DATA SYSTEM

Histologically, breast lesions may originate from the main lactiferous ducts (ductectasia, main duct papilloma, intraductal carcinoma), from small and terminal ducts (hyperplasia, peripheral duct papilloma, ductal carcinoma), lobules (cyst, fibroadenoma, adenosis, tumor phyllodes, lobular carcinoma), stroma (sarcoma), or unclassified origin (radial scarring).[2,18] The most important is breast carcinoma, and its early detection is of crucial importance.[2,26] Generally, other breast lesions are important because they put psychological strain on a woman, and because they should be differentiated from cancer.

US is indicated to evaluate palpable abnormalities and other breast symptoms, to evaluate abnormalities detected by mammography or breast MR imaging, and to evaluate breast implants.[23] US is also used for screening in specific groups

of women, as well as for the evaluation of axillary lymph nodes. It is an excellent modality for guiding interventional procedures.

In most countries, the terminology and classifications proposed by the American College of Radiology Breast Imaging-Reporting Data System (BI-RADS) are used in imaging reports.[27] Consistent and generally understood terminology and assessment categorization can help define the level of suspicion for malignancy, ease the communication between medical experts involved in breast cancer diagnosis and treatment, and help to evaluate the performance of the breast imaging unit. In a structured report, BI-RADS recommends first defining the background echotexture of the breast, then describing focal lesions using specific features and providing the assessment category that describes the level of suspicion about the abnormality seen.[27] Background patterns include homogeneous fatty background echotexture, homogeneous fibroglandular echotexture, and heterogeneous focal or diffuse background echotexture.

A mass is a space-occupying lesion that should be shown in 2 orthogonal projections. The shape, orientation, margins, boundary, echo pattern, and posterior acoustic features of masses should be evaluated. All features should be carefully analyzed, and the level of suspicion should be based on the most worrisome feature. Masses can be round, oval, or irregular. Benign lesions are usually oval, whereas cancers tend to be irregular, but it is not unusual for some cancers to be round or oval.[2,11,28] Orientation of the lesion with reference to the skin line is unique to US examination. Parallel lesions (wider than taller) are more likely benign, and vertical (taller than wider) are more likely malignant. The margins of a lesion in relation to the surrounding tissue can be circumscribed (well defined), with abrupt transition between the mass and the surrounding tissue, or noncircumscribed. Circumscribed lesions are usually round or oval. Noncircumscribed margins are indistinct, angular, microlobulated, or spiculated, and they raise a higher level of suspicion for malignancy. The sonographic appearance of margins depends on the lesion and on the resolution of the equipment used, which is especially important

with small lesions. The lesion boundary describes the transitional zone between the mass and the surrounding tissue. There can be an abrupt interface, with sharp demarcation of the lesion, as in simple cysts and fibroadenomas. On the other hand, some carcinomas present with an echogenic halo, when no sharp demarcation of the mass and surrounding tissue is possible. Echogenicity is compared with the patterns of adjacent tissues and in reference to known structures such as fat and glandular tissue. Simple cysts are anechoic, contain no internal echoes, and are darker than fat. A hyperechoic lesion has the same or higher echogenicity as fibroglandular tissue and higher echogenicity than fat; hypoechoic lesions are less echogenic than surrounding fat; isoechoic lesions approximate the echogenicity of the surrounding fat, and complex lesions contain anechoic (cystic) and echoic (solid) components. Distal acoustic phenomena should be observed: posterior shadowing, posterior enhancement, or no changes in the posterior echogenicity. Posterior enhancement suggests a benign lesion and is typical for cystic lesions. Posterior shadowing of different intensity suggests malignancy, and a true shadow must be present in 2 different scan planes. No change in posterior

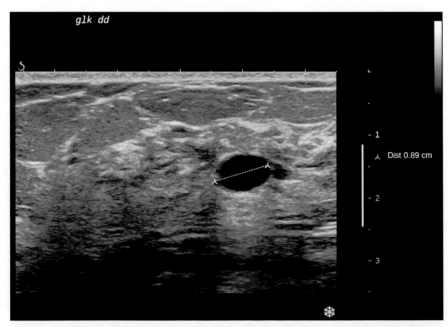

Fig. 5. B-mode image of the anechoic mass, with regular borders, clearly seen posterior wall, with refractory edge shadows and posterior acoustic enhancement. The lesion is darker compared with fat and contains no internal echoes. It is located within the parenchyma, and measures 9 mm in largest diameter. Typical US features of a simple cyst. Dist, distance.

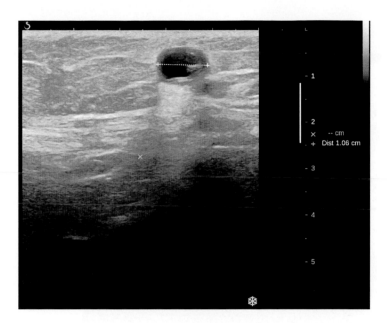

Fig. 6. B-mode image of the complicated cyst, with some internal echoes at the edge of the cyst and the thicker wall. Dist, distance.

echogenicity provides no diagnostic information because this pattern is seen in both benign and malignant lesions. Areas of acoustic shadowing or enhancement that do not originate from focal lesions commonly appear in dense fibrous breasts; with change of the transducer position, shadowing originating from benign fibrous tissue or Cooper ligaments may be eliminated (**Figs. 5–10**).[2,28]

The effects of the mass on the surrounding tissue include compression of the tissue with dilatation and infiltration of ducts, architectural distortion with obliteration of the anatomic tissue planes, straightening or thickening of the Cooper ligaments, skin thickening, skin retraction, or edema. Large calcifications, larger than 0.5 mm, present with dorsal acoustic shadowing.

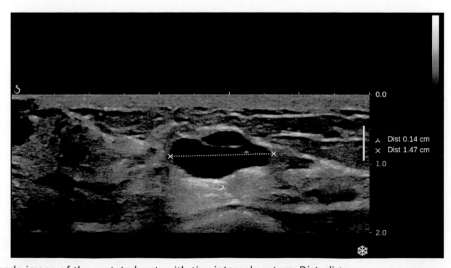

Fig. 7. B-mode image of the septated cyst, with tiny internal septum. Dist, distance.

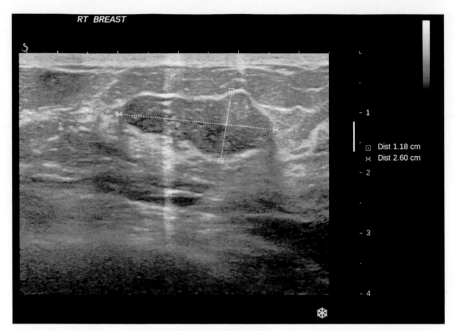

Fig. 8. B-mode image of the solid, horizontally located lesion, with regular, lobulated borders 2.6 × 1.2 cm in size. The lesion is only slightly more echogenic than fat, but hypoechoic to glandular parenchyma. It shows some posterior acoustic enhancement. Core biopsy finding: fibroadenoma. Lesion was initially categorized as BI-RADS 3, and is followed with US after biopsy as BI-RADS 2, benign lesion. Dist, distance.

Microcalcifications are difficult to visualize on US and too small to cause posterior shadowing. If visible with high-frequency transducers, microcalcification clusters present as multiple hyperechogenic foci either within the mass or within ducts. Although US is not used for the primary detection of microcalcifications, when suspicious microcalcifications have already been

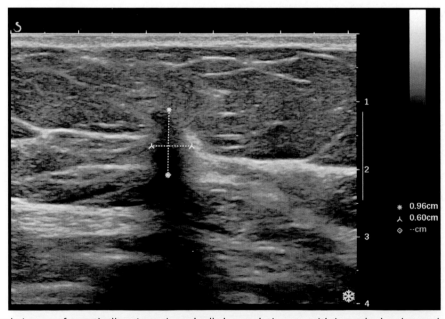

Fig. 9. B-mode image of a vertically oriented, markedly hypoechoic mass with irregular borders and distal acoustic shadow, located within glandular parenchyma. Anteroposterior diameter is 1 cm and laterolateral diameter 6 mm. Typical US image of a small invasive ductal cancer. Categorized as BI-RADS 5.

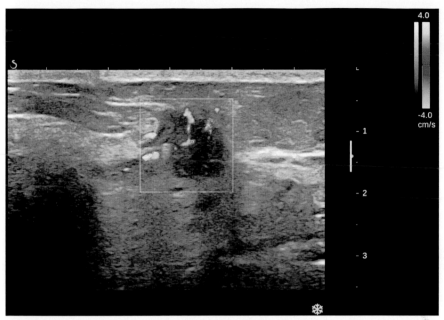

Fig. 10. Color Doppler shows irregular flow in a hypoechoic solid lesion, with irregular borders in the part of the lesion margins. This lesion does not show distal acoustic phenomena. Invasive ductal carcinoma.

diagnosed with mammography, focused US can be directed to the area observed on mammography. When US correlation is clearly present, the cluster can be subjected to US-guided biopsy. Some entities have unique sonographic presentations, such as clustered microcysts, complicated cysts, lesions in or on the skin, foreign bodies, and intramammary and axillary lymph nodes.[2,11,28]

Whenever possible, US should be correlated with mammographic and MR imaging findings. Based on all these features, the US report should contain 1 of the 6 final assessment categories and management recommendations. In category 0, additional imaging evaluation is indicated. Category 1 is for sonograms with no abnormality. Category 2 includes benign findings. Simple cysts are placed in this category, along with intramammary lymph nodes, breast implants, stable postsurgical changes, and fibroadenomas noted to be unchanged on successive US examinations. Category 3 includes probably benign findings. A solid mass with circumscribed margins, oval, and horizontal orientation (most likely a fibroadenoma) should have less than a 2% risk of malignancy. Nonpalpable complicated cysts and clustered microcysts might also be placed in this category for short-interval follow-up. The addition of elastographic findings may be useful because benign lesions are most often elastic, as opposed to cancers.[10,29–31] Lesions in category 4 have an intermediate probability of cancer, ranging from 3% to 94%. They can be stratified into additional groups of low, intermediate, or moderate likelihood of malignancy. In general, BI-RADS 4 lesions require tissue sampling, and needle biopsy can provide a histologic diagnosis. Included in this group are findings of a solid mass without all of the criteria for a fibroadenoma and other probably benign lesions. In category 5 (almost certainly malignant), the abnormality should have a 95% or higher risk of malignancy. With the increasing use of sentinel node imaging as a way of assessing nodal metastases and with the increasing use of neoadjuvant chemotherapy for large malignant masses or poorly differentiated masses, percutaneous imaging-guided core needle biopsy (CNB) can provide the histopathologic diagnosis. Category 6 is reserved for lesions with biopsy proof of malignancy before commencement of therapy.[27]

When US findings are correlated to mammography and MR imaging, the patient's position affects the lesion location, which may differ significantly between MR imaging performed in the prone position and US performed in the supine or lateral oblique position.[2,28]

BENIGN LESIONS OF THE BREAST

Hormonally induced secretion with retention results in the development of ectatic ducts and

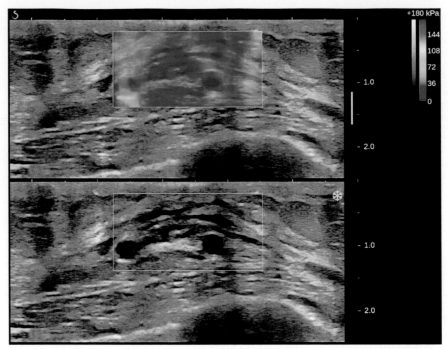

Fig. 11. B-mode and elastographic image of ductectasia. Dilated lactiferous ducts are visible as tubular anechoic structures behind the areole.

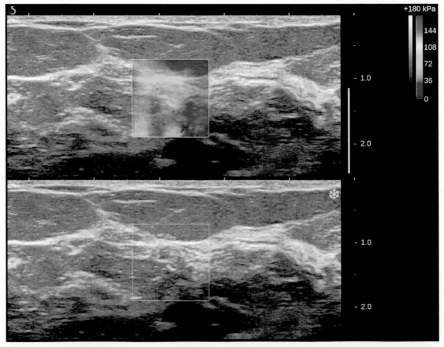

Fig. 12. B-mode and elastographic image of sclerosing adenosis; slightly inhomogeneous, slightly hypoechoic area within parenchyma, which is very elastic on sonoelastography. Diagnosis obtained by US-guided core biopsy.

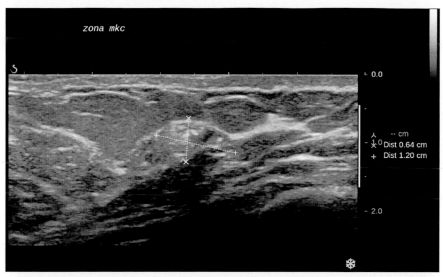

Fig. 13. B-mode image of inhomogeneous, slightly hyperechoic area with some internal echogenic foci corresponding to mammographically observed microcalcifications; core biopsy showed sclerosing adenosis. Dist, distance.

cysts. Proliferation of ductal and lobular epithelium causes different patterns and degrees of epithelial hyperplasia: adenosis, epithelosis, or atypical hyperplasia. Proliferative or hyperplastic changes are significant for their malignant potential, whereas nonproliferative fibrocystic changes have no malignant potential. More common benign breast lesions are cysts, sclerosing adenosis, fibroadenoma, ductectasia, intraductal papilloma or papillomatosis, or epithelial hyperplasia involving lobules or larger ducts. Less common benign conditions are lactational mastitis, lipomas, fat necrosis, foreign body granulomas, or sclerosing phlebitis (Mondor disease).[2,32]

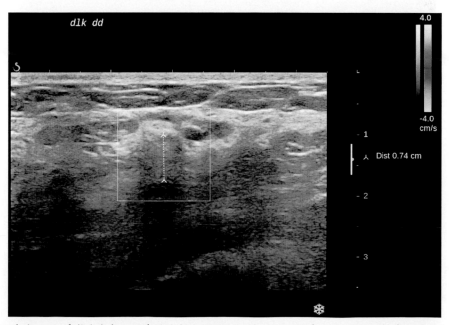

Fig. 14. B-mode image of slightly hypoechoic inhomogeneous lesion; core biopsy showed sclerosing adenosis and LCIS. Dist, distance.

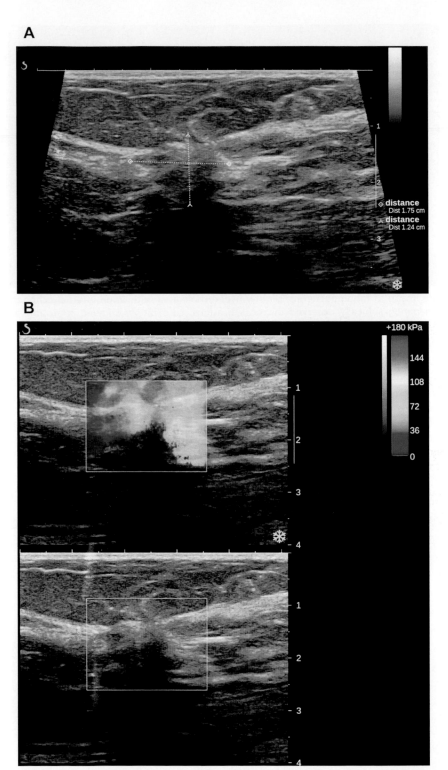

Fig. 15. (A) B-mode image of the radial scar; hypoechoic lesion with irregular borders. The same appearance can be seen in invasive cancer. The diagnosis was established with US-guided core biopsy. (B) The same patient as in (A); elastographic image of the radial scar showing slightly increased stiffness of the lesion.

Breast cysts occur commonly, and up to 50% of women in the age range between 30 and 40 years have solitary or multiple cysts.[2,20] US can show microcysts measuring 1 to 2 mm in diameter and simple or multiloculated macrocysts. In postmenopausal women, who are not receiving HRT, cysts are uncommon, and if detected, further evaluation is necessary. Special kinds of cysts are galactoceles and oil cysts. Galactoceles are retention cysts filled with milk that develop during pregnancy. Oil cysts are related to trauma or breast surgery, are filled with an oily, necrotic substance, and have typical peripheral eggshell calcifications. Simple cysts on US are round or oval, well-circumscribed anechoic masses with an abrupt interface to surrounding tissue, with bilateral refraction shadows and posterior acoustic enhancement.[2,20,33] The most important differentiating features of solid lesions are anechoic structure and capsulelike borders in cysts. If all criteria for a simple cyst are present, the diagnosis is reliable, and a BI-RADS 2 category is given.[2,27] Cysts show no internal color on elastography.[10] Septations in cysts should be distinguished from intracystic vegetation suspicious of malignancy by tissue sampling in case of doubt.

Adenosis, focal fibrosis, and epithelial hyperplasia are primarily histopathologic diagnoses.[32,33] Their US presentation is inconsistent and diverse. Hypoechoic, isolated, or multiple foci, which can be irregular or well circumscribed, are commonly observed, as well as solid or cystic lesions or hyperechoic areas of glandular tissue.[2,20,33] Sclerosing adenosis is the most common form of adenosis and is often associated with lesions such as fibroadenomas, papillomas, atypical lobular hyperplasia, and lobular carcinoma in situ (LCIS).[33] The relative risk of malignancy is increased by a factor of 1.5 to 2 (**Figs. 11–14**).

Radial scar is focal tubular proliferation developing around a fibrous elastoid center; because of its spiculations radiating outward, it resembles invasive cancer on mammography and US.[34] Areas of atypical hyperplasia, tubular, ductal (atypical ductal hyperplasia [ADH]), or lobular carcinoma can develop within the radial scar (**Fig. 15**).

Focal fibrosis is stromal proliferation associated with focal parenchymal atrophy, occurring in

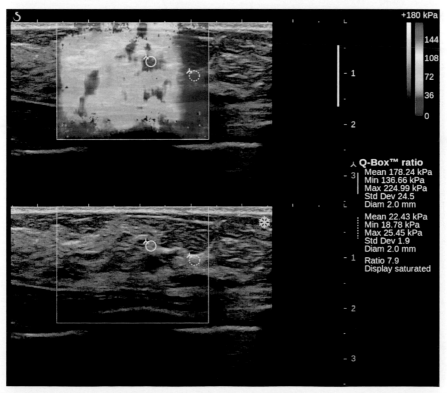

Fig. 16. B-mode and elastographic image of ADH showing a hypoechoic, irregular lesion, which is elastographically stiff (maximum elasticity value 225 kPa). The diagnosis was established with US-guided core biopsy. Diam, diameter; Max, maximum; Min, minimum; Std Dev, standard deviation.

younger women. It can produce hypoechoic focal lesions, with acoustic shadowing suspicious of malignancy.[2,20] Epithelial hyperplasia may be ductal, lobular, and atypical and increases the relative risk of malignancy by a factor of 4 to 5.[32,33] ADH is primarily observed in postmenopausal women, and when it is diagnosed in a biopsy specimen, the risk of underdiagnosing

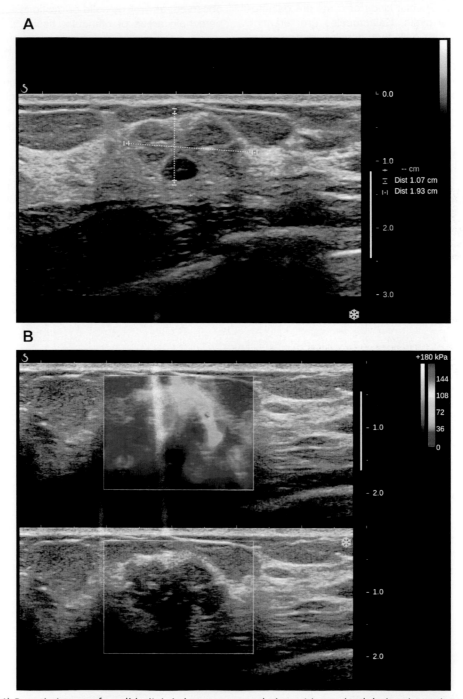

Fig. 17. (A) B-mode image of a solid, slightly heterogeneous lesion with regular, lobulated margins and absent distal acoustic phenomena. Dist, distance. (B) Shear-wave sonoelastographic image of the same lesion, which is soft. Core biopsy: fibroadenoma.

ductal carcinoma in situ (DCIS) exists, and a wider excisional biopsy should be considered.[35] Atypical lobular hyperplasia, on the other hand, corresponds with LCIS (Fig. 16).

Fibroadenomas are fibroepithelial mixed lesions, hormone-induced hyperplastic tumors of the lobular connective tissue, and the most common benign breast tumors.[33] The highest incidence occurs between 25 and 35 years of age. In women older than 40 years, the incidence decreases and the incidence of cancer increases. Therefore, all solid lesions in women older than 40 years, regardless of sonographic appearance, should be suspected for malignancy. Adult fibroadenomas found in young women have edematous stroma, whereas after menopause, stroma becomes sclerotic, and these lesions radiographically correspond to older fibroadenomas. Juvenile fibroadenomas generally occur in women younger than 20 years. They are large, grow fast, and are sometimes called giant fibroadenomas. Fibroadenomas are usually solitary, measuring about 1 to 2 cm and are seldom more than 4 cm in diameter. Multiple lesions are observed in 10% of patients. Most fibroadenomas present with typical benign sonographic features of round or oval, rarely lobulated contour, circumscribed borders, homogeneous hypoechoic internal pattern, bilateral refractive shadowing, posterior enhancement, horizontal orientation, and soft on elastography.[18,28,33] In involuted breasts with increasing fibrosis within the fibroadenoma, contour irregularities, and heterogeneous internal echoes, posterior acoustic shadowing caused by the calcifications may develop, and such lesions are difficult to differentiate from malignancies. Typical fibroadenomas are initially categorized as BI-RADS 3 and follow-up examinations at 6-month intervals are recommended, but in our practice, newly discovered lesions are further evaluated by tissue sampling, and then followed after the diagnosis is confirmed as a BI-RADS 2 lesion if unchanged.[2,20,32] It is not uncommon for a breast carcinoma to present as a well-circumscribed, smoothly marginated, horizontally oriented lesion (Figs. 17 and 18).

Papillomas are rare, benign fibroepithelial tumors located intraductally, and can cause watery,

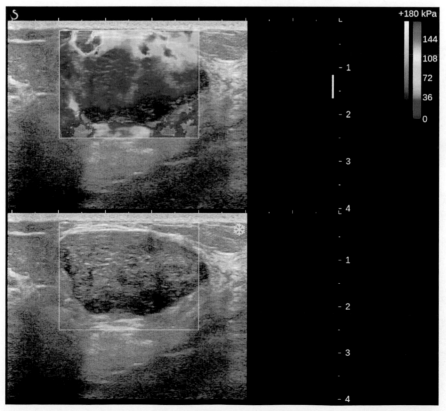

Fig. 18. B-mode and elastographic image of typical large fibroadenoma, with regular borders, hypoechoic echogenicity, and soft on elastography.

yellowish, brownish or bloody discharge, duct distension, or cyst formation. Three basic sonographic patterns are an intraductal mass with or without ductal dilatation, an intracystic mass, and a predominantly solid pattern with the intraductal mass totally filling the duct. Benign papillomas may have dense and coarse calcifications. Intraductal papillary neoplasms are highly vascular and may bleed spontaneously. Reliable differentiation between benign papilloma and papillary carcinoma is not possible on sonography and requires further diagnostic evaluation (**Fig. 19**).[2,32,33]

Hamartomas are abnormal collections of tissues normally found in the breast, such as parenchyma, smooth muscle, and fat. They are surrounded by a pseudocapsule and are completely benign. The sonographic appearance is of smoothly marginated, well-defined, horizontally oriented lesions. Hypoechoic fat islands, separated by hyperechoic septa, can be identified within the nodule. The diagnosis can be made only by excision biopsy.[2,33]

Other benign tumors are rare: lipoma, leiomyoma, neurofibroma, chondroma, osteoma,

A

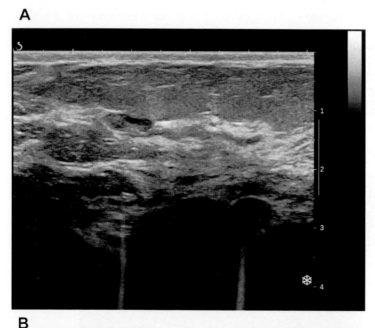

B

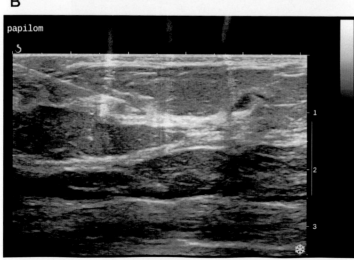

Fig. 19. (*A*) B-mode image of a small intraductal lesion of mixed internal echogenicity; (*B*) Needle during core biopsy in the lesion. Papilloma.

angioma, epithelial and dermoid cysts, and so forth. They mostly present as smoothly outlined, oval or round structures and are difficult to distinguish from fibroadenomas by imaging alone (**Fig. 20**).[2,33]

Subacute and chronic mastitis develop after inadequate therapy for the acute forms and present with formation of abscesses and sometimes fistulas. Sonographically, skin thickening, changes in echogenicity of parenchyma and subcutaneous tissue, dilated ducts with hypoechoic content, and fibrosis with acoustic shadowing are seen. Abscesses usually present as irregularly circumscribed, low-echogenicity lesions with internal echoes surrounded by a hyperechoic rim of demarcation and edema. They may be difficult to differentiate from malignancy and tissue sampling is then necessary (**Figs. 21 and 22**).[2,33]

Pseudoangiomatous stromal hyperplasia is also not an uncommon diagnosis acquired on core biopsy of inhomogeneous, usually hypoechoic areas within the breast parenchyma (**Fig. 23**).

MALIGNANT LESIONS OF THE BREAST

Carcinomas in situ are neoplasms without penetration of the basement epithelial membrane. They mark an increased risk of development of a malignant disease. Two types of in situ carcinomas are DCIS, and LCIS.[2] DCIS develops from lactiferous ductal epithelium and is often multifocal. Five types differ in differentiation and malignant potential; comedo DCIS is the less differentiated type, which progresses into invasive carcinoma in about 50% of cases. Better differentiated types turn into invasive cancer in 20% to 30% of cases.[36] LCIS arises in ductolobular units of breast parenchyma, but frequently involves extralobular ducts as well. Half of patients have multicentric LCIS, and one-third bilateral. LCIS has less malignant potential than DCIS and is not considered a true carcinoma but rather a severe epithelial atypia. Generally, LCIS lesions are not sonographically recognizable.[2,18]

The increased use of screening mammography has led to a marked increase in the number of diagnosed DCIS. Most DCIS are detected by mammographically visible microcalcifications.[37] Sonography is not the first choice imaging modality for diagnosing and staging carcinomas in situ because US is inferior to mammography for the detection of suspicious microcalcifications. US features of DCIS include hypoechoic irregular mass, ductal abnormalities, and architectural distortions. In our experience, in more than 70% of DCIS, hyperechoic foci can be found on US, either within a mass or within a duct, representing microcalcification clusters visible on

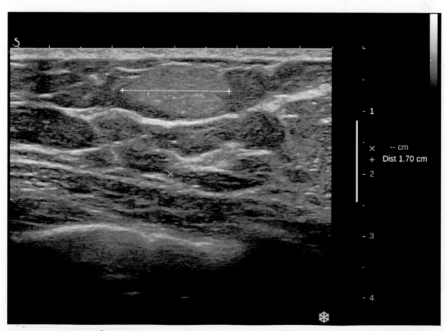

Fig. 20. B-mode image of homogeneous, hyperechoic, horizontally positioned lesion with regular margins located within the fat; typical image of lipoma. Dist, distance.

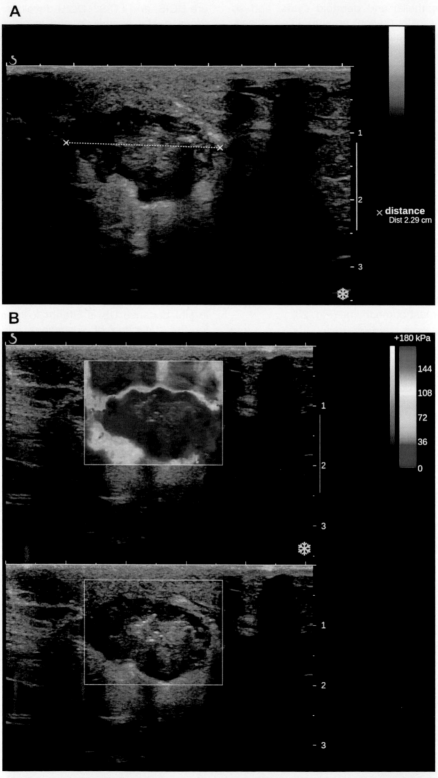

Fig. 21. (A) B-mode image of a palpable lesion in a 50-year-old woman that appears solid, inhomogeneous, dominantly hypoechoic, with irregular margins. (B) Elastographic image of the same lesion showing a soft lesion and stiff surroundings. Biopsy showed breast abscess.

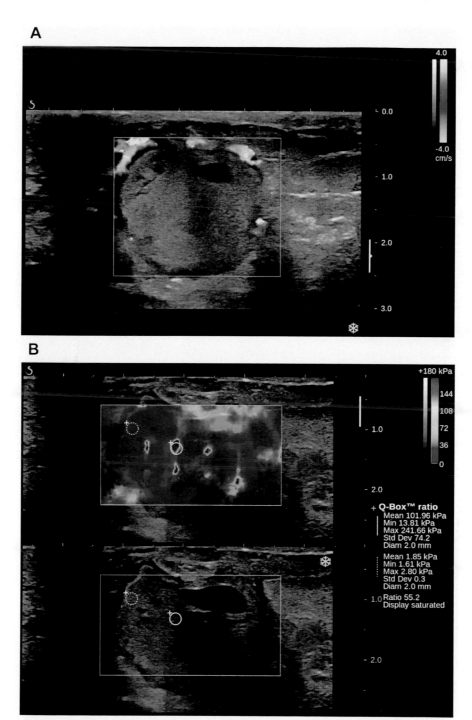

Fig. 22. Color Doppler image (*A*) of a large lesion that appears solid but avascular, with a hypervascular margin. On sonoelastography (*B*), the lesion is soft. Biopsy showed breast abscess. Diam, diameter; Max, maximum; Min, minimum; Std Dev, standard deviation.

mammography, usually larger than 10 mm. When those changes are visible on US, performing a biopsy under sonographic guidance is an option (**Figs. 24–26**).[38–40]

Invasive breast cancers are divided into invasive ductal carcinoma (IDC), arising from ducts, and invasive lobular carcinoma (ILC), arising from lobules. Some IDCs show distinct patterns of growth

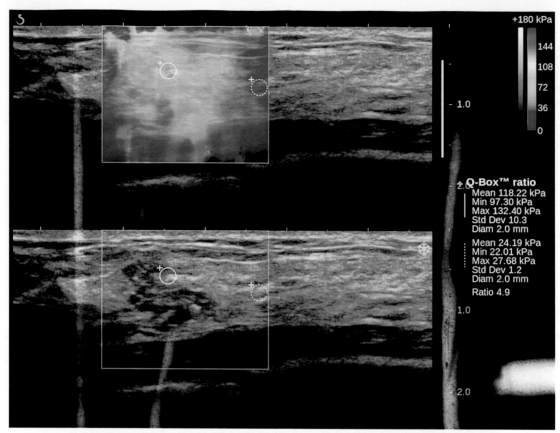

Fig. 23. Inhomogeneous dominantly anechoic lesions appearing as a cluster of septated cysts within the breast parenchyma. Core biopsy: pseudoangiomatous stromal hyperplasia. Diam, diameter; Max, maximum; Min, minimum; Std Dev, standard deviation.

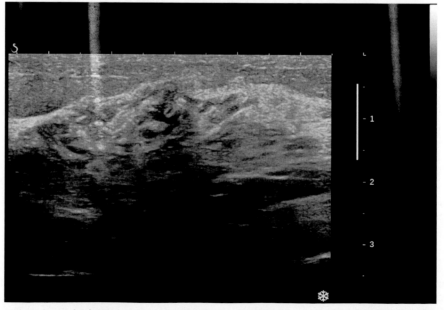

Fig. 24. Hypoechoic irregular lesion with appearance of ductal dilatation and abnormalities within echogenic parenchyma; core biopsy and final histopathology: DCIS.

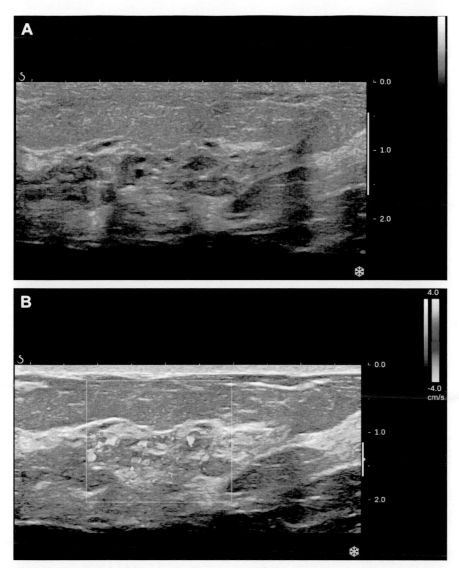

Fig. 25. B-mode (*A*), color Doppler (*B*) and sonoelastography (*C*) showing irregular hypoechoic area with tubular channels, which is hypervascular on color Doppler and stiff on elastography. Core biopsy and final histopathology: DCIS. Diam, diameter; Max, maximum; Min, minimum; Std Dev, standard deviation.

and cellular morphology and are called IDC of special types; most (60% to 80%) are considered to be of no special type (not otherwise specified).[41,42] ILC comprises 10% to 15% of invasive breast cancers and they are often multicentric and bilateral.[43] Medullary, mucinous, tubular, and papillary carcinoma are infrequent (2%). The treatment and survival for all cancer types depend on the stage of the disease at the time of detection, so early diagnosis is of utmost importance.[2,41] US is also used to evaluate clinically symptomatic patients and those with abnormal screening results to

help direct further procedures, as well as for preinterventional staging of the disease.[28]

According to a study by Stavros and colleagues in 1995,[44] solid breast lesions can be characterized as malignant or benign from B-mode US features: malignant features include vertical orientation, spiculation, marked hypoechogenicity, angular margins, posterior acoustic shadowing, and microcalcifications, whereas benign features include gentle lobulations, ellipsoid shape, homogeneous echotexture, thin capsule, and horizontal orientation. Although it is generally assumed that

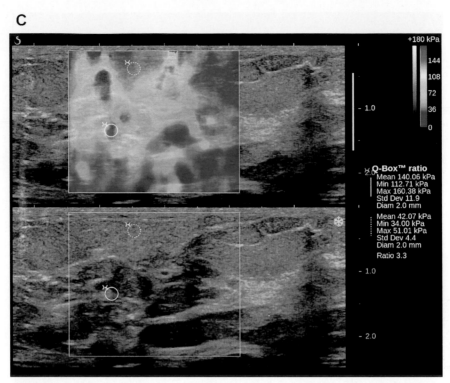

Fig. 25. (continued)

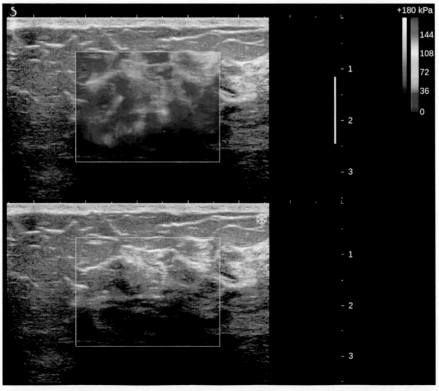

Fig. 26. B-mode and sonoelastography of hypoechoic inhomogeneous area within the parenchyma, which is soft on elastography. Core biopsy: LCIS.

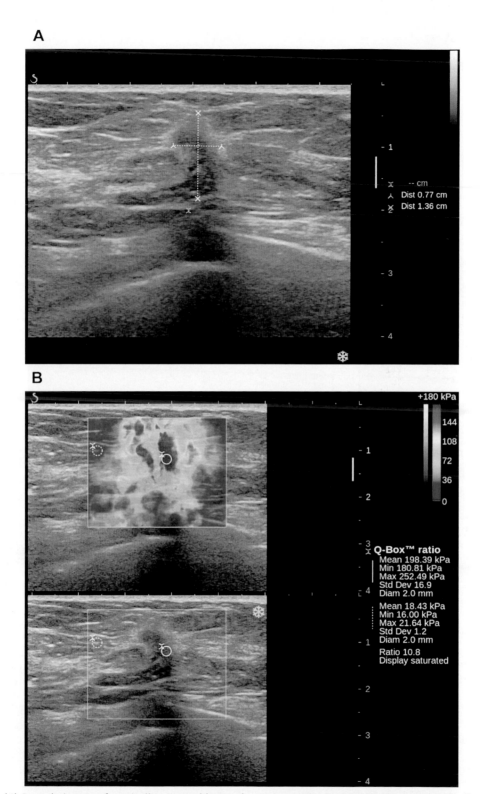

Fig. 27. (*A*) B-mode image of vertically oriented hypoechoic mass with irregular borders; IDC. Dist, distance. (*B*) Shear-wave sonoelastography of the same lesion shows a very stiff lesion with maximum elasticity value of 252 kPa, 10 times higher than the surrounding fat. Diam, diameter; Max, maximum; Min, minimum; Std Dev, standard deviation.

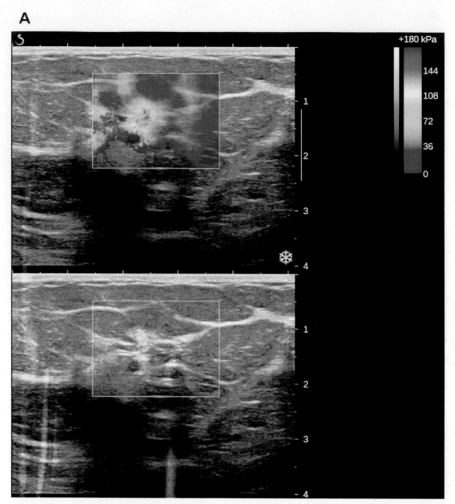

Fig. 28. (*A, B*) B-mode image of a small, hyperechoic irregular lesion, which is relatively atypical for IDC but sonoelastography shows a very stiff lesion, coded in reddish colors, with maximum elasticity value of 148 kPa. Core biopsy and final histopathology showed IDC. Diam, diameter; Max, maximum; Min, minimum; Std Dev, standard deviation.

sonographic features of irregular margins, hypoechogenicity, vertical orientation and others allow relatively straightforward differentiation of invasive cancers from benign lesions, it is often not accurate. There is a considerable overlap between benign and malignant US features, which requires correlation with mammography, MR imaging, and often, image-guided biopsy.[2,28] Some lesions invisible on mammography may be visualized on US, and even small, impalpable carcinomas can be seen, especially in mammographically dense breasts.[21,22] Up to 25% of malignant lesions can present as well-circumscribed nodular lesions, sometimes mimicking fibroadenomas. Even very invasive and aggressive cancers, such as triple-negative breast cancers, may have benign features in terms of lesions with well-circumscribed, regular margins and horizontal orientation.[45,46] Medullary and mucinous cancers may often present as hypoechoic, oval, well-circumscribed masses, which may look like dense cysts with some internal echoes on US.[47] Therefore, neither the absence of malignant sonographic features nor the presence of benign features can be evaluated other than from mammographic findings, clinical examinations, and MR findings in selected cases.

Posterior acoustic shadowing is also considered as strongly suggestive of malignancies. It is likely a consequence of an extensive fibrotic reaction, and the fibrotic tissue is absorbing the sound beam.[2,28] Only a few benign lesions, such as

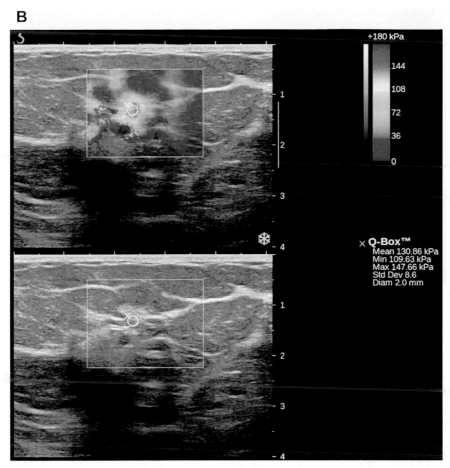

Fig. 28. (*continued*)

extensively fibrosed or calcified fibroadenomas, can mimic this finding, but they are usually reliably diagnosed on mammography. Some carcinomas, on the other hand, present no significant posterior shadowing, and some (medullary and mucinous carcinomas) can even have posterior acoustic enhancement. Many carcinomas present heterogeneous internal echoes, but this is an even less specific feature. As a result of local invasion and extensive reactive fibrosis, most malignant lesions distort normal breast tissue architecture. Many carcinomas are very stiff, which can be quantified using sonoelastography.[10,30,31]

High-resolution US is helpful in assessing intraductal spread and multifocality of breast cancer, although it cannot compete with MR imaging.[18,28] IDC is more easily visualized with US, whereas the less common ILC, because of its diffuse and multicentric growth pattern, is sometimes inconspicuous or visible only when large.[43] US is useful for the detection of enlarged axillary

lymph nodes, and color Doppler is helpful to evaluate patterns of vascularization of lymph nodes (**Figs. 27–36**).[14,15]

Focused second-look US is important for lesions detected on contrast-enhanced MR imaging. Up to 71% of MR-detected lesions are visible on second-look focused US, and enhancing MR masses are seen more commonly by US than non–mass enhancement.[48–52] Detectability by US is related to the lesion size on MR imaging, and 86% of masses larger than 1.5 cm are seen on US.[50] When US findings correlate with MR-detected lesion, the higher the likelihood that the lesion is malignant; these lesions should be subjected to US-guided biopsy.[51,52]

Fine-needle aspiration cytology (FNAC), CNB, and vacuum-assisted biopsy (VAB) are performed to improve the specificity of breast examination and to avoid unnecessary interventions in benign breast lesions. US-guided procedures are

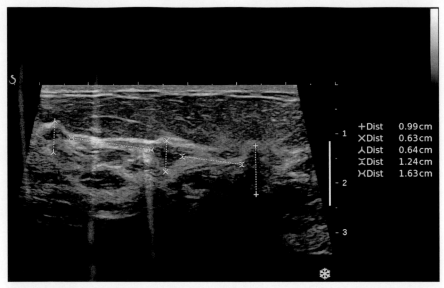

Fig. 29. B-mode trapezoid (fan-shaped) image of multicentric IDC, clearly showing 3 separate hypoechoic irregular subcentimetric invasive lesions within the same breast lobule. The distance (Dist) between lesions is 1.2 and 1.6 cm.

performed in real time, allowing constant visualization and modification of the needle path and optimal positioning of the needle to obtain an adequate specimen from the lesion. The accuracy of the aspiration/biopsy depends on the size, location, and morphology of the lesion, on the accuracy of targeting, needle diameter, and the number of needle passes.[2,18,53,54] FNAC uses fine 20-gauge to 25-gauge almost atraumatic needles, but evaluation of the acquired material is difficult. The results are dependent on the skill of the cytopathologist, and because a tissue

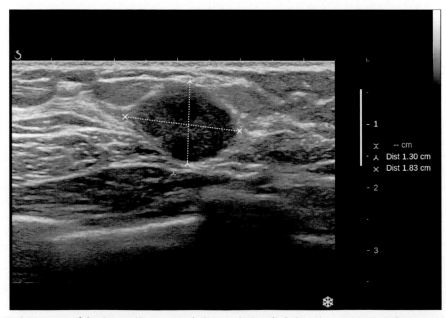

Fig. 30. B-mode image of horizontally oriented, hypoechoic, slightly inhomogeneous lesion, without distal acoustic shadow or enhancement, with only minimally irregular margins, 1.8 × 1.3 cm in size. Core biopsy and final histopathology showed triple-negative IDC. Dist, distance.

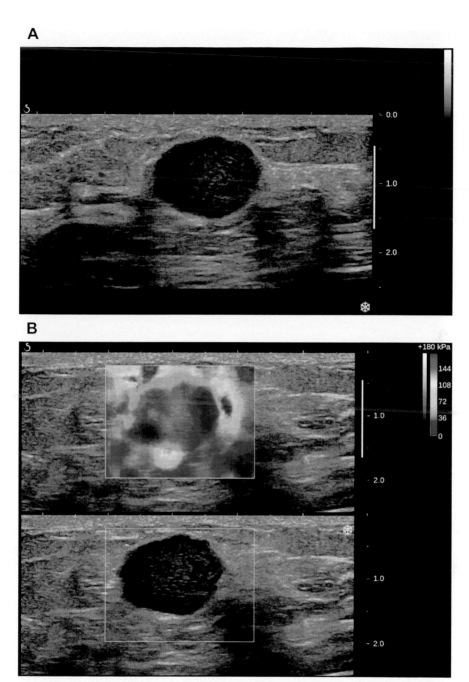

Fig. 31. (*A, B*) B-mode image (*A*) and sonoelastography (*B*) of hypoechoic, solid, horizontally oriented mass, with slight posterior acoustic enhancement and mostly regular margins, which is soft on elastography but has stiff margins. Mostly benign B-mode features. Core biopsy and final histopathology showed medullary cancer.

sample is not obtained, the type of lesion cannot be determined. FNAC can be used to evaluate complicated and symptomatic simple cysts, and to aspirate lymph nodes in proximity to axillary vessels. A negative FNAC result cannot exclude malignancy with suspicious imaging findings.[53] CNB is superior to FNAC in terms of higher sensitivity, specificity, and accuracy. CNB is performed using a 14-gauge needle mounted on a spring-acting puncture device.

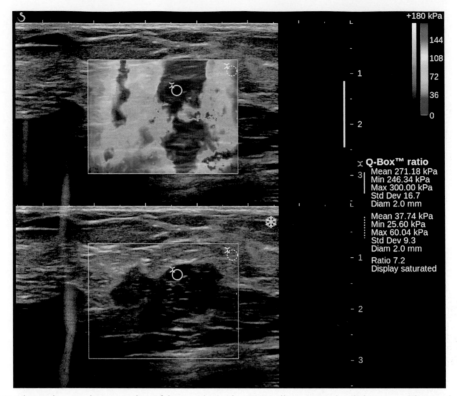

Fig. 32. B-mode and sonoelastography of hypoechoic, horizontally oriented solid mass with regular margins, with relatively benign grayscale features. However, the lesion is stiff on elastography. Core biopsy and final histopathology showed mucinous cancer. Diam, diameter; Max, maximum; Min, minimum; Std Dev, standard deviation.

Two or more passes are needed with needle advancement of at least 15 mm for adequate specimen retrieval. A cylinder of target tissue obtained by CNB allows a complete histologic diagnosis. Its sensitivity is 92% to 98% and specificity up to 100%.[2,53] VAB uses larger needles, usually 11 gauge or 8 gauge, which are inserted into the lesion, and the specimen is then taken with a device that simultaneously aspirates blood and debris from the area around the lesion. Larger cylinders of tissue are obtained, which allow accurate histologic diagnosis.[54] VAB has even higher sensitivity and specificity than CNB[54,55] Preoperative wire localization of lesions can be performed under US guidance, with the purpose of accurate surgical removal of impalpable or deeply positioned breast lesions (**Figs. 37** and **38**).

BREAST US AFTER RADIATION THERAPY AND AFTER SURGERY

Postoperative changes in breasts often have imaging features similar to malignant lesions. Scars are visible after all surgical procedures. Architectural distortion, edema, thickening of the skin, fluid collection, and dystrophic calcifications may be seen. Most changes regress spontaneously within the year after surgery. Radiation therapy causes more pronounced changes, which tend to persist longer, and are visible on US and mammography. Edema presents as a diffusely decreased echogenicity and loss of normal tissue differentiation. Hematomas and seromas present as irregularly marginated hypoechoic lesions, which with time become more distinctly demarcated and can develop internal echoes. Acute fat necrosis generally appears as irregularly marginated hypoechoic lesions, with a varying degree of distal acoustic shadowing. These lesions are sonographically difficult to differentiate from malignancies, which makes clinical examination and correlation of US findings to MR imaging important. US is an excellent modality for biopsy guidance in these patients. The thoracic wall after mastectomy should be examined by US. Tumor recurrence can be visualized, as well as infiltration of intercostal muscles, pectoral muscle, or pleura. US enables evaluation

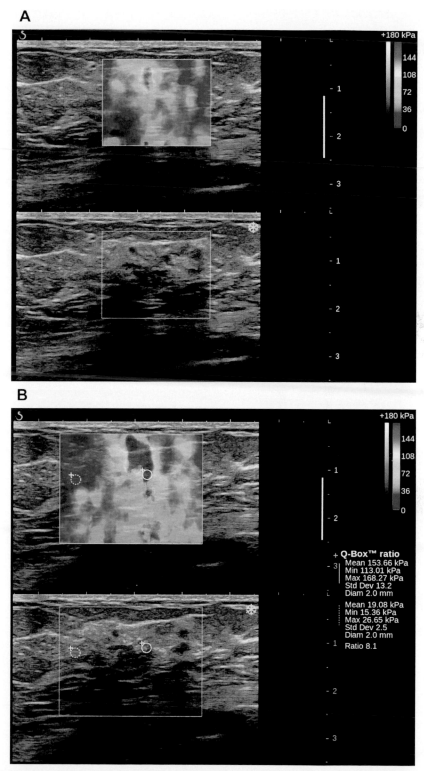

Fig. 33. (A, B) B-mode and sonoelastography of almost inconspicuous irregular, heterogeneous lesion, with mixed echogenicity and lack of distal acoustic features, which is stiff on elastography. Core biopsy and final histopathology showed ILC. Diam, diameter; Max, maximum; Min, minimum; Std Dev, standard deviation.

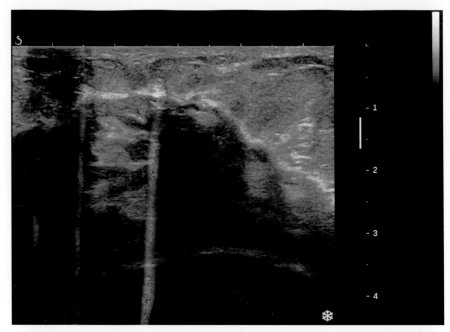

Fig. 34. B-mode image of 2 markedly hypoechoic large masses with distal acoustic shadowing; ILC. Different presentation compared with the patient in Fig. 33.

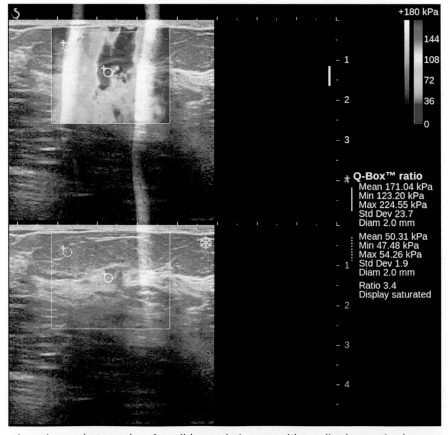

Fig. 35. B-mode and sonoelastography of small hypoechoic mass without distal acoustic phenomena, which is stiff on elastography. ILC. Diam, diameter; Max, maximum; Min, minimum; Std Dev, standard deviation.

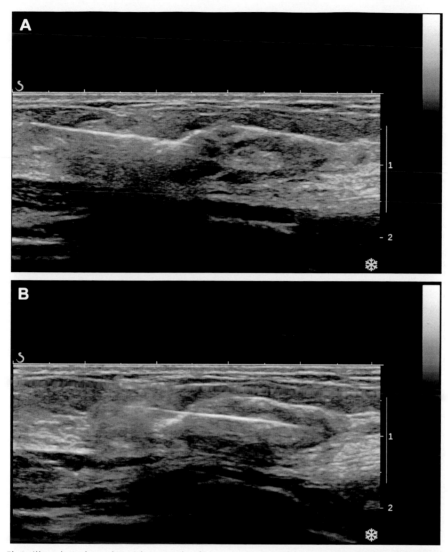

Fig. 36. (A, B) Axillary lymph node with central echogenic sinus and hypoechoic cortex. The passage of needle during fine-needle aspiration is clearly visible.

of the depth of infiltration and of the relation of the lesion to the bones, pleura, and blood vessels. US is used also for the visualization of implants placed after subcutaneous mastectomy and skin-flaps after mastectomy.[2,18]

Radiation therapy induces fibrosis, with a consequent dense appearance of the breast on mammography. Radiation fibrosis results in increased echogenicity of the parenchyma and the whole breast, thickening of the skin, and distortion of the normal parenchymal architecture. Edema and skin thickening usually regress over a 2-year period. If skin thickening is observed after

previous regression, tumor recurrence should be considered. Tumor recurrence after conservative treatment may resemble the primary tumor morphologically, but it may also have peculiar features. The diagnosis requires US-guided biopsy. US is also useful for the follow-up of hematoma and seroma and for the detection of abscesses (**Figs. 39–41**).[2,18]

US IN THE SCREENING ALGORITHM

Mammographic breast cancer screening is performed for decades, beginning at the age of 40

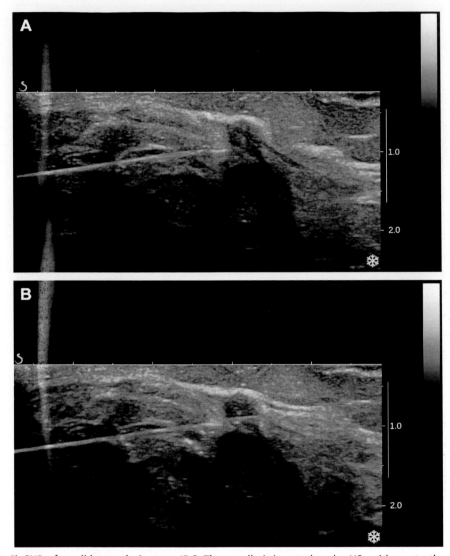

Fig. 37. (A, B) CNB of small hypoechoic mass; IDC. The needle is inserted under US guidance to the edge of the lesion (A), and after firing, the passage of needle is clearly visible on US (B), confirming sample retrieval from the proper position.

or 50 years.[56] Mammography has well-known limitations in women with very dense breasts, and the addition of US to mammography can improve the overall sensitivity of imaging, because it enables the diagnosis of an additional 2.3 to 4.6 of mammographically occult breast cancers per 1000 women.[26,57,58] In some US states, it is now mandatory to inform women about their breast density and to advise them to perform additional screening with US.[59,60] Automated whole-breast US has recently been developed as an alternative to handheld US for screening, in which a standardized set of images is obtained. More than 3000 images in sagittal, coronal, and transverse planes are obtained and are available for later review with 3D reconstructions by radiologists. The patients have to be recalled for additional US examination to review indeterminate findings of automated whole-breast US, and more studies are needed to assess the clinical use of automated US compared with the traditional handheld systems.[61–63]

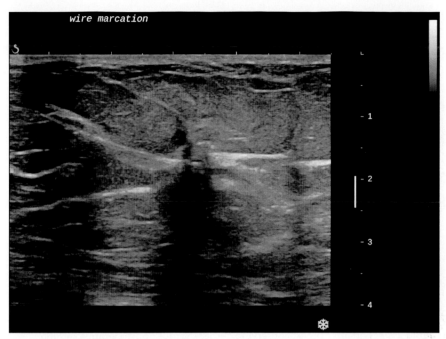

Fig. 38. Marcation wire inserted under US guidance into a small hypoechoic impalpable mass (tubular cancer) preoperatively, so that the surgeon can excise the impalpable lesion with certainty. The tip of the wire within the lesion is clearly seen.

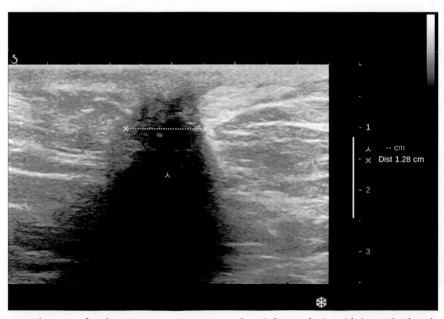

Fig. 39. Postoperative scar after breast-conserving surgery. Scar is hypoechoic, with irregular borders, and distal acoustic shadow, difficult to differentiate by US from local recurrence or residual tumor. Dist, distance.

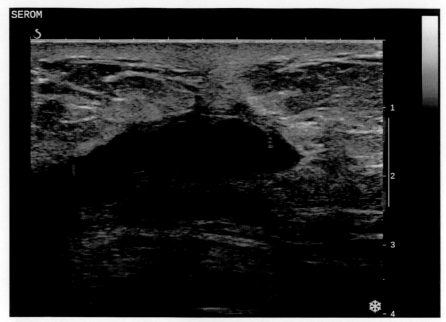

Fig. 40. Large liquid collection after breast-conserving surgery for IDC; postoperative seroma.

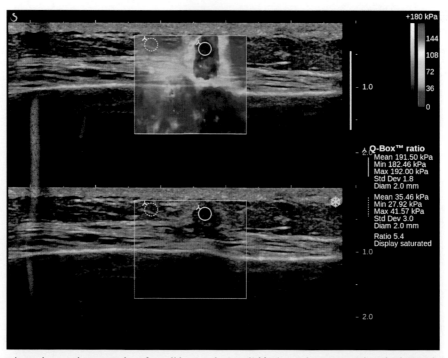

Fig. 41. B-mode and sonoelastography of small hypoechoic solid lesion subcutaneously, which developed 10 years after mastectomy for IDC. The lesion is very stiff on sonoelastography, with maximum elasticity value of 192 kPa. Recurrence of IDC after 10 years at the thoracic wall after mastectomy. Diam, diameter; Max, maximum; Min, minimum; Std Dev, standard deviation.

REFERENCES

1. Weinstein SP, Conant EF, Sehgal C. Technical advances in breast ultrasound imaging. Semin Ultrasound CT MR 2006;27(4):273–83.

2. Brkljačić B, Huzjan-Korunić R, Pavić L. Ultrasound of the breast. In: Kurjak A, Chervenak F, editors. Donald School textbook of ultrasound in obstetrics and gynaecology. New Delhi (India): Jaypee; 2007. p. 950–70.

3. Brkljačić B, Čikara I, Ivanac G, et al. Ultrasound-guided bipolar radiofrequency ablation of breast cancer in inoperable patients: a pilot study. Ultraschall Med 2010;31:156–62.

4. Kremkau FW. Sonography principles and instruments. 8th edition. St Louis (MO): Elsevier Saunders; 2011.

5. Athanasiou A, Tardivon A, Ollivier L, et al. How to optimize breast ultrasound. Eur J Radiol 2009; 69(1):6–13.

6. Stafford RJ, Whitman GJ. Ultrasound physics and technology in breast imaging. Ultrasound Clin 2011;6(3):299–312.

7. Zhao QL, Ruan LT, Zhang H, et al. Diagnosis of solid breast lesions by elastography 5-point score and strain ratio method. Eur J Radiol 2012;81(11): 3245–9.

8. Stachs A, Hartmann S, Stubert J, et al. Differentiating between malignant and benign breast masses: factors limiting sonoelastographic strain ratio. Ultraschall Med 2013;34(2):131–6.

9. Bercoff J, Tanter M, Fink M. Supersonic shear imaging: a new technique for soft tissue elasticity mapping. IEEE Trans Ultrason Ferroelectr Freq Control 2004;51(4):396–409.

10. Ivanac G, Hrkać Pustahija A, Huzjan Korunić R, et al. Shear-wave elastographic values of benign and malignant breast lesions and surrounding tissue. Official Proceedings of the 13th Congress oft he World Federation for Ultrasound in Medicine and Biology. Ultrasound Med Biol 2011;37(8S):S45–6.

11. Sadigh G, Carlos RC, Neal CH, et al. Ultrasonographic differentiation of malignant from benign breast lesions: a meta-analytic comparison of elasticity and BIRADS scoring. Breast Cancer Res Treat 2012;133:23–35.

12. Barr RG. Sonographic breast elastography. J Ultrasound Med 2012;31:773–83.

13. Chadha M, Young A, Geraghty C, et al. Image guidance using 3D ultrasound (3D-US) for daily positioning of lumpectomy cavity for boost irradiation. Radiat Oncol 2011;6:45.

14. Cosgrove DO, Kedar RP, Bamber JC, et al. Breast diseases: color Doppler US in differential diagnosis. Radiology 1993;189:99–104.

15. Rizzatto G. Towards a more sophisticated use of breast ultrasound. Eur Radiol 2001;11:2425–35.

16. Birdwell RL, Ikeda DM, Jeffrey SS, et al. Preliminary experience with power Doppler imaging of solid breast masses. AJR Am J Roentgenol 1997; 169(3):703–7.

17. Gokalp G, Topal U, Kizilkaya E. Power Doppler sonography: anything to add to BI-RADS US in solid breast masses? Eur J Radiol 2009;70(1):77–85.

18. Heywang-Koebrunner SH, Dershaw DD, Schreer I. Diagnostic breast imaging. Stuttgart (Germany): Thieme; 2001.

19. Teubner J. Echomammography: technique and results. In: Friedrich M, Sickles EA, editors. Radiological diagnosis of breast diseases. Berlin: Springer-Verlag; 2000. p. 181–220.

20. Kopans DB. Ultrasound and breast evaluation. In: Kopans DB, editor. Breast imaging. Philadelphia: Lippincott-Raven; 1998. p. 439–41.

21. Crystal P, Strano SD, Scharynski S, et al. Using sonography to screen women with mammographically dense breasts. AJR Am J Roentgenol 2003; 181(1):177–82.

22. Buchberger W, Niehoff A, Obrist P, et al. Clinically and mammographically occult breast lesions: detection and classification with high-resolution sonography. Semin Ultrasound CT MR 2000;21(4):325–36.

23. ACR practice guideline for the performance of a breast ultrasound examination. 2011. Available at: http://www.acr.org./Quality-Safety/Standards-Guidelines/Practice-Guidelines-by-Modality/Ultrasound. Accessed January 6, 2014.

24. Kopans DB. The altered breast: pregnancy. Lactation. Biopsy, mastectomy, radiation, and implants. In: Kopans DB, editor. Breast imaging. 2nd edition. Philadelphia: Lippincott-Raven; 1998. p. 445–69.

25. Roubidoux MA, Wilson TE, Orange RJ, et al. Breast cancer in women who undergo screening mammography: relationship of hormone replacement therapy to stage and detection method. Radiology 1998;208:725–8.

26. Kolb TM, Lichy J, Newhouse JH. Comparison of the performance of screening mammography, physical examination, and breast US and evaluation of factors that influence them: an analysis of 27,825 patient evaluations. Radiology 2002;225(1):165–75.

27. Mendelson EB, Baum JK, Berg WA, et al. Breast imaging reporting and data system. BIRADS: ultrasound. Reston (VA): American College of Radiology; 2003.

28. Hooley RJ, Scoutt LM, Philpotts LE. Breast ultrasonography: state of the art. Radiology 2013;268(3): 642–59.

29. Berg WA, Cosgrove DO, Dore CJ, et al. Shear-wave elastography improves the specificity of breast US: the BE1 multinational study of 939 masses. Radiology 2012;262(2):435–49.

30. Evans A, Whelehan P, Thomson K, et al. Invasive breast cancer: relationship between shear-wave

elastographic findings and histologic prognostic factors. Radiology 2012;263(3):673–7.

31. Cosgrove DO, Berg WA, Dore CJ, et al. Shear wave elastography for breast masses is highly reproducible. Eur Radiol 2012;22(5):1023–32.

32. Kriger N, Hiatt RA. Risk of breast cancer after benign breast diseases: variation by histologic type, degree of atypia, age at biopsy, and length of follow-up. Am J Epidemiol 1992;135:619–31.

33. Hughes LE, Mansel RE, Webster DJ. Benign disorders and diseases of the breast: concepts and clinical management. London: Bailliere Tindall; 1989.

34. Adler DD. Imaging evaluation of spiculated masses. In: Friedrich M, Sickles EA, editors. Radiological diagnosis of breast diseases. Berlin: Springer-Verlag; 2000. p. 137–48.

35. Rao A, Parker S, Ratzer E, et al. Atypical ductal hyperplasia of the breast diagnosed by 11-gauge directional vacuum-assisted biopsy. Am J Surg 2002;184:534–7.

36. Izumori A, Takebe K, Sato A. Ultrasound findings and histological features of ductal carcinoma in situ detected by ultrasound examination alone. Breast Cancer 2010;17(2):136–41.

37. Holland R, Hendriks JH. Microcalcifications associated with ductal carcinoma in situ: mammographic-pathologic correlation. Semin Diagn Pathol 1994; 11:181–92.

38. Park JS, Park YM, Kiem EK, et al. Sonographic findings of high-grade and non-high-grade ductal carcinoma in situ of the breast. J Ultrasound Med 2010;29(12):1687–97.

39. Nagashima T, Hashimoto H, Oshida K, et al. Ultrasound demonstration of mammographically detected microcalcification in patients with ductal carcinoma in situ of the breast. Breast Cancer 2005;12:216–20.

40. Uematsu T. Non-mass-like lesions on breast ultrasonography: a systematic review. Breast Cancer 2012;19:295–301.

41. Sainsbury JR, Anderson TJ, Morgan DA. ABC of breast diseases: breast cancer. BMJ 2000;321: 745–50.

42. Page DL. Special types of invasive breast cancer, with clinical implications. Am J Surg Pathol 2003; 27:832–5.

43. Kim SH, Cha ES, Park CS, et al. Imaging features of invasive lobular carcinoma: comparison with invasive ductal carcinoma. Jpn J Radiol 2011;29(7): 475–82.

44. Stavros AT, Thickman D, Rapp CL, et al. Solid breast nodules: use of sonography to distinguish between benign and malignant lesions. Radiology 1995;196(1):123–34.

45. Dogan BE, Turnbull LW. Imaging of triple-negative breast cancer. Ann Oncol 2012;23:23–9.

46. Kojima Y, Tsunoda H. Mammography and ultrasound features of triple-negative breast cancer. Breast cancer 2011;18(3):146–51.

47. Liu H, Tan H, Cheng Y, et al. Imaging findings in mucinous breast carcinoma and correlating factors. Eur J Radiol 2011;80(3):706–12.

48. Abe H, Schmidt RA, Shah RN, et al. MR-directed ("second-look") ultrasound examination for breast lesions detected initially on MRI: MR and sonographic findings. AJR Am J Roentgenol 2010; 194(2):370–7.

49. Demartini WB, Eby PR, Peacock S, et al. Utility of targeted sonography for breast lesions that were suspicious on MRI. AJR Am J Roentgenol 2009; 192(4):1128–34.

50. Meissnitzer M, Dershaw DD, Lee CH, et al. Targeted ultrasound of the breast in women with abnormal MRI findings for whom biopsy has been recommended. AJR Am J Roentgenol 2009; 193(4):1025–9.

51. Candelaria R, Fornage BD. Second-look US examination of MR-detected breast lesions. J Clin Ultrasound 2011;39(3):115–21.

52. Cargognin G, Girardi V, Calciolari C, et al. Utility of second-look ultrasound in the management of incidental enhancing lesions detected by breast MR imaging. Radiol Med 2010;115(8):1234–45.

53. Bauer M, Tontsch P, Schulz-Wendtland R. Fine-needle aspiration and core biopsy. In: Friedrich M, Sickles EA, editors. Radiological diagnosis of breast diseases. Berlin: Springer; 2000. p. 291–8.

54. Obenauer S, Fischer U, Baum F, et al. Indications for percutaneous stereotactic vacuum core biopsy of the breast. Radiologe 2002;42(1):11–8.

55. Meloni GB, Dessole S, Becchere MP, et al. Ultrasound-guided mammotome vacuum biopsy for the diagnosis of impalpable breast lesions. Ultrasound Obstet Gynecol 2001;18:520–4.

56. Bleyer A, Welch HG. Effect of three decades of screening mammography on breast-cancer incidence. N Engl J Med 2012;367:1998–2005.

57. Berg WA, Zhang Z, Lehrer D, et al. Detection of breast cancer with addition of annual screening ultrasound or a single screening MRI to mammography in women with elevated breast cancer risk. JAMA 2012;307(13):1394–404.

58. Berg WA, Blume JD, Cormack JB, et al. Combined screening with ultrasound and mammography vs. mammography alone in women at elevated risk of breast cancer. JAMA 2008;299(18):2151–63.

59. Hooley RJ, Greenberg KL, Stackhouse RM, et al. Screening US in patients with mammographically dense breasts: initial experience with Connecticut Public Act 09-41. Radiology 2012;265(1): 59–69.

60. Leconte I, Feger C, Galant C, et al. Mammography and subsequent whole-breast sonography of

nonpalpable breast cancers: the importance of radiologic breast density. AJR Am J Roentgenol 2003;180(6):1675–9.

61. Kaplan SS. Clinical utility of bilateral whole-breast US in the evaluation of women with dense breast tissue. Radiology 2001;221(3):641–9.

62. Kelly KM, Dean J, Lee SJ, et al. Breast cancer detection: radiologists' performance using

mammography with and without automated whole-breast-ultrasound. Eur Radiol 2010;20(11): 2557–64.

63. Chang JM, Moon WK, Cho N, et al. Breast cancer initially detected by hand-held ultrasound: detection performance of radiologists using automated breast ultrasound data. Acta Radiol 2011; 52(1):8–14.

Sonography of Testis

S. Boopathy Vijayaraghavan, MD, DMRD

KEYWORDS

- Sonography • Testis • Ultrasonography • Scrotum

KEY POINTS

- Ultrasonography is the modality of choice for the evaluation of the scrotum.
- Sonography has come to be the first and primary modality for imaging the testis because there has been marked improvement in the resolution of the equipment and it is easily available, quicker, and cost-effective.
- Sonographic diagnosis of various pathologies of testis are described.

Videos of whirlpool sign on gray-scale and color Doppler imaging, tracking the cord from inguinal region to up to testis, laparoscopy of intra-abdominal testis with spermatic cord coming into abdomen from inguinal canal, and peristalsis in the small bowel loop accompany this article at http://www.ultrasound.theclinics.com/

SONOGRAPHY OF SCROTUM

Ultrasonography is the modality of choice for the evaluation of the scrotum. It shows testicular abnormalities, peritesticular abnormalities such as varicocele, and epididymal disorders. It also helps to visualize the changes caused secondary to distal vasal obstruction.

Technique

The ultrasonography examination should begin with the patient in a supine position. The scrotum is supported by a towel between the thighs. A towel is used to cover the penis, which is placed over the abdomen to keep it out of the scanning field. A generous amount of gel is applied to the scrotum to avoid artifacts caused by scrotal hair. The examination is started on the asymptomatic side. A high-frequency probe of 7 to 12 MHz with short focal zone and large footprint is used to accommodate the length of the testis in a single image. The testis and the epididymis are examined separately in longitudinal and transverse planes. The study is done using gray-scale, color, and spectral Doppler techniques.

Normal Sonographic Anatomy

The normal testis is an ovoid or slightly rounded structure. It is homogeneously granular with uniformly distributed medium-level echoes (similar to thyroid echotexture) (**Fig. 1**). Both the testes are symmetric in size, shape, and echotexture, so it is important to compare the testes side by side on a split screen. The volume of the testis is calculated by the ellipsoidal formula (length × width × height × 0.51). Total testicular volume (both testes) of greater than 30 mL and a single testicular volume of 12 to 15 mL are generally considered as normal.[1] The mediastinum testis is a linear echogenic strand that runs craniocaudally within the testis. The rete testis at the mediastinum testis is sometimes seen as a hypoechoic area in the posterosuperior aspect of the testis in a transverse section. The epididymis has 3 parts: head, body, and tail. Scanning from the lateral aspect of the scrotum may allow visualization of the entire epididymis (**Fig. 2**). The body and tail are better appreciated in the presence of hydrocele. The head of the epididymis is isoechoic or slightly more echogenic than the testis. It is about 10 to

The author has nothing to disclose.

Sonoscan: Ultrasonic Scan Centre, 15B Venkatachalam Road, R.S. Puram, Coimbatore, Tamil Nadu 641 002, India

E-mail addresses: sonoscan@vsnl.com; sboopathy@eth.net

Ultrasound Clin 9 (2014) 429–456

http://dx.doi.org/10.1016/j.cult.2014.03.005

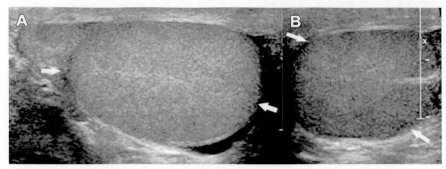

Fig. 1. Longitudinal (*A*) and transverse (*B*) scan of the normal testis (*arrows*) showing the uniform granular appearance.

12 mm in diameter. The body and tail of epididymis are isoechoic or slightly less echogenic than the head. On color Doppler study, fine vessels coursing through the normal testis are seen and intratesticular flow is seen to be symmetric on both sides (**Fig. 3**). There is normally minimal flow or no flow in the epididymis (**Fig. 4**).

SONOGRAPHY OF TESTIS
Introduction

Sonography has come to be the first and primary modality for imaging the testis because there has been marked improvement in the resolution of the equipment and it is easily available, quicker, and cost-effective. Before imaging, knowledge of the clinical details of the patient is essential.

Tunica Albuginea Cyst

Tunica albuginea cyst is usually an incidental finding or a palpable nodule in the testis. The cause is unknown. It is single or multiple and varies in size from 2 to 30 mm. The mean age at presentation is 40 years but it may be seen in patients in their 50s and 60s.[2] Tunica albuginea cyst is usually located along the anterior superior or lateral surface of the testis.[3] On ultrasonography, it is seen

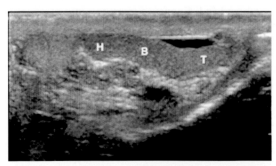

Fig. 2. Longitudinal scan of posterolateral aspect of testis showing the head (H), body (B), and tail (T) of normal epididymis.

as a small, round, or oval anechoic lesion on the surface of the testis with smooth thin walls and clear fluid; typical characteristics of a simple cyst (**Fig. 5A**). They may occasionally have internal echoes (see **Fig. 5B**) or septations,[3] or rarely calcification of the wall. The typical location differentiates it from intratesticular or paratesticular lesions. It is easiest to locate them on ultrasonography by directing the patient to point to the palpable nodule. Sometimes they are multiple (see **Fig. 5C**).

Tunica Vaginalis Cyst

Tunica vaginalis cyst is rare. It arises from the parietal or visceral layer of the tunica vaginalis and may be single or multiple. On ultrasonography, it is seen as a simple anechoic structure but occasionally can have internal echoes or septations.[3]

Intratesticular Cysts

Intratesticular cyst is seen incidentally during ultrasonography, because they are asymptomatic and nonpalpable. The origin is not clear. It is postulated that they result from an anomalous efferent duct, obstruction of the spermatic duct, or postinflammatory cystic dilatation of the duct.[4] It is usually single but can be multiple. It can be seen anywhere in the testis but is most common close to the mediastinum. On ultrasonography, it is seen as a well-defined, round, or oval anechoic lesion. The rim is usually echogenic (**Fig. 6**).[5] The cyst rarely shows internal echoes.

Ectasia of the Rete Testis

Ectasia of the rete testis is a benign condition resulting from obstruction of the vas. Other possible causes include cryptorchidism; mechanical compression of epididymis or spermatic cord by surgical, neoplastic, or infectious processes; and ischemia-induced or hormone-induced atrophic alteration to the tubules.[6] The causes may not be

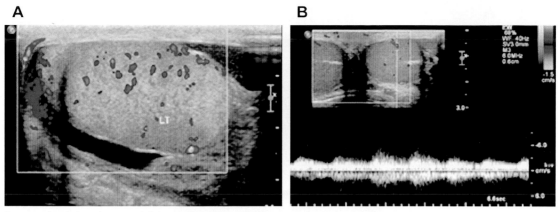

Fig. 3. Color (*A*) and spectral (*B*) Doppler study of the normal testis. LT, left testis.

apparent in some patients. On ultrasonography, it is seen as widening of mediastinum testis by tubular fluid-filled structures (**Fig. 7**). If ectasia is caused by obstruction of vas deferens, there can be associated epididymal cysts. It resembles intratesticular varicocele, from which it can be differentiated by color Doppler study with Valsalva maneuver. Ectasia of rete testis of a milder degree is seen in patients who are more than 50 years of age and in whom it is not associated with obstruction.

Testicular Microlithiasis

Testicular microlithiasis is characterized by multiple (more than 5) small, brightly echogenic dots of 1 to 2 mm in 1 section of testis (**Fig. 8**A). Its prevalence ranges from 0.1% to 9%.[7] Microlithiasis can vary in number and distribution pattern. The diffuse microlithiasis gives a starry-sky appearance to the parenchyma of the testis (see **Fig. 8**B). Testicular microlithiasis (TM) has been categorized into 2 histologic types of intratesticular microcalcifications. The first is the hematoxylin body consisting of amorphous calcific debris,

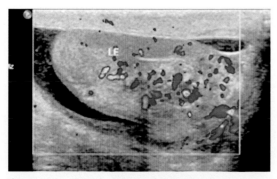

Fig. 4. Color Doppler study of normal left epididymis (LE) showing sparse flow.

which is associated with germ cell tumors and thought to be the result of a rapid cell turnover. The second is laminated calcifications, which are found in association with germ cell tumors, cryptorchid testes, and otherwise normal testes.[8] The risk of developing a tumor is not yet clearly defined, but seems to be greater with large numbers of microcalcifications (see **Fig. 8**C). Recent studies show a lower incidence of associated germ cell tumors and no interval development of tumor in longer-term follow-up. Recent literature suggests that both TM and testicular germ cell tumor may be caused by a common defect, such as tubular degeneration, and TM may therefore be considered as a marker for such abnormalities (premalignant lesion). Given the association with germ cell tumor, it is prudent to follow up patients who have TM with physical examination and ultrasonography at least annually and to encourage self-examination.[7]

Segmental Testicular Infarction

Segmental testicular infarction is an infrequent testicular disorder rarely described in the radiological literature and is usually diagnosed after orchidectomy.[9] The predisposing factors for segmental infarction include polycythemia, intimal fibroplasia of the spermatic artery, sickle cell disease, hypersensitivity angiitis, polyarteritis nodosa, thromboangiitis obliterans, arterial embolism, and trauma, although most cases are still considered to be idiopathic.[10] The theory of reduced blood flow (usually caused by venous thrombosis) to certain areas of testicular tissue functioning as end organs explains the pathogenesis of segmental testicular infarction in most cases.[11] It can also be seen as a result of torsion-detorsion sequence.[12] This condition normally affects patients between 20 and 40 years of age, although

A

B

C

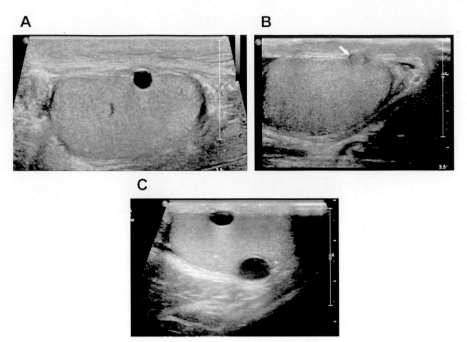

Fig. 5. (A) The tunica albuginea cyst is on the surface with smooth thin walls and clear fluid. (B) A tunica albuginea cyst with internal echoes (arrow). (C) Multiple tunica albuginea cysts.

it has occasionally been reported in neonates.[13] The clinical presentation is nonspecific and usually heralded by acute scrotal pain and swelling. A few cases with recurrent testicular pain have also been reported; this sometimes provides an important clue to diagnosis.[11] On ultrasonography, segmental testicular infarction is seen as an irregular echo-poor area in the testis. On color Doppler study, there is absence of flow in this area (Fig. 9). The evolving intratesticular abscess may mimic segmental testicular infarction. History of acute onset of symptoms suggests segmental testicular infarction, whereas laboratory evidence of infection suggests abscess. Sometimes follow-up scan may be necessary, which reveals fluid in the abscess.

Mumps Orchitis

Mumps orchitis is a rare condition of the testis. Patients present with painful swelling of the testis, along with parotitis or shortly after it. On ultrasonography the testis appears globally swollen and echo poor. On color Doppler study, there is marked hyperemia in the testis (Fig. 10). The epididymis is normal. The association with parotitis makes the diagnosis simple and specific.

Henoch-Schönlein Purpura

In Henoch-Schönlein purpura, testis is rarely involved because of vasculitis. Patients present with painful swelling of the testis, either along with purpura or shortly after it, or without purpura.

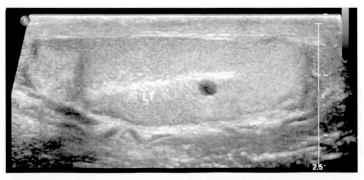

Fig. 6. Intratesticular cyst with thin walls and clear fluid close to the mediastinum.

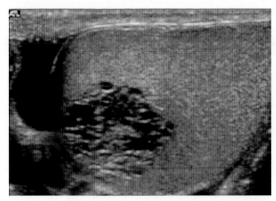

Fig. 7. Ectasia of rete testis, seen as widening of mediastinum by tubular cystic structures.

On ultrasonography, the testis is swollen and echo poor. On color Doppler study, there is intense hyperemia in the testis (**Fig. 11**). The appearance mimics mumps orchitis but there is no association with parotitis. It rarely results in focal infarcts, which are seen as focal, echo-poor areas lacking flow on color Doppler study.

Testicular Abscess

Testicular abscess is usually a complication of epididymo-orchitis. It may also occur as a complication of testicular torsion, testicular hemorrhage, and secondary to trauma or superadded infection of a necrotic tumor. It may also be associated with systemic infections such as mumps, smallpox, typhoid, scarlet fever, and tuberculosis.[14] Patients usually present with an acutely painful, swollen scrotum and often have an increased white blood cell count and fever. They may have diabetes mellitus, human immunodeficiency virus infection, or other immunosuppressive conditions. On ultrasonography scan, it appears as a complex, heterogeneous fluid collection, with shaggy, irregular walls, intratesticular location, low-level internal echoes, and occasionally hypervascular margins (**Fig. 12**).[15] Gas may be present, which is seen as bright specular reflectors and shadowing.[16] It may extend outwardly, rupturing the tunica vaginalis and draining outside (**Fig. 13**), and may produce a fistulous formation on the overlying scrotal skin. A chronic or partially treated abscess may be difficult to distinguish clinically and sonographically from a testicular tumor (**Fig. 14**).

Adrenal Rests in Testis

Adrenal rests in testis is caused by increased adrenocorticotrophic hormone (ACTH) in congenital adrenal hyperplasia, adrenogenital syndrome, or

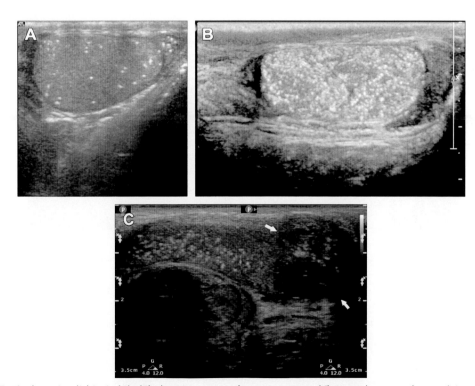

Fig. 8. Testicular microlithiasis (A), (B) showing starry sky appearance. (C) Irregular mass (arrows) in testis with microlithiasis.

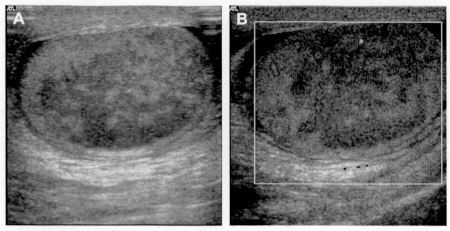

Fig. 9. Segmental infarction of testis seen as an irregular echo-poor area involving lower two-thirds of testis (*A*). On color Doppler study there is no flow (*B*) seen in the lesion.

Addison disease. In these conditions glucocorticoids synthesis is defective. As a result there is increased ACTH, which prevents involution of aberrant adrenal rests in the testes. These intratesticular nodules of adrenal rests can enlarge gradually, thereby destroying the testicular parenchyma, which results in low testosterone production and infertility. These lesions are not premalignant and tend to regress with hormone replacement.[17] On ultrasonography they appear as rounded, heterogeneous, solid masses that are multifocal in origin. They may be bilateral. They usually originate near the hilum and extend peripherally (**Fig. 15**). On color Doppler study, the masses show normal, hypovascularity or hypervascularity. The vessels course through the masses, which differentiates the condition from tumors.[18]

Torsion of the Testis

Torsion of the testis presents as acute painful scrotum. Acute scrotal pain can have diverse causes. The most important objective of treatment is to rule in or rule out testicular torsion. It requires immediate intervention to avoid infarction of the affected testis.[19] In contrast, if torsion can be

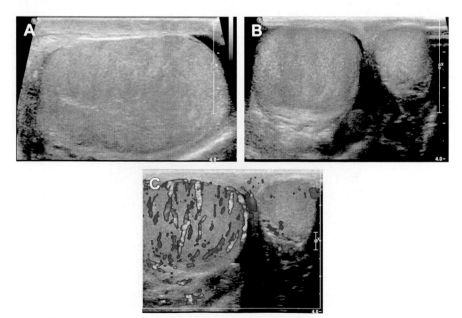

Fig. 10. Mumps orchitis. (*A, B*) Swollen echo-poor right testis. (*C*) Color Doppler study shows hyperemia of right testis.

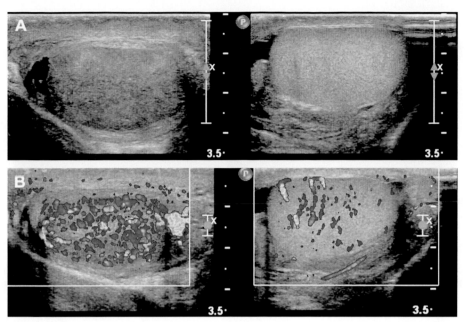

Fig. 11. Henoch-Schönlein purpura. (A) Echo-poor right testis and normal left testis. (B) Color Doppler study shows hyperemia of the right testis.

confidently ruled out, unnecessary surgical intervention can be avoided. Until recently, a sonographic study of acute scrotum has been focused on the evaluation of the testis, epididymis, and scrotal wall on gray-scale sonography and study of the intratesticular vascular flow by color Doppler imaging.[20–28] Sonographic signs of torsion have been described as swollen, echo-poor testis and epididymis with absent flow on color Doppler study (Fig. 16A, B). However, there are

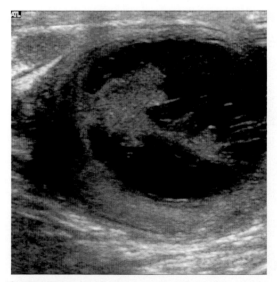

Fig. 12. Testicular abscess seen as an irregular complex heterogeneous fluid collection in testis.

situations that may show inconclusive results on color Doppler studies. The torsion-detorsion phenomenon may show testicular hyperemia, mimicking an inflammatory process.[28,29] There are reports of spermatic cord torsion with preserved perfusion of the testis on color Doppler studies.[22,30–33] Arce and colleagues[34] and Baud and colleagues[24] concluded that all these pitfalls occur because of indirect evaluation of a condition that is caused elsewhere. Hence, they proposed to study the spermatic cord directly because torsion occurs there. Baud and colleagues[24] and Kalfa and colleagues[35] studied the full length of the spermatic cord, including the inguinal canal, and described a spiral twist of the cord at the external inguinal ring that was diagnostic of torsion, irrespective of the color Doppler findings in the testis. This sign had a high sensitivity and specificity and the rate of unnecessary surgery was 0%. The same sign was elicited by the author with a real-time modification in the form of downward movement of the transducer along the spermatic cord to look for the whirlpool sign (Video 1).[12] The mass of torsion of the cord had the appearance of a doughnut, a target, a snail shell, or a storm on a weather map (Fig. 17). The movement of the transducer in a downward direction perpendicular to the axis of this mass brought on the whirlpool sign. The whirlpool mass can be seen in various locations: just distal to the external ring, above or posterior to the testis, and in the inguinal canal if the testis is undescended. The angle at

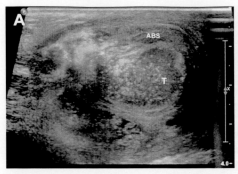
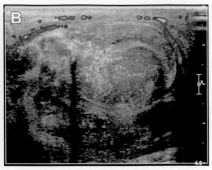

Fig. 13. Ruptured testicular abscess. (*A*) Collapsed irregular testis (T) with abscess (ABS) around it. (*B*) Color Doppler study shows flow around the abscess.

which it is best seen also varies. In complete torsion, the whirlpool sign is seen only on gray-scale sonography with absent intratesticular flow on color Doppler imaging (see **Fig. 16**C, D, Video 2). In incomplete torsion, there is flow in the vessels of the whirlpool mass, distal to it, and in the testis (**Fig. 18**). The whirlpool sign is seen on gray-scale as well as color Doppler imaging (see Video 1). The incomplete torsion probably explains the cases mentioned in earlier reports as missed torsion or torsion with preserved testicular perfusion, and the whirlpool sign helps in diagnosis of torsion in such patients. Hence, the real-time whirlpool sign is the most definitive sign of torsion because it has 100% specificity and sensitivity.

The following algorithm is suggested for sonography in a case of acute scrotal pain:

1. When the clinical history and physical examination are sufficiently alarming and unequivocal for testicular torsion and sonography is not possible immediately, surgical exploration is done without any imaging.
2. When there are unequivocal sonographic features of testicular torsion showing total absence of intratesticular blood flow, torsion of the testicular appendage, and acute idiopathic scrotal edema, then the patient is treated accordingly.
3. When symmetric or asymmetric arterial flow is seen in the testis, the spermatic cord is studied in detail to look for the whirlpool sign. The real-time whirlpool sign is the most specific sign of both complete and incomplete testicular torsion.

Intermittent Testicular Torsion

Intermittent testicular torsion (ITT) or a torsion-detorsion sequence is a clinical syndrome defined by a history of unilateral scrotal pain of sudden onset and of short duration that resolves

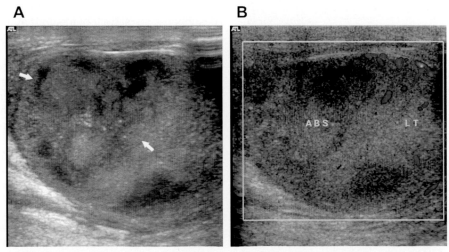

Fig. 14. (*A*) Evolving abscess seen as an irregular echo-poor area (*arrows*) in testis mimicking tumor. (*B*) Color Doppler study shows no flow.

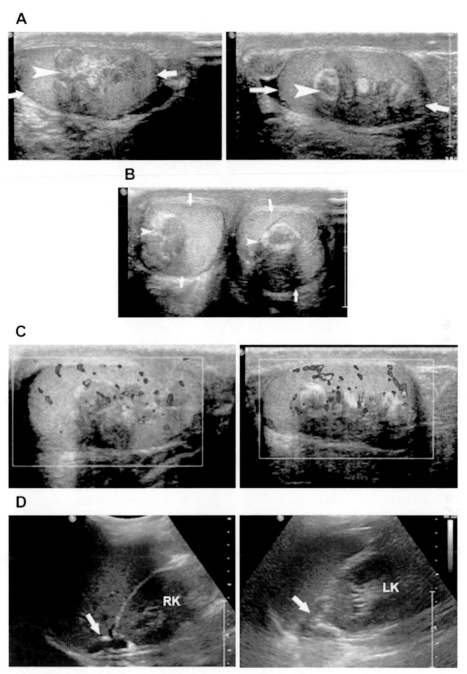

Fig. 15. Adrenal rests in the testis. Longitudinal (*A*) and transverse (*B*) images of both testes (*arrows*) showing multiple rounded heterogeneous solid masses (*arrowheads*) in both testes. (*C*) Color Doppler image shows vessels coursing through the masses. (*D*) Coronal scan of both adrenals (*arrows*) showing bilateral adrenal hyperplasia. LK, left kidney; RK, right kidney.

spontaneously.[36] The natural history of ITT varies. Some patients may have acute torsion at a later date, which is shown by the observation that up to half of patients with acute torsion report previous episodes of testicular pain.[37] Some patients have continued attacks that, if lasting long enough,

can result in ischemic damage to the testis, although definite evidence of this is lacking.[38–40]

The sonographic features of this syndrome depend on the time between sonography and the event, the severity of the torsion, and the duration of the event.[12] If patients report after a few days of

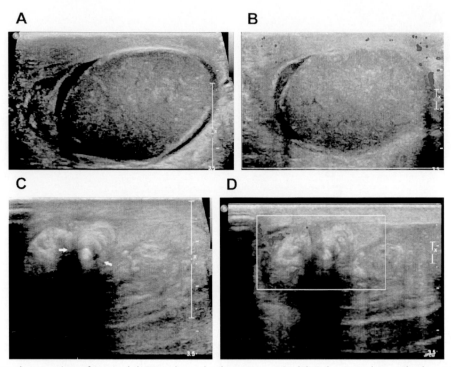

Fig. 16. Complete torsion of testis. (*A*) An enlarged echo-poor testis. (*B*) Color Doppler study shows absence of intratesticular flow. (*C*) Oblique section of the spermatic cord shows the mass of whirlpool (*arrows*) on gray scale. (*D*) Color Doppler study shows absence of flow in the mass, indicating occlusion of vessels.

a mild event, the sonographic findings may be normal. If they report within a few hours after severe torsion and complete detorsion, the testis will be slightly swollen and hypoechoic, and the spermatic cord will be straight. There is hyperemia of the testis on color Doppler imaging (**Fig. 19**). The same features are also seen in acute epididymo-orchitis. The differentiation of ITT and epididymo-orchitis in this situation is only clinical. One useful and consistent sonographic finding in ITT is the horizontal lie of the testis.[37,41] Some of these patients with a torsion-detorsion sequence showing testicular hyperemia and mimicking epididymo-orchitis have testicular atrophy later.[39] The third group of patients with ITT, who have severe torsion with complete detorsion and report early, reveal sonographic features of segmental testicular infarction.[42] The horizontally placed testis reveals focal hypoechoic areas that lack blood flow, with the rest of the testis showing a normal echo pattern (**Fig. 20**). These areas with a normal echo pattern either show normal blood flow in sparse arteries or show hyperemia. The epididymis may show increased blood flow. Although polycythemia, sickle cell anemia, and acute angiitis have been linked to segmental infarction, the cause of most reported cases is unknown,[13,42–44] and these were probably cases of

ITT. The differential diagnosis of this condition can be severe epididymo-orchitis with suppuration. These two conditions can be differentiated by the presence of clinical features of infection seen in epididymo-orchitis, and the history of acute pain with spontaneous relief, a history of a previous episode, and a horizontal testicular axis in ITT. If ITT is diagnosed, ipsilateral orchidopexy should be performed along with prophylactic contralateral orchidopexy to preserve the normal testis because of the high association of future contralateral torsion.[41] When these differentiating features are absent, the patients need active follow-up. This follow-up is essential because ITT is a possibility. The challenges of clinical decision making in these patients lie in the recognition that there is no definitive diagnostic test to confirm ITT. Only by halting the pattern of recurrent pain can the diagnosis be made, albeit retrospectively.[40] When there is a clinical history typical of ITT and a horizontal testicular axis, bilateral orchidopexy is done.

Trauma

Scrotal trauma is common and usually results from traffic accidents, sports injury, or direct perineal injury with compression of the scrotum against

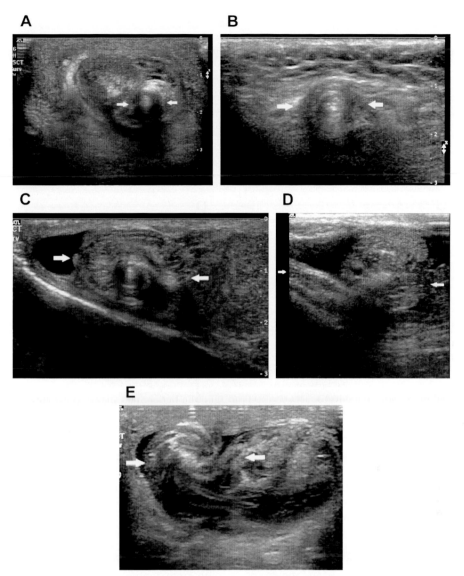

Fig. 17. Various appearances of a whirlpool mass (*between arrows*) on static images resembling a doughnut (*A*), a target with concentric rings (*B*), a snail shell (*C*), a snail (*D*), and a storm on a weather map (*E*).

the pubic bone.[45] Trauma can result in contusion, hematoma, hematocele, fracture, or rupture of the testis. Untreated testicular injuries may result in ischemic atrophy, chronic pain, or secondary infection.[45,46] Immediate surgical intervention is not necessary in all cases. Testicular rupture needs immediate treatment because up to 90% of ruptured testicles can be saved if surgery is performed within 72 hours; however, less than half of these procedures are performed within 72 hours.[47,48] In contrast, a conservative watchful approach can be adopted in intratesticular hematoma. Clinical diagnosis is often impossible because of marked scrotal pain and swelling and therefore ultrasonography with color Doppler is

essential to establish the diagnosis, evaluate the extent of damage, and predict possible complications.[45] The role of ultrasonography is crucial, especially in the case of blunt trauma to (1) confirm or exclude testicular rupture, (2) to differentiate soft tissue hematomas from hematocele, and (3) provide follow-up of patients undergoing conservative therapy.

On ultrasonography, intratesticular hematoma appears echogenic in the immediate phase. However, it is usually seen as an echo-poor area that mimics a tumor (**Fig. 21**). The history of trauma is useful to differentiate it from tumor. However, it has to be a significant trauma, because most patients relate any symptom of the scrotum to a trivial

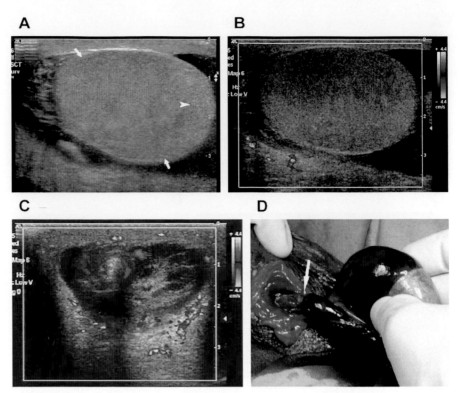

Fig. 18. Incomplete torsion of the testis. (*A*) Longitudinal scan of a horizontally placed testis showing a large hypoechoic area (*arrows*) in the upper two-thirds of the testis and a normal echo pattern (*arrowhead*) in the lower third. (*B*) Color Doppler image showing no flow in the hypoechoic area with a few vessels seen in the poles. (*C*) Color Doppler image of the whirlpool mass showing the visualized vessels going around the central axis. (*D*) Ischemic testis with the segmental infarction of the upper two-thirds and torsion of the spermatic cord (*arrow*).

incident of trauma, which may be misleading. Color Doppler study helps to differentiate tumors from hematoma. Tumors show increased blood flow, whereas hematoma does not show any flow. The most useful sign is the temporal change in appearance of hematoma on follow-up scan. In testicular rupture, the testis shows an irregular or indistinct contour. A breach in the continuity of the tunica albuginea confirms the diagnosis (**Fig. 22**). When there is extreme fragmentation of the testis, sonography shows a heterogeneous mass in the scrotum without any testislike structure. Color Doppler study shows flow in the fragments of parenchyma of testis and absence of flow in ischemic areas and hematoma. Most patients show hematocele around the testis, which is seen as solid echogenic mass without any flow on color Doppler in the immediate phase. Later, it is seen as echogenic and septated fluid (see **Fig. 22**).

Undescended Testis or Cryptorchidism

Undescended testis, also known as cryptorchidism, refers to the condition in which the testis fails to reach the scrotum. The testis develops intraabdominally and moves toward the scrotum during fetal development. The descent of testis into the scrotum normally occurs by the ninth month of gestational age or a few weeks after birth. The descent may be arrested at any level along the path from the retroperitoneum to the scrotum. Although most patients with nonpalpable testis present during childhood, there are a few patients who present in adulthood with infertility. The descent of the testes is important for normal spermatogenesis. Progressive germ cell damage occurs in undescended testis secondary to increased temperature at its extrascrotal location and untreated postpubertal undescended testis may be devoid of germ cells. In bilateral cryptorchidism, the rate of paternity is approximately 50% but unilateral condition results in little, if any, impairment of fertility.[49] Other complications of undescended testis are testicular malignancy, torsion, and inguinal hernia. The rationale of management of this condition is to place the testis in the scrotum to maximize its potential for spermatogenesis, screen for occurrence of malignancy, or to remove a nonviable testis.

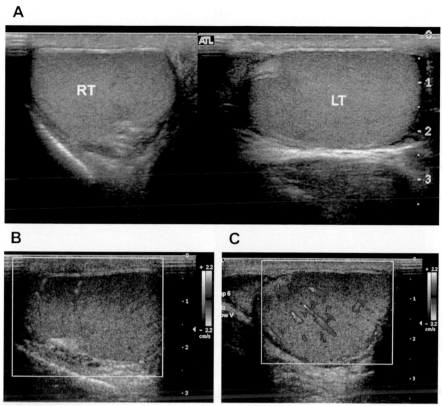

Fig. 19. ITT. (*A*) Transverse scan of a scrotum showing the short axis of the right testis (RT) and long axis of the left testis (LT) indicating the horizontally placed left testis. The left testis is slightly hypoechoic compared with the right testis. (*B*) Color Doppler image of the right testis showing a normal flow pattern. (*C*) Color Doppler image showing increased flow in the left testis.

Preoperative localization of the testis by an imaging study is beneficial, because it can modify the surgical procedure. The aims of an imaging method are therefore (1) to localize the testis, including ectopic locations; (2) to establish whether the testis is viable or atrophic; and (3) to establish whether the testis is absent. On clinical examination, 80% of undescended testes are palpable and do not need any imaging investigation. The other 20% of undescended testes are nonpalpable.[50,51] Nonpalpable testis (NPT) is caused by undescended canalicular or abdominal testis, or rarely by absent, ectopic, or atrophic testis.

In the past, imaging was targeted toward visualizing the testis and hence there was difficulty in visualizing the atrophic, absent, or ectopic testis, which resulted in low sensitivity and specificity of the imaging method.[52,53] Tracking the spermatic cord is a new technique to locate the testis.[54] The spermatic cord, being an accompanying structure of the testis, helps to locate the testis. The high resolution of modern ultrasonography scanners helps to visualize the spermatic cord in the inguinal canal. On a transverse scan of the inguinal region, it is seen as an oval echogenic structure with a few round echo-poor areas, representing the vas deferens and vessels (**Fig. 23**). It is seen anteromedial to the common femoral vessels. When it is seen, it can be traced down as shown in Video 3. The visualization and tracing of the cord helps to locate the NPT in the following ways:

1. When the cord is visualized, it can be traced down, which can lead to a testis of normal size located either in the inguinal canal (**Fig. 24**) or in the scrotum.
2. The visualized cord can be traced to an ectopic testis, which otherwise would not have been detected. Ectopic testis is a condition in which the testis is located outside the path of its descent. It can be found in the (1) superficial inguinal pouch, (2) anterior abdominal wall, (3) prepenile region, (4) perineal region (**Fig. 25**), and (5) femoral region.[55,56] In all these situations, the spermatic cord is seen in the inguinal canal and it acts as a guide to the ectopic testis. Transverse testicular ectopia is a condition in

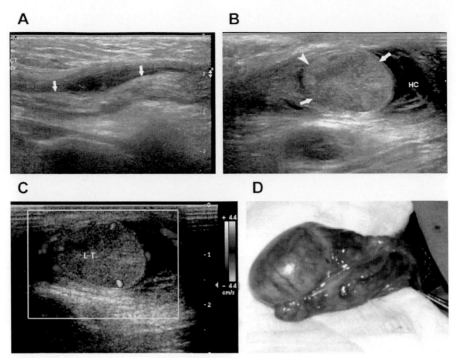

Fig. 20. Segmental testicular infarction. (*A*) Longitudinal scan of the straight spermatic cord (*arrows*). (*B*) Longitudinal scan showing a transverse section of a swollen testis with a large hypoechoic area (*arrows*) in the lower part and a normal echo pattern (*arrowhead*) in the upper part. There is a septated hydrocele (HC). (*C*) Color Doppler image showing lack of flow in the hypoechoic area with a few vessels in the periphery of the left testis (LT). (*D*) Ischemic testis with segmental infarction.

which both gonads migrate toward the same hemiscrotum. The testis may lie in the opposite hemiscrotum (**Fig. 26**A), in the opposite inguinal canal (see **Fig. 26**B), or at the opposite deep inguinal ring. Transverse testicular ectopia may be a feature in persistent müllerian duct syndrome, in which there are persistent or rudimentary müllerian duct structures. It is caused by a defect in either the synthesis of, or the receptor for, müllerian-inhibiting substance. Although virilization generally remains unaffected in these patients, infertility is common.[57]

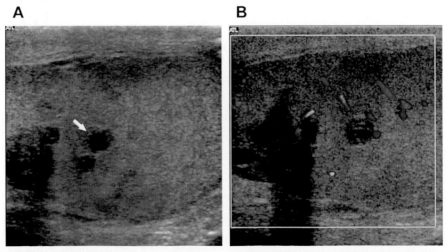

Fig. 21. Intratesticular hematoma. (*A*) Gray-scale image of the testis showing echo-poor area in upper part of the testis (*arrow*). (*B*) Color Doppler shows no flow in this area.

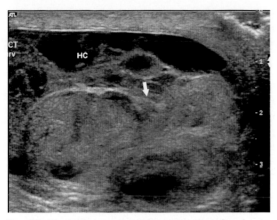

Fig. 22. Testicular rupture. Irregular ill-defined contour with a breach (*arrow*) in the tunica albuginea. There is hematocele (HC) around the testis.

3. Tracing the visualized cord leads to an atrophic testis in the canal or scrotum that otherwise can be easily missed because of its small size. The smallest atrophic testis can be 3 to 4 mm in length. Such a small testis can be missed on routine ultrasonography, but, with the technique of tracking the spermatic cord, it can

easily be identified and confirmed. The atrophic testes may have varied appearance: echo poor, echogenic, or showing central/egg shell calcification (**Fig. 27**).

4. The cord can be looped in the inguinal canal in ascended testis in which the returning loop can be traced to the intra-abdominal testis. Ascended testis is defined as a condition in which the testis is initially thought to be normally descended but is later found to be outside the scrotum.[58] Hence, there are 2 sections of the cord because of looping of the cord in the inguinal canal. The testis is seen in an intra-abdominal location (**Fig. 28**, Video 4).

5. If the testis is not visualized in spite of the spermatic cord being visualized in the inguinal canal, it indicates a vanished testis. Vanished testis occurs when the testis has descended into the scrotum but has atrophied totally because of torsion or an ischemic event during prenatal or early postnatal life. In this situation, the spermatic cord is seen in the inguinal canal, but, when tracked down, it does not lead to a testis. Ultrasonography predicts vanished testis accurately.

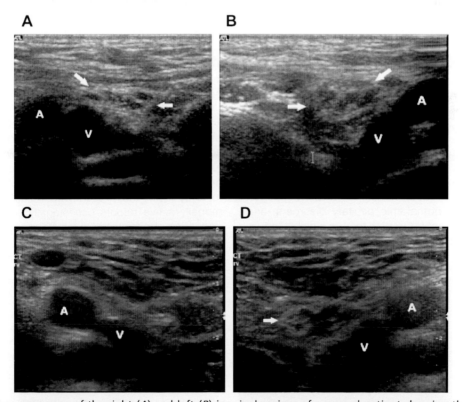

Fig. 23. Transverse scan of the right (*A*) and left (*B*) inguinal regions of a normal patient showing the oblique section of spermatic cord (*arrows*) anteromedial to the common femoral artery (A) and vein (V). (*C, D*) Similar sections in a patient with a right NPT revealing a nonvisualization of the spermatic cord on right side and normal cord (*arrow*) on left side.

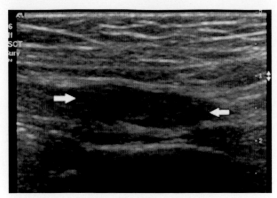

Fig. 24. Oblique section showing the testis (*arrows*) in the inguinal canal.

6. If the spermatic cord is not visualized in the inguinal canal, it rules out an extra-abdominal location of the testis and the search can be extended up to look for an abdominal, retroperitoneal, or pelvic location of the testis (**Fig. 29**). If necessary, a lower-frequency probe can be used. The intra-abdominal testis is differentiated from a bowel loop by the presence of peristalsis in the bowel (Video 5) and the mobility of the testis.

Thus high-resolution ultrasonography, with the technique of tracking the spermatic cord, is a cost-effective and sensitive preoperative imaging method in NPT. It is useful in selecting the ideal therapeutic surgical approach and avoiding diagnostic laparoscopy in most patients (**Fig. 30**).

Testicular Atrophy

Testicular atrophy is associated with reduced spermatogenesis and a reduction in fertility. Atrophy may occur following previous inflammation, ischemia, trauma, torsion, liver cirrhosis, estrogen treatment, hypothalamic pituitary disorders, and aging. On ultrasonography, there is a global reduction in the volume of the testis. A decrease in both

testicular reflectivity and vascularity are common findings. The epididymis usually appears normal.[1]

TESTICULAR NEOPLASMS

Testicular neoplasm accounts for only 1% of all malignancies in men and it is the most common cancer in men aged 20 to 35 years of age. Lymphoma, spermatocytic seminoma, and metastases occur in patients between 50 and 70 years of age. There is a low incidence in children caused by yolk sac tumors and teratomas.[59,60]

Testicular tumors are categorized into germ cell and non–germ cell tumors. Germ cell tumors arise from spermatogenic cells and constitute 95% of testicular neoplasms. They are almost always malignant. Germ cell tumors are divided into seminomatous germ cell tumors and nonseminomatous germ cell tumors (NSGCTs). Seminomas are more common and less aggressive than nonseminomatous tumors.[61] Mixed germ cell tumors are common among NSGCTs. Non–germ cell primary tumors of the testis derive from the sex cords (Sertoli cells) and stroma (Leydig cells). These tumors are malignant in only 10% of cases. Other rare tumors are lymphoma, leukemia, and metastases.[60]

Various risk factors for testicular cancer are cryptorchidism, prior testicular tumor, positive family history, infertility, testicular dysgenesis, TM, and Klinefelter syndrome. Risk of malignancy is high both in cryptorchid testis and contralateral normal testis.[62]

The most common manifestation is a painless scrotal mass. Other symptoms include a sensation of heaviness or fullness in the lower abdomen or scrotum. Only 10% of patients present with a painful mass caused by hemorrhage or infarction[63] that may initially be misdiagnosed as orchitis. Only a minority of patients present with metastases. Hormonally active tumors occasionally present with endocrine abnormalities such as precocious puberty and gynecomastia.[60,63]

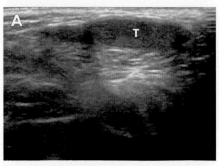
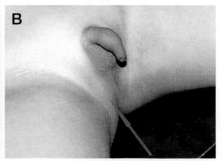

Fig. 25. Perineal testis. (*A*) The testis (T) in subcutaneous plane in the perineum posterolateral to the scrotum. (*B*) The site of the located testis (*arrow*).

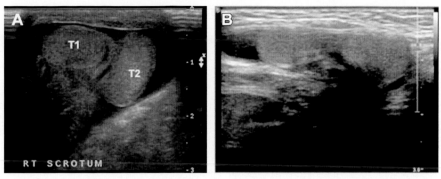

Fig. 26. Transverse testicular ectopia. (*A*) Both testes (T1 and T2) in the right side of scrotum. (*B*) Image showing both testes in the same inguinal canal.

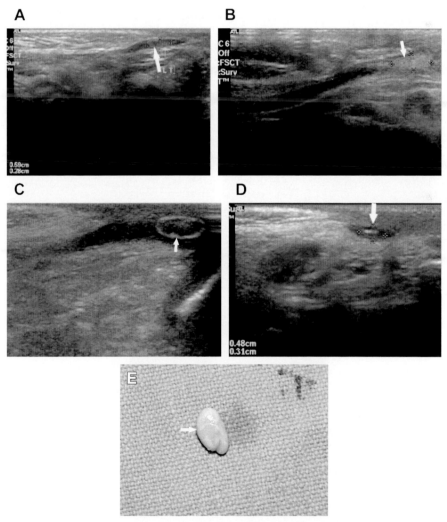

Fig. 27. Varying appearance of atrophic testis (*arrows*). (*A*) Echo-poor testis. (*B*) Echogenic testis. (*C*) Egg shell calcification. (*D*) Central calcification. (*E*) An atrophic testis removed at exploration.

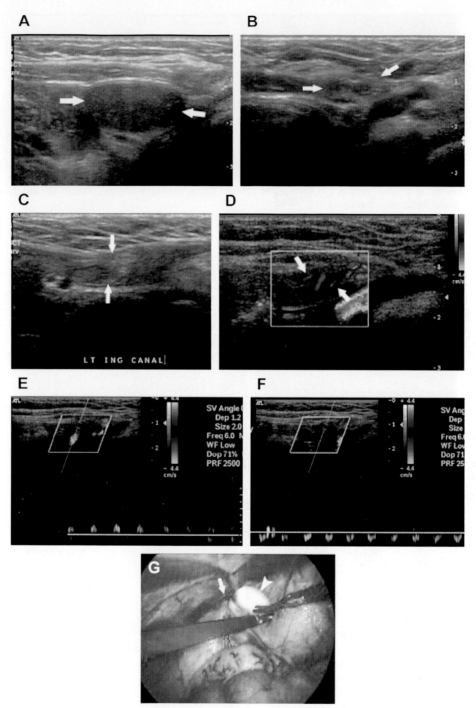

Fig. 28. Ascended testis. (*A*) Oblique scan of the lower abdomen showing the intra-abdominal testis (*arrows*). (*B*) Transverse and (*C*) longitudinal section of inguinal region showing the 2 loops (*arrows*) of the spermatic cord in the inguinal canal. (*D*) Color Doppler image showing the testicular artery (*arrows*) in the 2 loops of the cord confirming the looping of the cord. (*E, F*) Spectral Doppler images of testicular artery in the 2 loops showing flow in opposite directions. (*G*) Laparoscopic picture shows the intra-abdominal testis (*arrowhead*) with spermatic cord (*arrow*) emerging out of the internal ring.

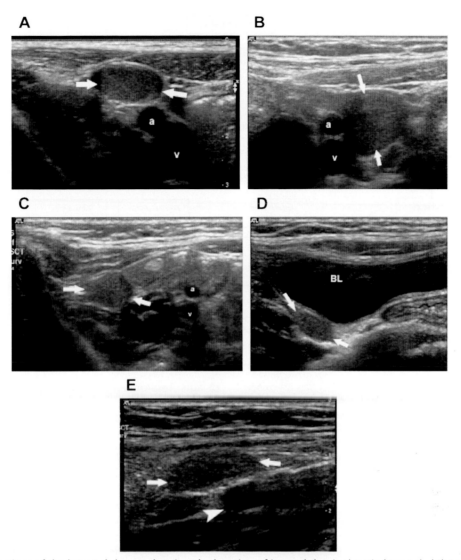

Fig. 29. Sections of the lower abdomen showing the location of intra-abdominal testis (*arrows*). (*A*) Anterior, (*B*) medial, and (*C*) lateral to external iliac vessels (a and v). (*D*) Testis is located along the right side wall of pelvis and (*E*) anterior to the bifurcation of the common iliac artery (*arrowhead*). BL, urinary bladder.

Tumor markers play an important adjunct role in the diagnosis, prognosis, and follow-up of testicular germ cell tumors. β-Human chorionic gonadotrophin (β-HCG) is significantly increased in nearly all patients with pure and mixed choriocarcinoma. In 10% to 25% of patients, seminomas are also associated with an increased β-HCG level. The alpha-fetoprotein is increased in yolk sac tumors and mixed germ cell tumors with yolk sac component. The alpha-fetoprotein level is never increased in patients with pure seminoma,[64] which provides a useful tool to distinguish pure seminoma and nonseminomatous germ cell tumors. Concentrations of tumor markers that are persistently increased or increasing indicate residual or recurrent disease.[60] Increased tumor markers significantly increase the positive predictive value of ultrasonography findings but, in contrast, a negative serologic diagnosis does not affect the ultrasonography diagnosis.[65]

Seminoma is the most common germ cell tumor and occurs in men aged 20 to 40 years. Pure seminoma accounts for 35% to 50% of all germ cell tumors and is sometimes a component of mixed germ cell tumors.[60] It can be bilateral. Seminoma is the most common tumor associated with cryptorchidism. There are 3 subtypes of seminomas: typical seminomas account for 85%; anaplastic seminomas for 5% to 10%; and spermatocytic seminomas for 4% to 6%. Spermatocytic

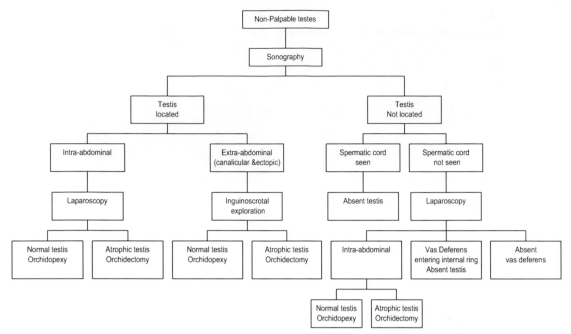

Fig. 30. Algorithm for management of nonpalpable testis after sonography using the tracking cord technique.

seminoma occurs in older men and has an excellent prognosis. On gray-scale sonography, seminoma appears as a homogeneous echo-poor lesion varying in size from a small nodule (**Fig. 31**) to a large mass that totally replaces the testis causing diffuse enlargement (**Fig. 32**). Other rare features are multinodularity, in which all the nodules are in continuity (**Fig. 33**),[60] and cystic changes caused by dilated rete testis or liquefaction necrosis (**Fig. 34**).[66] Seminomas are usually confined by the tunica albuginea and rarely extend to peritesticular structures.[46] About 20% of patients show retroperitoneal lymphadenopathy (**Fig. 35**) and hematological metastases. Seminoma is less aggressive and has a good prognosis because it is radiosensitive.

NSGCTs are mostly of mixed type with various histologic patterns like teratomas, embryonal carcinoma, yolk sac tumor, and choriocarcinoma.[67] Seminoma can also be a component of mixed germ cell tumors and, when it is present, the tumor is treated as NSGCT. Unlike seminomas, NSGCTs are very aggressive with frequent metastases. The macroscopic and ultrasonographic appearance of these tumors show a varied pattern with heterogeneous echotexture, irregular or ill-defined margins, cystic components, echogenic foci caused by calcification, hemorrhage, and fibrosis.[66] Tumor invasion of tunica albuginea is common and distorts the contour of the testis (**Fig. 36**). Pure embryonal carcinoma is rare and mixed teratocarcinoma is common in patients from 25 to 35 years

of age. Teratomas can occur in any age group. Pure teratomas occur in children and are mostly benign, whereas immature and malignant teratomas can occur in adults. Cystic changes with echogenic foci caused by calcification, cartilage, fat, and keratin debris are common (**Fig. 37**). Pure yolk sac tumor is common in children less than 2 years of age, whereas in adults it is mostly seen as part of mixed germ cell tumor in which alpha-fetoprotein is significantly increased.[61,63] On ultrasonography, it is seen as a predominantly solid mass with heterogeneous echo pattern and anechoic spaces (**Fig. 38**).[4,68,69] Choriocarcinoma shows extensive hemorrhagic necrosis that, on sonography, appears as mixed cystic and solid areas. Hematological metastases are more common with choriocarcinoma.

Burned-out testicular tumor is the condition in which primary tumor metastasizes and then burns out, leaving metastases in the retroperitoneum without any apparent source. It is usually a teratocarcinoma or choriocarcinoma. It occurs secondary to rapid tumor growth, resulting in the tumor outstripping its blood supply with subsequent tumor regression. The sonographic features are small echo-poor mass, echogenic foci, or atrophic testis.[46,60,70]

Sex cord stromal tumors include 4% of all testicular tumors. Ninety percent of these tumors are benign. The prevalence is higher in the pediatric age group.[63] Approximately 30% of patients have endocrinopathy secondary to secretion of

A

B

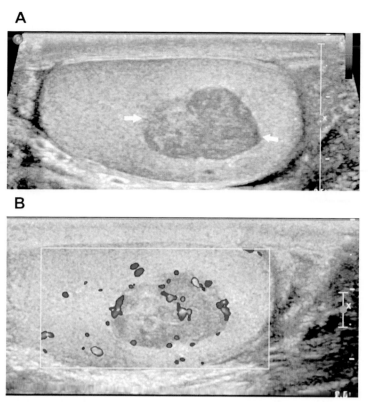

Fig. 31. Seminoma of testis. (*A*) Gray-scale and (*B*) color Doppler images of the testis showing an echo-poor mass (*arrows*) with flow in the mass.

androgens or estrogens by the tumor. The endocrinopathy may manifest as precocious virilization, gynecomastia, or decreased libido. Their sonographic appearance is variable and is indistinguishable from that of germ cell tumors. They do not have any specific sonographic appearance but sometimes appear as well-defined hypoechoic lesions (**Fig. 39**).[46,60]

Lymphomas constitute 5% of all testicular tumors but the incidence increases to 25% after the age of 50 years.[46,71] It is the most common

testicular tumor in men aged more than 60 years. It is almost exclusively diffuse non-Hodgkin B-cell type. Secondary lymphoma is more common than primary lymphoma. Lymphoma is the most common bilateral testicular tumor. Gray-scale ultrasonography shows homogeneously echo-poor testes (**Fig. 40**) or multifocal echo-poor lesions of various sizes.[72,73] Sometimes striated echo-poor bands with parallel echogenic lines radiating peripherally from the mediastinum testis are seen and they represent blood vessels

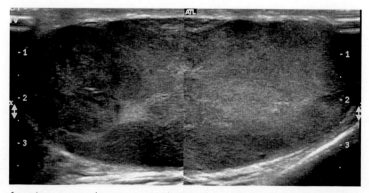

Fig. 32. Seminoma of testis seen as a large mass replacing the testis causing diffuse enlargement of the testis.

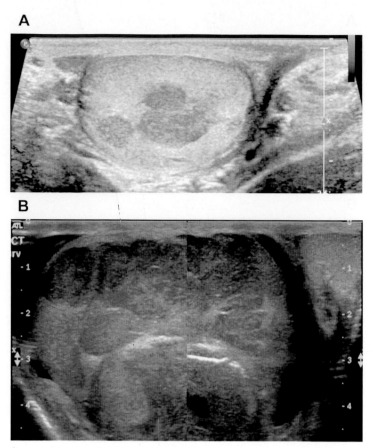

Fig. 33. Seminoma of testis. (*A, B*) Multinodular appearance of seminoma in 2 patients. The nodules are seen in continuity.

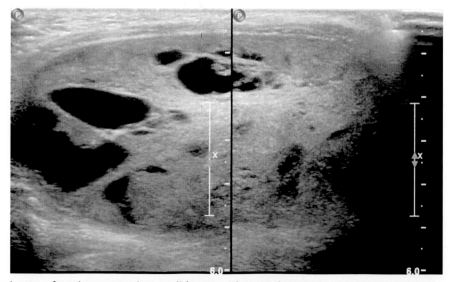

Fig. 34. Seminoma of testis seen as a large solid mass with necrotic areas.

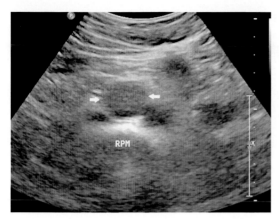

Fig. 35. Transverse scan of midabdomen showing an enlarged metastatic para-aortic lymph node (*arrows*) from seminoma of testis.

traversing the lesion.[4] Patient age and bilateralism are the important factors in favoring the diagnosis. Primary leukemia of the testis is rare. However, the testis is a common site of acute lymphoblastic leukemia recurrence in children, with 80% of patients being in bone marrow remission.[74,75] A blood-testis barrier limiting the effect of chemotherapeutic agents in the testes explains the persistence of leukemia in the testes after remission.[67] Testicular metastases are rare and the common primary tumors are prostate, lung, malignant melanoma, colon, and renal carcinoma.

Ultrasonography is the first and most common technique for the evaluation of testicular tumors. Magnetic resonance imaging provides additional information only in selected cases and computed tomography is used only for staging. No imaging technique can provide histologic diagnosis.[65] Some benign conditions like hematoma, infarction, and orchitis mimic neoplasm, so follow-up examination is necessary in equivocal cases.[60] In most intratesticular lesions, the differentiation between benign and malignant lesions and the type of malignancy can be made only by histopathologic examination. The role of ultrasonography in these lesions is to provide a provisional diagnosis of benign or malignant lesions, because the management can vary from just a follow-up scan or testis-sparing surgery to inguinal orchidectomy. This diagnosis is made possible to a great extent by a combination of clinical and ultrasonographic features:

1. Age distribution for testicular malignancy is fairly characteristic. The peak incidence of testicular cancer is between 25 and 35 years of age.[4] Some types of tumors (mainly lymphoma, spermatocytic seminoma, and metastasis) occur later in life (50–70 years). The third and much less pronounced peak, which occurs in children, is caused by yolk sac tumors and teratomas.

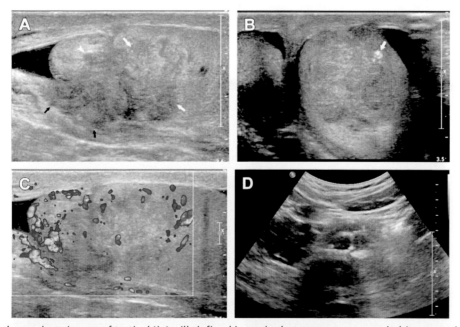

Fig. 36. Embryonal carcinoma of testis. (*A*) An ill-defined irregular heterogeneous mass (*white arrows*) in the upper pole with infiltration of the head of epididymis (*arrowhead*) and the spermatic cord (*black arrows*). (*B*) Transverse scan of the mass showing calcification (*arrow*). (*C*) Color Doppler image shows flow in the mass. (*D*) Transverse scan of retroperitoneum shows a metastatic para-aortic lymph node.

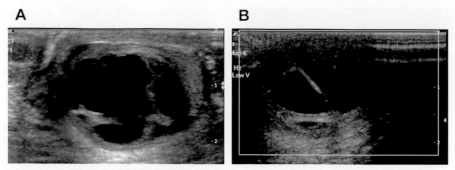

Fig. 37. Teratoma of testis. (*A*) The testis in a child showing a solid and cystic mass. (*B*) Color Doppler image shows flow the solid areas.

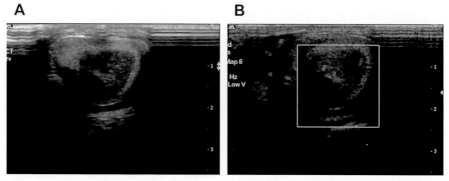

Fig. 38. Yolk sac tumor (*A*) seen as a solid heterogeneous mass in the testis of a child. (*B*) Color Doppler shows flow in the tumor.

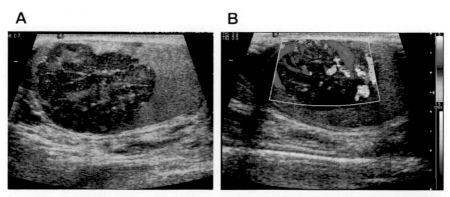

Fig. 39. Leydig cell tumor. (*A*) The testis of a 35-year-old man showing a well-defined irregular echo-poor lesion in upper part. (*B*) Color Doppler shows increased flow in the mass. (*Courtesy of* Dr R. Subramaniam, DMRD, Salem, India.)

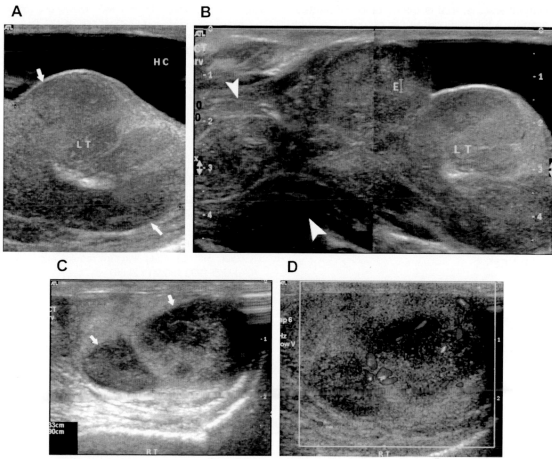

Fig. 40. Lymphoma of testis. (*A*) Large multifocal echo-poor mass (*arrows*) in the left testis (LT) and hydrocele (HC) around it. (*B*) The mass infiltrates the epididymis (E) and the spermatic cord (*arrowheads*). (*C*) The right testis of the same patient showing 2 echo-poor masses (*arrows*) that show increased flow on color Doppler study (*D*).

2. Presence of risk factors as described previously points more to a malignant lesion.
3. Symptoms may help to differentiate between benign and malignant lesions to some extent. Although malignant lesions present as a painless swelling or dull scrotal pain, most benign conditions present with acute pain.
4. Role of tumor markers is discussed earlier.
5. Features of sonography:
   a. The primary goal of ultrasonography examination in the diagnosis of testicular neoplasm is to determine whether a mass is intratesticular or extratesticular because most extratesticular masses are benign and intratesticular masses are more likely to be malignant.[46,67]
   b. Most malignant lesions are focal, solid, and echo poor compared with normal testicular parenchyma, and most benign lesions are cystic.
   c. The third useful feature is the presence of normal testicular parenchyma, which

suggests malignancy. In orchitis and trauma, normal tissue is not visible and, even if visible, it is usually edematous and abnormal.
   d. The fourth feature is irregularity of shape of the testis, which is seen in malignancy.
   e. The fifth finding is associated extratesticular features like involvement of epididymis, which suggests benign epididymo-orchitis or Koch infection.
   f. Presence of hydrocele is more common in benign condition like orchitis or trauma.
   g. A mass in the testis with TM suggests malignancy.
   h. Color Doppler shows increased flow in most malignant lesions.[76]
   i. It is crucial to do an abdominal scan to detect metastatic retroperitoneal lymphadenopathy, which indicates that the lesion in the testis is malignant.

There is considerable overlap of the ultrasonographic features described earlier in benign and malignant lesions; that is the limitation of ultrasonography. A follow-up scan can be useful in such a situation.

ACKNOWLEDGMENTS

The author thanks Dr Sathiya Senthil and Dr G. Swapna for their assistance in preparing this article; Mr Srambical Sreedharan, EDP, for technical assistance; and Mrs Padma Ramesh for secretarial assistance. The author also thanks all his clinical colleagues for their cooperation.

SUPPLEMENTARY DATA

Video related to this article can be found online at http://dx.doi.org/10.1016/j.cult.2014.03.005.

REFERENCES

1. Sidhu PS. Diseases of the testis and epididymis. In: Baxter GM, Sidhu PS, editors. Ultrasound of the urogenital system. Stuttgart (Germany): Thieme; 2006. p. 153–80.

2. Chou SJ, Liu HY, Fu YT, et al. Cysts of the tunica albuginea. Arch Androl 2004;50(2):89–92.

3. Dogra VS, Gottlieb RH, Rubens DJ, et al. Benign intratesticular cystic lesions: US features. Radiographics 2001;21(Spec No):S273–81.

4. Oyen RH. Scrotal ultrasound. Eur Radiol 2002; 12(1):19–34.

5. Rubenstein RA, Dogra VS, Seftel AD, et al. Benign intrascrotal lesions. J Urol 2004;171(5):1765–72.

6. Colangelo SM, Fried K, Hyacinthe LM, et al. Tubular ectasia of the rete testis: an ultrasound diagnosis. Urology 1995;45(3):532–4.

7. Kim B, Winter TC 3rd, Ryu JA. Testicular microlithiasis: clinical significance and review of the literature. Eur Radiol 2003;13(12):2567–76.

8. Bach AM, Hann LE, Hadar O, et al. Testicular microlithiasis: what is its association with testicular cancer? Radiology 2001;220(1):70–5.

9. Fernandez-Perez GC, Tardaguila FM, Velasco M, et al. Radiologic findings of segmental testicular infarction. AJR Am J Roentgenol 2005;184(5): 1587–93.

10. Sriprasad S, Kooiman GG, Muir GH, et al. Acute segmental testicular infarction: differentiation from tumour using high frequency colour Doppler ultrasound. Br J Radiol 2001;74(886):965–7.

11. Sharma SB, Gupta V. Segmental testicular infarction. Indian J Pediatr 2005;72(1):81–2.

12. Vijayaraghavan SB. Sonographic differential diagnosis of acute scrotum: real-time whirlpool sign, a key sign of torsion. J Ultrasound Med 2006;25(5): 563–74.

13. Costa M, Calleja R, Ball RY, et al. Segmental testicular infarction. BJU Int 1999;83(4):525.

14. Akin EA, Khati NJ, Hill MC. Ultrasound of the scrotum. Ultrasound Q 2004;20(4):181–200.

15. Dogra V, Bhatt S. Acute painful scrotum. Radiol Clin North Am 2004;42(2):349–63.

16. Woodward PJ, Schwab CM, Sesterhenn IA. From the archives of the AFIP: extratesticular scrotal masses: radiologic-pathologic correlation. Radiographics 2003;23(1):215–40.

17. Nagamine WH, Mehta SV, Vade A. Testicular adrenal rest tumors in a patient with congenital adrenal hyperplasia: sonographic and magnetic resonance imaging findings. J Ultrasound Med 2005;24(12): 1717–20.

18. Howlett DC, Jones AJ, Saunders AJ. Case of the month. Painless testicular nodularity in a young man. Br J Radiol 1997;70(839):1195–6.

19. Kass EJ, Stone KT, Cacciarelli AA, et al. Do all children with an acute scrotum require exploration? J Urol 1993;150(2 Pt 2):667–9.

20. Burks DD, Markey BJ, Burkhard TK, et al. Suspected testicular torsion and ischemia: evaluation with color Doppler sonography. Radiology 1990; 175(3):815–21.

21. Paltiel HJ, Connolly LP, Atala A, et al. Acute scrotal symptoms in boys with an indeterminate clinical presentation: comparison of color Doppler sonography and scintigraphy. Radiology 1998;207(1): 223–31.

22. Kravchick S, Cytron S, Leibovici O, et al. Color Doppler sonography: its real role in the evaluation of children with highly suspected testicular torsion. Eur Radiol 2001;11(6):1000–5.

23. Aso C, Enriquez G, Fite M, et al. Gray-scale and color Doppler sonography of scrotal disorders in children: an update. Radiographics 2005;25(5): 1197–214.

24. Baud C, Veyrac C, Couture A, et al. Spiral twist of the spermatic cord: a reliable sign of testicular torsion. Pediatr Radiol 1998;28(12):950–4.

25. Patriquin HB, Yazbeck S, Trinh B, et al. Testicular torsion in infants and children: diagnosis with Doppler sonography. Radiology 1993;188(3): 781–5.

26. Middleton WD, Middleton MA, Dierks M, et al. Sonographic prediction of viability in testicular torsion: preliminary observations. J Ultrasound Med 1997;16(1):23–7 [quiz: 29–30].

27. Wilbert DM, Schaerfe CW, Stern WD, et al. Evaluation of the acute scrotum by color-coded Doppler ultrasonography. J Urol 1993;149(6):1475–7.

28. Middleton WD, Siegel BA, Melson GL, et al. Acute scrotal disorders: prospective comparison of color Doppler US and testicular scintigraphy. Radiology 1990;177(1):177–81.

29. Ralls PW, Larsen D, Johnson MB, et al. Color Doppler sonography of the scrotum. Semin Ultrasound CT MR 1991;12(2):109–14.

30. Bentley DF, Ricchiuti DJ, Nasrallah PF, et al. Spermatic cord torsion with preserved testis perfusion: initial anatomical observations. J Urol 2004;172(6 Pt 1): 2373–6.

31. Steinhardt GF, Boyarsky S, Mackey R. Testicular torsion: pitfalls of color Doppler sonography. J Urol 1993;150(2 Pt 1):461–2.

32. Allen TD, Elder JS. Shortcomings of color Doppler sonography in the diagnosis of testicular torsion. J Urol 1995;154(4):1508–10.

33. Ingram S, Hollman AS, Azmy A. Testicular torsion: missed diagnosis on colour Doppler sonography. Pediatr Radiol 1993;23(6):483–4.

34. Arce JD, Cortes M, Vargas JC. Sonographic diagnosis of acute spermatic cord torsion. Rotation of the cord: a key to the diagnosis. Pediatr Radiol 2002;32(7):485–91.

35. Kalfa N, Veyrac C, Baud C, et al. Ultrasonography of the spermatic cord in children with testicular torsion: impact on the surgical strategy. J Urol 2004; 172(4 Pt 2):1692–5 [discussion: 1695].

36. Creagh TA, McDermott TE, McLean PA, et al. Intermittent torsion of the testis. BMJ 1988;297(6647): 525–6.

37. Kamaledeen S, Surana R. Intermittent testicular pain: fix the testes. BJU Int 2003;91(4):406–8.

38. Schulsinger D, Glassberg K, Strashun A. Intermittent torsion: association with horizontal lie of the testicle. J Urol 1991;145(5):1053–5.

39. Sellu DP, Lynn JA. Intermittent torsion of the testis. J R Coll Surg Edinb 1984;29(2):107–8.

40. Stillwell TJ, Kramer SA. Intermittent testicular torsion. Pediatrics 1986;77(6):908–11.

41. Eaton SH, Cendron MA, Estrada CR, et al. Intermittent testicular torsion: diagnostic features and management outcomes. J Urol 2005;174(4 Pt 2): 1532–5 [discussion: 1535].

42. Ledwidge ME, Lee DK, Winter TC 3rd, et al. Sonographic diagnosis of superior hemispheric testicular infarction. AJR Am J Roentgenol 2002;179(3):775–6.

43. Baratelli GM, Vischi S, Mandelli PG, et al. Segmental hemorrhagic infarction of testicle. J Urol 1996; 156(4):1442.

44. Bird K, Rosenfield AT. Testicular infarction secondary to acute inflammatory disease: demonstration by B-scan ultrasound. Radiology 1984;152(3):785–8.

45. Muttarak M, Lojanapiwat B. The painful scrotum: an ultrasonographical approach to diagnosis. Singapore Med J 2005;46(7):352–7 [quiz: 358].

46. Dogra VS, Gottlieb RH, Oka M, et al. Sonography of the scrotum. Radiology 2003;227(1):18–36.

47. Jeffrey RB, Laing FC, Hricak H, et al. Sonography of testicular trauma. AJR Am J Roentgenol 1983; 141(5):993–5.

48. Lupetin AR, King W 3rd, Rich PJ, et al. The traumatized scrotum. Ultrasound evaluation. Radiology 1983;148(1):203–7.

49. Edey AJ, Sidhu PS. Male infertility: role of imaging in the diagnosis and management. Imaging 2008; 20:139–46.

50. Elder JS. The undescended testis. Hormonal and surgical management. Surg Clin North Am 1988; 68(5):983–1005.

51. MacKinnon AE. The undescended testis. Indian J Pediatr 2005;72(5):429–32.

52. Cain MP, Garra B, Gibbons MD. Scrotal-inguinal ultrasonography: a technique for identifying the non-palpable inguinal testis without laparoscopy. J Urol 1996;156(2 Pt 2):791–4.

53. Nijs SM, Eijsbouts SW, Madern GC, et al. Nonpalpable testes: is there a relationship between ultrasonographic and operative findings? Pediatr Radiol 2007;37(4):374–9.

54. Vijayaraghavan SB. Sonographic localization of nonpalpable testis: tracking the cord technique. Indian J Radiol Imaging 2011;21(2):134–41.

55. Hutcheson JC, Snyder HM 3rd, Zuniga ZV, et al. Ectopic and undescended testes: 2 variants of a single congenital anomaly? J Urol 2000;163(3): 961–3.

56. Rao PL, Gupta V, Kumar V. Anterior abdominal wall–an unusual site for ectopic testis. Pediatr Surg Int 2005;21(8):687–8.

57. Gutte AA, Pendharkar PS, Sorte SZ. Transverse testicular ectopia associated with persistent Mullerian duct syndrome - the role of imaging. Br J Radiol 2008;81(967):e176–8.

58. Rusnack SL, Wu HY, Huff DS, et al. The ascending testis and the testis undescended since birth share the same histopathology. J Urol 2002;168(6):2590–1.

59. Carkaci S, Ozkan E, Lane D, et al. Scrotal sonography revisited. J Clin Ultrasound 2010;38(1):21–37.

60. Woodward PJ, Sohaey R, O'Donoghue MJ, et al. From the archives of the AFIP: tumors and tumor-like lesions of the testis: radiologic-pathologic correlation. Radiographics 2002;22(1):189–216.

61. Frush DP, Sheldon CA. Diagnostic imaging for pediatric scrotal disorders. Radiographics 1998; 18(4):969–85.

62. Howlett DC, Marchbank ND, Sallomi DF. Pictorial review. Ultrasound of the testis. Clin Radiol 2000; 55(8):595–601.

63. Ulbright T, Amin M, Young R. Tumors of the testis, adnexa, spermatic cord, and scrotum. Washington, DC: Armed Forces Institute of Pathology; 1999.

64. Javadpour N. Current status of tumor markers in testicular cancer. A practical review. Eur Urol 1992;21(Suppl 1):34–6.

65. Isidori AM. Neoplastic intratesticular lesions. In: Isidori AM, Lenzi A, editors. Scrotal ultrasound. Morphological and functional atlas. Genova, Italy: Accademia Nazionale di Medicina; 2008. p. 49–50.

66. Schwerk WB, Schwerk WN, Rodeck G. Testicular tumors: prospective analysis of real-time US

patterns and abdominal staging. Radiology 1987; 164(2):369–74.

67. Geraghty MJ, Lee FT Jr, Bernsten SA, et al. Sonography of testicular tumors and tumor-like conditions: a radiologic-pathologic correlation. Crit Rev Diagn Imaging 1998;39(1):1–63.

68. McEniff N, Doherty F, Katz J, et al. Yolk sac tumor of the testis discovered on a routine annual sonogram in a boy with testicular microlithiasis. AJR Am J Roentgenol 1995;164(4):971–2.

69. Thava V, Cooper N, Egginton JA. Yolk sac tumour of the testis in childhood. Br J Radiol 1992;65(780):1142–4.

70. Hamm B. Differential diagnosis of scrotal masses by ultrasound. Eur Radiol 1997;7(5):668–79.

71. Basu S, Howlett DC. High-resolution ultrasound in the evaluation of the nonacute testis. Abdom Imaging 2001;26(4):425–32.

72. Emura A, Kudo S, Mihara M, et al. Testicular malignant lymphoma; imaging and diagnosis. Radiat Med 1996;14(3):121–6.

73. Mazzu D, Jeffrey RB Jr, Ralls PW. Lymphoma and leukemia involving the testicles: findings on gray-scale and color Doppler sonography. AJR Am J Roentgenol 1995;164(3):645–7.

74. Rayor RA, Scheible W, Brock WA, et al. High resolution ultrasonography in the diagnosis of testicular relapse in patients with acute lymphoblastic leukemia. J Urol 1982;128(3):602–3.

75. Heaney JA, Klauber GT, Conley GR. Acute leukemia: diagnosis and management of testicular involvement. Urology 1983;21(6):573–7.

76. Horstman WG, Melson GL, Middleton WD, et al. Testicular tumors: findings with color Doppler US. Radiology 1992;185(3):733–7.

Ultrasonography of the Scrotum: Extratesticular

Nirvikar Dahiya, MD*, Maitray D. Patel, MD, Christine O. Menias, MD

KEYWORDS

- Ultrasonography • Extratesticular • Epididymis • Scrotum • Testes

KEY POINTS

- Extratesticular lesions are mostly benign.
- Adenomatoid tumor of the epididymis is the most common solid extratesticular tumor.
- Differentiating between a spermatocele and an epididymal cyst is not clinically relevant.
- Sperm granuloma is an entity to consider more strongly in patients with previous vasectomy.
- When evaluating a suspected palpable lesion with ultrasonography, the examiner should palpate the lesion to ascertain firmness and help direct the examination.
- By virtue of the ascending nature of the infection, epididymitis may be limited to the epididymal tail, so sonographic evaluation of suspected acute epididymitis must carefully evaluate this region.
- Evaluation of suspected hernias and varicoceles usually requires provocative maneuvers; having the patient do a Valsalva maneuver may be sufficient, but in some cases upright positioning will be needed to better demonstrate the abnormality.

INTRODUCTION

The extratesticular scrotal structures consist of the epididymis, spermatic cord, and enveloping fascia, derived as the testis descends during its embryologic development through the abdominal wall into the scrotal sac. The epididymis is a crescent-shaped structure that lies along the posterior border of the testis, connecting the efferent seminiferous tubules in the testis to the vas deferens.

The efferent ductules pierce through the tunica albuginea of the testis and coalesce to form the head of the epididymis. The ductules then merge as they travel along the edge of the testis, forming the body and the tail of the epididymis, which is attached to the lower pole of the testes by loose areolar tissue. The tail continues onward as the vas deferens. The vas deferens loops superiorly in the spermatic cord to meet the duct from seminal vesicle and forms the ejaculatory duct, which connects to the urethra.[1,2] Knowledge of this anatomic course is valuable in understanding the retrograde progression of infection along the same pathway, which occurs in epididymo-orchitis.

The spermatic cord contains blood vessels (including the interconnected network of small veins, the pampiniform plexus), nerves, lymphatics, and connective tissue apart from the vas deferens.

High-resolution ultrasonography with color or power Doppler is the imaging modality of choice for patients with scrotal abnormalities. It has also demonstrated good reliability in differentiating between intratesticular and extratesticular lesions.[3–5]

Furthermore, ultrasonography is helpful in characterizing extratesticular lesions as cystic or solid, which is an important feature to consider when evaluating these lesions. Most extratesticular lesions are benign, although approximately 5% are malignant.

Disclosures: None.

Department of Radiology, Mayo Clinic, 5777 East Mayo Boulevard, Phoenix, AZ 85054, USA

* Corresponding author. Department of Radiology, Mayo Clinic, 5777 East Mayo Boulevard, Phoenix, AZ 85054.

E-mail address: dahiya.nirvikar@mayo.edu

Ultrasound Clin 9 (2014) 457–469

http://dx.doi.org/10.1016/j.cult.2014.03.002

TECHNIQUE AND SONOGRAPHIC ANATOMY

Although a detailed examination technique has been described elsewhere in this issue in the article "Sonography of Testis" by Vijayaraghavan, a few key points that enable improved evaluation of the extratesticular components are reviewed along with review of the normal sonographic anatomy of these structures.

- The initial task in evaluation of extratesticular anatomy is to identify the head of the epididymis (globus major) generally at the superior aspect of the testes; this is usually best achieved in the longitudinal plane (**Fig. 1**).
- While the head of the epididymis is kept in view at the superior aspect of the field of view, the bottom part of the transducer is gently rotated in a lateral or medial direction with the intention of locating the body (corpus) and the tail (globus minor) of the epididymis, thereby laying the epididymis out as one long crescent-shaped structure (**Fig. 2**).
- Sonographically, the epididymis is isoechoic or slightly more echogenic than the testis, with slightly coarse echotexture. The head measures approximately 10 to 12 mm in diameter. The body and tail tend to be slightly less echogenic than the head, and measure less than 4 mm in diameter.
- The transducer is then moved inferiorly to facilitate evaluation of the tail region and to visualize the epididymodeferential loop, where the tail of the epididymis with its convoluted tubules transforms into the vas deferens (**Fig. 3**).
- The vas deferens can then be traced up superiorly into the spermatic cord area and again evaluated in longitudinal and transverse planes. The vas in transverse plane generally has a doughnut appearance, is noncompressible, and measures less than 0.5 mm (**Fig. 4**).[6]

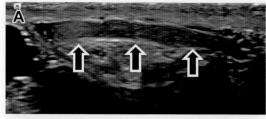

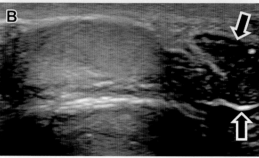

Fig. 2. Normal body and tail of epididymis. (*A*) Longitudinal sonogram of the body of the epididymis (*arrows*). (*B*) Oblique sonogram showing the convoluted tail of the epididymis (*between arrows*).

- Additional sweeps are made along the medial and lateral aspect of the testes to evaluate for any masses or fluid collections.
- Doppler is used to evaluate for the presence or absence of vascularity. It is particularly useful for documenting flow within the epididymis and for evaluating varicocele.

EXTRATESTICULAR LESIONS
Hydrocele, Hematocele, and Pyocele

Hydroceles, hematoceles, and pyoceles are collections of fluid, blood, and pus that are entrapped between the visceral and parietal layer of the tunica vaginalis, known as the scrotal sac. The visceral layer of the tunica vaginalis blends imperceptibly with the tunica albuginea.[7]

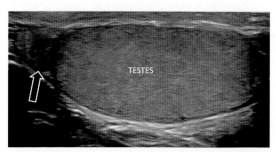

Fig. 1. Normal head of epididymis. Longitudinal sonogram showing the testes and the head of the epididymis (*arrow*).

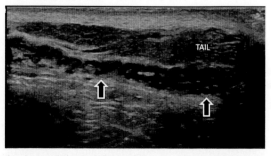

Fig. 3. Epididymodeferential loop. The epididymodeferential loop is the point where the tail of the epididymis leads into a convoluted tubule that represents the vas deferens (*arrows*). The vas deferens makes a 180° turn to course cephalad at this junction.

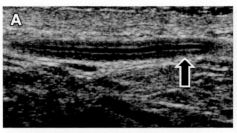
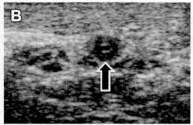

Fig. 4. Vas deferens. Longitudinal (*A*) and transverse (*B*) sonograms of the vas deferens (*arrows*) at the root of the scrotum within the spermatic cord. The vas deferens looks like a tram track in longitudinal plane, with thick hypoechoic walls and central anechoic lumen; It looks like a doughnut in the transverse plane, with a targetoid appearance.

A small amount of fluid in the scrotal sac is a normal finding, identified on ultrasonography in up to 86% of asymptomatic men.[8]

Most congenital hydroceles are formed by passive collection of fluid formed in the peritoneal cavity, and resolve by 18 months of age following complete closure of the processus vaginalis.

Acquired hydroceles can be secondary to inflammation, trauma, or tumor. Uncomplicated hydrocele is easily visualized by ultrasonography, and is generally anechoic (**Fig. 5**) or with few low-level echoes from cellular debris or cholesterol crystals (**Fig. 6**).[9]

Hematoceles (**Fig. 7**), usually attributable to trauma, and pyoceles (**Fig. 8**) caused by infection have internal echoes, often with multiple septations, loculations, and occasional mural calcifications.

Varicocele

Varicocele is the term for dilated veins in the pampiniform venous plexus, which has been described as feeling like a "bag of worms" on physical examination. The veins of the pampiniform plexus normally range from 0.5 to 1.5 mm in diameter, with the main draining vein usually measuring up to 2 mm in diameter. Historically, varicoceles have been grouped into categories based on detection method; varicoceles greater than 5 mm in diameter are invariably large enough to be felt on physical examination, and are called clinical varicoceles. Subclinical varicocele is the term applied to the condition whereby pampiniform plexus veins are enlarged but not readily palpable. Although there is some debate among experts, generally a subclinical varicocele is considered to be present when the pampiniform plexus veins measure more than 2.5 mm in diameter at rest or more than 3 mm in diameter with Valsalva or other provocative maneuvers, such as with standing.[10] Venous dilatation in a varicocele is usually limited to the pampiniform plexus, but can extend into the testis (often in the setting of testicular atrophy), which has been termed an intratesticular varicocele.

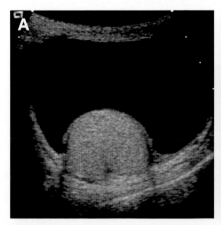
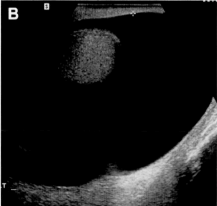

Fig. 5. Large hydrocele. (*A, B*) Sonogram of the left scrotal sac with the transducer along the anterior scrotal wall (*A*) and posterior scrotal wall (*B*), showing a large hydrocele enveloping much of the testes, except for the bare area that anchors the testis to the scrotal wall.

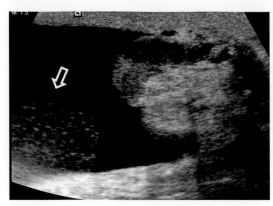

Fig. 6. Hydrocele with low-level internal echoes (*arrow*) from cellular debris or cholesterol crystals.

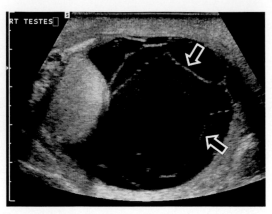

Fig. 7. Hematocele. Thin septations (*arrows*) traverse the fluid collection representing fibrin strands.

Primary varicoceles are invariably caused by gonadal vein reflux related to valvular incompetency, resulting in venous engorgement and dilatation. Doppler is useful to reveal reflux on Valsalva, and this can be augmented by performing the examination in standing position. Primary varicoceles are more common on the left because of the anatomic relationship of left spermatic vein draining into the left renal vein at an angle that facilitates reflux, whereas the anatomy of the right spermatic vein enables it to drain into the inferior vena cava at an acute angle that is less prone to the development of reflux (**Fig. 9**).[11]

Secondary varicoceles occur as a result of obstruction of venous flow in the spermatic vein; this may occur as a result of extrinsic pressure on the vein owing to multiple causes including severe hydronephrosis, abdominal or retroperitoneal masses or neoplasms, and inguinal hernias. The presence of a unilateral right-sided varicocele should prompt consideration of the underlying cause, and may justify imaging examination of the inguinal region and retroperitoneum to evaluate for masses or malignancy (**Fig. 10**).

Scrotal Hernia

A hernia into the scrotal sac can present as an extratesticular scrotal mass. On ultrasonography, the appearance of peristalsing bowel loops, with their characteristic conniventes or haustrations, helps in making the diagnosis (**Fig. 11**). However, scrotal hernias may only contain herniated mesenteric or omental fat (**Fig. 12**), which can be difficult to distinguish from a fatty tumor of the spermatic cord (usually a lipoma); in such cases, diligent sonographic evaluation using provocative maneuvers such as Valsalva can assist in the diagnosis by causing telescoping movement of the hernia contents.[12]

Solid Extratesticular Lesions

The most common extratesticular scrotal tumor is the adenomatoid tumor, which is a benign tumor originating from connective tissue (mesothelial origin). Adenomatoid tumors account for 30% of all extratesticular masses, usually seen in men between the ages of 20 and 50 years.[1,2]

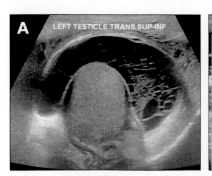
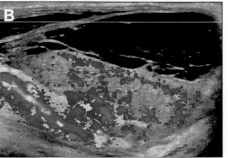

Fig. 8. Pyocele. Gray-scale (*A*) and color Doppler (*B*) images show a swollen testis (*A*) and hypervascular epididymis (*B*) surrounded by fluid in the scrotal sac containing multiple thin internal septations. In this clinical setting of epididymo-orchitis, this most likely represents a pyocele.

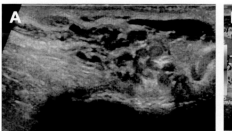
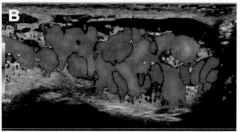

Fig. 9. Varicocele. Gray-scale image (A) at rest and color Doppler image (B) during Valsalva show dilated paratesticular veins that show augmented venous flow during Valsalva, reflecting gonadal vein reflux in a varicocele.

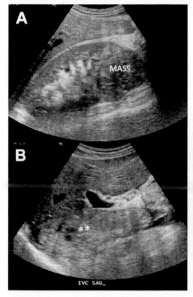
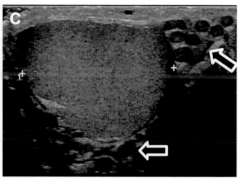

Fig. 10. Right-side varicocele. (A) Mass lesion in lower pole of right kidney. (B) Infiltration of inferior vena cava (IVC) by thrombus (double asterisk). (C) Dilated veins along the posterior and medial aspect of right testis secondary to thrombus within the IVC (arrows).

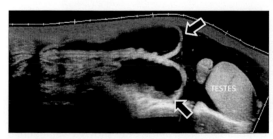

Fig. 11. Hernia. Longitudinal sonogram of the scrotum shows the testis inferiorly, displaced by fluid-filled bowel loops and fluid (arrows), surgically confirmed to be incarcerated inguinal hernia.

These tumors are frequently located in the tail of the epididymis, although they can also originate elsewhere in the epididymis, in the spermatic cord, or the testicular tunica. The tumors are mostly unilateral, solitary, and well defined, and have a myriad of sonographic appearances, although most of those arising in the epididymis are hypoechoic, well-circumscribed, round or oval masses (**Fig. 13**A), usually with some internal vascularity demonstrable with color Doppler. Adenomatoid tumors arising from the testicular tunica are usually lenticular in shape (see **Fig. 13**B), are often hyperechoic, and may show diminished vascularity.[13] The location of these tunical adenomatoid tumors on the surface of the testis can simulate peripheral testicular tumors or make it seem like the mass is invading the adjacent testes even though these tumors are not invasive, reflecting their benign histology.

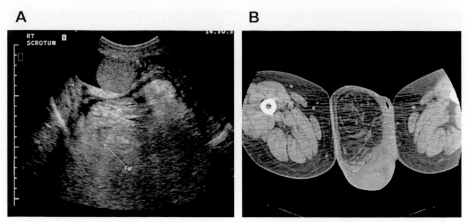

Fig. 12. Hernia fat. Scrotal hernia containing hyperechoic omentum/mesentery (*A*), confirmed as fat on computed tomography (CT) (*B*).

Among extratesticular masses, lipomas are relatively common, arising from the spermatic cord. The sonographic appearance of these lipomas is similar to those seen elsewhere in the body, usually being hyperechoic or showing hyperechoic striations. Spermatic cord lipomas tend to be positioned laterally within the spermatic cord. When large, it is difficult to differentiate a benign lipoma from a liposarcoma (**Fig. 14**).[14]

Other benign tumors include fibromas (**Fig. 15**), hemangiomas, leiomyomas (**Fig. 16**), and neurofibromas.

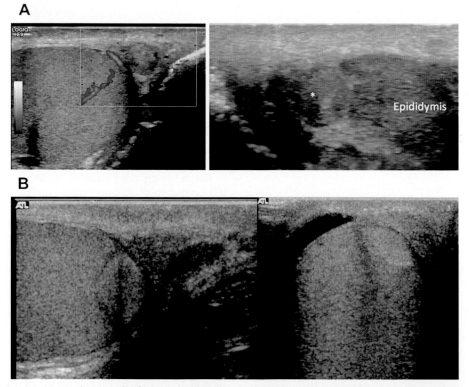

Fig. 13. (*A*) Adenomatoid tumor. (*Left*) Gray-scale with color Doppler sonogram of the testis shows a well-defined slightly heterogeneous lesion at the inferior extratesticular location with no internal vascularity. (*Right*) The mass (*asterisk*) is located within the tail of the epididymis. (*B*) Adenomatoid tumor from tunica. Both images (*left and right*) show longitudinal and transverse views of the testes with a lenticular hyperechoic mass lesion that was an adenomatoid tumor arising from the tunica albuginea.

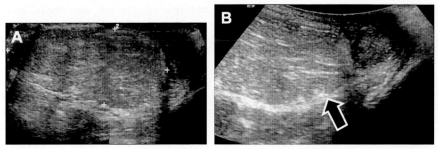

Fig. 14. Liposarcoma. Gray-scale longitudinal sonograms (*A, B*) of the left inguinal canal and scrotum show a large echogenic mass (*arrow*) with poorly defined margins.

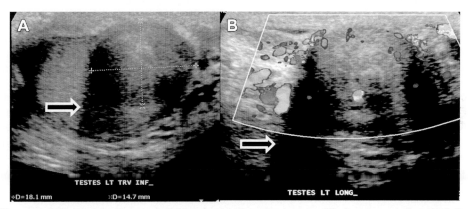

Fig. 15. Fibroma of the tunica. Gray-scale (*A*) and color Doppler images (*B*) show a round, well-defined round lesion within the tunica albuginea with mass effect on the testes. Minimal vascularity is present. There is significant sound attenuation (*arrows*) with distal shadowing.

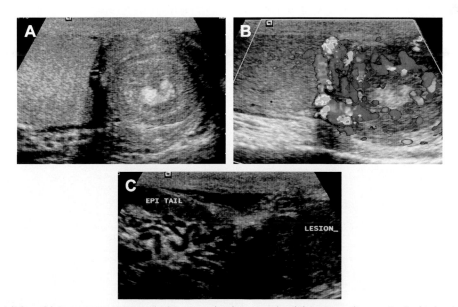

Fig. 16. Epididymal leiomyoma. Gray-scale (*A, C*) and color Doppler (*B*) images show a typical whorled appearance of an extratesticular leiomyoma. The proximity of the leiomyoma with the rest of the epididymal (epi) tail is shown in *C*.

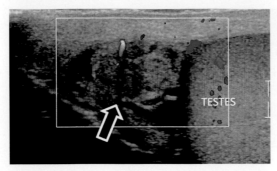

Fig. 17. Papillary cystadenoma. This slightly lobulated, mixed echotexture solid mass (*arrow*) in the head of the epididymis with internal vascularity proved to be a papillary cystadenoma on pathology.

Extratesticular papillary cystadenoma is a rare entity that can be seen in patients with von Hippel–Lindau disease. Two-thirds of men with papillary cystadenoma have von Hippel–Lindau disease (**Fig. 17**). These tumors may range in size from 1 to 5 cm and are usually solid.[15]

Primary extratesticular scrotal malignant neoplasms include fibrosarcoma, liposarcoma, histiocytoma, and lymphoma. Extratesticular scrotal metastases are rare. Children may present with rhabdomyosarcoma.[16]

Sperm granulomas are benign epididymal lesions that arise as a granulomatous reaction to extravasation of spermatozoa into the soft tissue surrounding the epididymis. These lesions may be painful and can be associated with prior infection, trauma, or vasectomy. These granulomas typically appear on ultrasonography as a solid heterogeneous mass with demonstrable internal vascularity (**Fig. 18**).

Fibrous pseudotumor is a rare reactive fibrous proliferation in the epididymis and/or tunica vaginalis. These masses can be hyperechoic or hypoechoic; suggestive features include the paucity or absence of internal vascularity and substantial sound attenuation (**Fig. 19**).

Adrenal rests that hypertrophy in patients with congenital adrenal hyperplasia are also rare lesions that characteristically show substantial sound attenuation. Although most of these adrenal rests are intratesticular in location, they can also be seen as an extratesticular mass. The combination of hypoechoic intratesticular and extratesticular lesions, especially when sound attenuating, should raise suspicion for adrenal rests, which only occur in patients with congenital adrenal hyperplasia (**Fig. 20**).

Focal Cystic Lesions

Cystic structures are commonly found in the epididymis, seen in 20% to 40% of asymptomatic subjects.[8] Spermatoceles, representing dilated fluid-filled spaces containing spermatozoa, are common, and are caused by obstruction and subsequent dilatation of an epididymal tubule. These lesions are usually located in the head of the epididymis and usually exhibit low-level internal echoes, which can appear to be constantly moving (**Fig. 21**). Spermatoceles can become large, filling the scrotal sac and thereby being confused with a large hydrocele. One helpful sonographic feature to consider when trying to distinguish a large spermatocele (**Fig. 22**) from a hydrocele is to observe whether the fluid collection envelops the testis (as would be seen with a hydrocele) or whether it exerts mass effect on the testis (which would be predictive of a spermatocele).

Epididymal cysts are also common. These cysts do not contain spermatozoa, and therefore do not have internal echoes; otherwise, the sonographic distinction between epididymal cysts and spermatoceles often cannot be made. Differentiation is not so important clinically, and the terms have been used interchangeably historically while describing the findings.

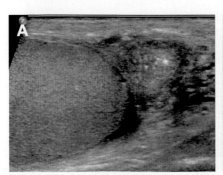
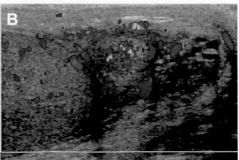

Fig. 18. Sperm granuloma. Gray-scale (*A*) and color Doppler (*B*) longitudinal views through the scrotum show a slightly heterogeneous lesion in the tail of the epididymis.

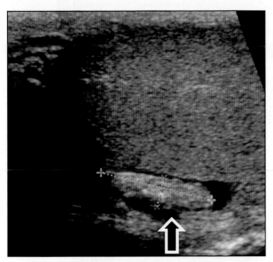

Fig. 19. Extratesticular fibrous pseudotumor. Sagittal sonogram shows an elongated hyperechoic paratesticular nodule denoted with electronic calipers (*arrow*).

Cysts can arise from the tunica albuginea, and are usually small in size and variable in number. These cysts are less common than testicular cysts, with an incidence estimated at 0.3%. Cysts of the tunica albuginea are benign, and their significance lies only in that they raise suspicion for testicular neoplasm on physical examination.[8,17,18]

Acute Epididymitis

Acute epididymitis is the most common cause of acute scrotal pain in adult men. The infection usually results from retrograde spread of an organism from the prostate or bladder via the vas deferens. As a result, the process typically begins in the epididymis (often the tail), before involving the epididymis globally (**Fig. 23**), and may subsequently progress to involve the testis (epididymo-orchitis) (**Fig. 24**). Gonococci and *Chlamydia* are the common cause of epididymitis in men younger than 35 years; in older men, *Escherichia coli*, other coliforms, and *Pseudomonas* species are more common pathogens.[2,18,19]

The universal sonographic feature of epididymitis and epididymo-orchitis is hyperemia of the affected structures; in fact, the increased color flow shown with color Doppler can precede any gray-scale abnormalities, with one study demonstrating a normal gray-scale examination in 20% of cases of epididymitis.[20] On gray-scale ultrasonography, epididymitis usually shows enlargement and decreased echogenicity of the epididymis, although with application of increasing transducer frequencies using newer technology it is increasingly common to find substantial heterogeneity in echogenicity of the inflamed epididymis. Epididymal enlargement is typically diffuse, but can be focal in 20% to 30% of cases.[20] Because of the "ascending" course of the infection, focal

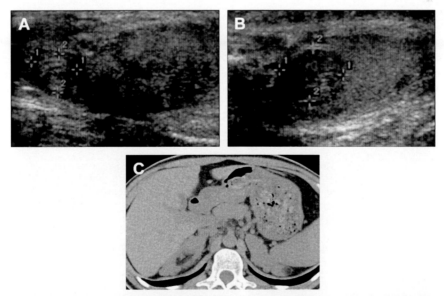

Fig. 20. Adrenal rests. Sagittal sonograms of the right hemiscrotum (*A, B*) show a round, slightly hypoechoic mass adjacent to the testis (*A*) and another mass in the testis (*B*), which are characteristic of adrenal rests in a patient with congenital adrenal hyperplasia; axial CT (*C*) shows lobulated enlarged adrenal glands in the same patient.

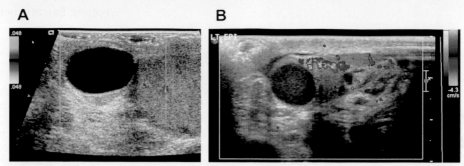

Fig. 21. Small epididymal cyst. (*A*) Long section through the head of the epididymis shows a well-defined, nonvascular, anechoic cyst consistent with an epididymal cyst. (*B*) Oblique color Doppler image of the left epididymis shows a small, round mass with low-level internal echoes but without internal flow, indicating a cyst. This cyst could be a spermatocele or epididymal cyst, but the presence of low-level internal echoes would make a spermatocele more likely.

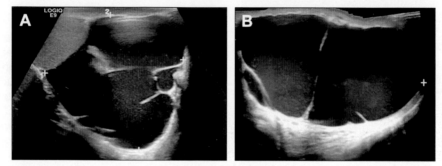

Fig. 22. Spermatocele. Transverse (*A*) and sagittal (*B*) sonograms of the left hemiscrotum show a large multiseptated fluid collection with low-level echoes adjacent to the testis, which is partially shown on image *A*. The fluid does not envelop the testis, as one would expect for a hydrocele. In a patient without a history of trauma or infection, the appearance of this extratesticular large cyst is characteristic of a cluster of spermatoceles.

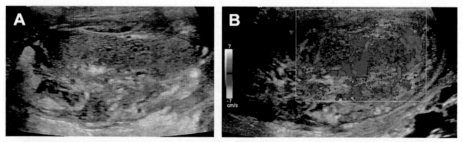

Fig. 23. Epididymitis. Oblique sonogram (*A*) shows an enlarged and heterogeneous epididymis, with hyperemia shown on color Doppler imaging (*B*). There are no focal avascular areas to indicate abscess formation.

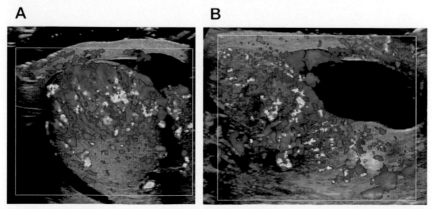

Fig. 24. Epididymo-orchitis. Color Doppler images centered on the testis (*A*) and the enlarged epididymis (*B*) show profuse hyperemia reflecting inflammatory changes in this patient with epididymo-orchitis. The adjacent reactive hydrocele and coexisting skin thickening are common associated findings.

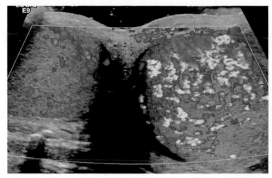

Fig. 25. Thick scrotal skin. Transverse color Doppler image of the scrotum shows enlargement and hyperemia of the left testis compared with the right. Scrotal wall thickening is also shown, with hyperemia overlying the inflamed left testis.

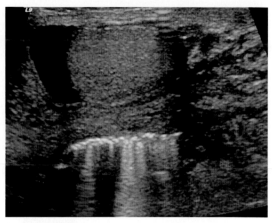

Fig. 27. Fournier gangrene. Scrotal sonogram in a diabetic patient with Fournier gangrene shows prominent scrotal wall thickening posteriorly and laterally; the echogenic area with so-called dirty shadowing represents gas that has developed in the affected area.

epididymitis tends to involve the tail of the epididymis. With progression of the inflammation to the testis, the testis becomes diffusely enlarged and hypoechoic. Other findings can include a reactive hydrocele and skin thickening (**Fig. 25**).[21]

Severe infections can lead to the development of focal testicular or epididymal abscesses (**Fig. 26**) or generalized intratunical pyohydroceles. These collections may merit prompt surgical intervention in an attempt to prevent more extensive intrascrotal necrosis. These abscesses appear as focal complex fluid collections with internal echogenic material and debris. Gas formation is uncommon. Color Doppler sonography can be of assistance in identifying nonvascularized hypoechoic areas with peripheral vascularity within inflamed intrascrotal tissue suspicious for developing abscess.

Fournier gangrene (**Fig. 27**) is a necrotizing fasciitis that may occur in immunocompromised individuals or diabetics. Ultrasonography may be able to show the necrotic areas in the skin and the presence of gas manifesting as hyperechoic foci with dirty distal shadowing.

Chronic Epididymitis

Patients with granulomatous infection can present with a hard nontender mass that is shown to be due to an enlarged epididymis on ultrasonography (**Fig. 28**). Historically this has been seen in patients with chronic tuberculous infection of the epididymis, but granulomatous epididymitis is now sometimes seen as a subacute infection in men who have been treated for bladder carcinoma with intravesicular bacillus Calmette-Guérin. The epididymis may demonstrate calcifications, and

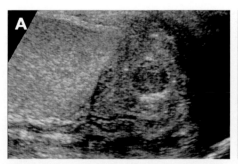
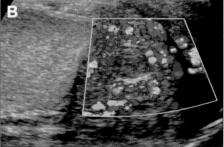

Fig. 26. Epididymal abscess. Longitudinal sonogram (*A*) of the epididymal tail shows it to be diffusely enlarged with a central round area of altered echogenicity. Color Doppler imaging (*B*) shows the increased vascularity of the enlarged epididymal tail reflecting epididymitis; the central avascular area is a small abscess that has developed.

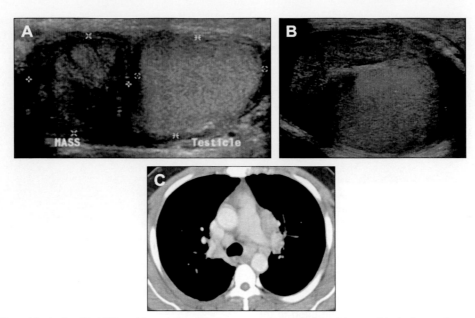

Fig. 28. Sarcoidosis. Sagittal (*A*) and transverse (*B*) sonograms in a patient with sarcoidosis show a heterogeneous extratesticular mass involving the epididymis. There was no hyperemia with color Doppler (not shown). This chronic finding was consistent with granulomatous changes in this patient, who had mediastinal adenopathy on CT (*C*).

the inflammatory process can involve the adjacent testicular parenchyma. Advanced cases can lead to development of an abscess that can involve adjacent structures and extend superiorly to involve the root of the scrotum (**Fig. 29**).[22]

Postvasectomy Epididymis

The epididymis after vasectomy may appear somewhat enlarged with ductal ectasia (**Fig. 30**).

In addition, there may be development of sperm granulomas and cysts.[23]

Scrotal Pearls

Scrotal pearls are extratesticular loose bodies that lie within the scrotal sac, sometimes calcified (**Fig. 31**). A prior episode of torsion of the appendix of the testis or epididymis can serve as a nidus for development of a scrotal pearl. These pearls can also be secondary to inflammation of the tunica vaginalis; the presence of a hydrocele facilitates detection of these clinically insignificant

Fig. 29. Tuberculosis of scrotum. Scrotal cold abscess (*arrows*) in a known case of tuberculosis of the scrotum. The infection does not respect the boundaries between the testes and the epididymis (epi) and involves both.

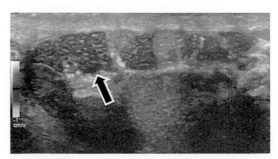

Fig. 30. Postvasectomy appearance of the epididymis with dilated tubules and a heterogeneous echogenicity (*arrow*).

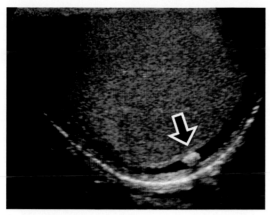

Fig. 31. Scrotal pearl. Transverse sonogram shows a small echogenic scrotal pearl (*arrow*) adjacent to the testis within the normal amount of fluid within the scrotal sac. In the absence of fluid in the scrotal sac, these small scrotal pearls may not be recognized, blending in with the adjacent scrotal wall.

structures, which may otherwise blend imperceptibly with other paratesticular structures.

REFERENCES

1. Ulbright TM, Amin MB, Young RH. Miscellaneous primary tumors of the testis, adnexa, and spermatic cord. In: Rosai J, Sobin LH, editors. Atlas of tumor pathology, fasc 25, ser 3. Washington, DC: Armed Forces Institute of Pathology; 1999. p. 235–366.
2. Bostwick DG. Spermatic cord and testicular adnexa. In: Bostwick DG, Eble JN, editors. Urologic surgical pathology. St Louis (MO): Mosby; 1997. p. 647–74.
3. Carroll BA, Gross DM. High-frequency scrotal sonography. AJR Am J Roentgenol 1983;140:511–5.
4. Benson CB, Doubilet PM, Richie JP. Sonography of the male genital tract. AJR Am J Roentgenol 1989; 153:705–13.
5. Rifkin MD, Kurtz AB, Pasto ME, et al. Diagnostic capabilities of high-resolution scrotal ultrasonography: prospective evaluation. J Ultrasound Med 1985;4:13–9.
6. Middleton WD, Dahiya N, Naughton CK, et al. High-resolution sonography of the normal extrapelvic vas deferens. J Ultrasound Med 2009;28(7):839–46.
7. Middleton WD, Thorne DA, Melson GL. Color Doppler ultrasound of the normal testis. AJR Am J Roentgenol 1989;152(2):293–7.
8. Leung ML, Gooding GA, Williams RD. High-resolution sonography of scrotal contents in asymptomatic subjects. AJR Am J Roentgenol 1984;143:161–4.
9. Gooding GA, Leonhardt WC, Marshall G, et al. Cholesterol crystals in hydroceles: sonographic detection and possible significance. AJR Am J Roentgenol 1997;169(2):527–9.
10. Pilatz A, Altinkilic B, Köhler E, et al. Color Doppler ultrasound imaging in varicoceles: is the venous diameter sufficient for predicting clinical and subclinical varicocele? World J Urol 2011;29(5):645–50.
11. Beddy P, Geoghegan T, Browne RF, et al. Testicular varicoceles. Clin Radiol 2005;60(12):1248–55.
12. Bhosale PR, Patnana M, Viswanathan C, et al. The inguinal canal: anatomy and imaging features of common and uncommon masses. Radiographics 2008;28(3):819–35.
13. Patel MD, Silva AC. MRI of an adenomatoid tumor of the tunica albuginea. Am J Roentgenol 2004;182(2): 415–7.
14. Rosenberg R, Williamson MR. Lipomas of the spermatic cord and testis: report of two cases. J Clin Ultrasound 1989;17:670–4.
15. Choyke PL, Glenn GM, Walther MM, et al. von Hippel-Lindau disease: genetic, clinical, and imaging features. Radiology 1995;194:629–42.
16. Powell BL, Craig JB, Muss HB. Secondary malignancies of the penis and epididymis: a case report and review of the literature. J Clin Oncol 1985;3: 110–6.
17. Tammela TL, Karttunen TJ, Mattila SI, et al. Cysts of the tunica albuginea—more common testicular masses than previously thought? Br J Urol 1991; 68(3):280–4 PubMed PMID: 1913070. [Tammela, 91, Br J Urol].
18. Holden A, List A. Extratesticular lesions: a radiological and pathological correlation. Australas Radiol 1994;38:99–105.
19. Feld R, Middleton WD. Recent advances in sonography of the testis and scrotum. Radiol Clin North Am 1992;30:1033–51.
20. Horstman WG, Middleton WD, Melson GL. Scrotal inflammatory disease: color Doppler US findings. Radiology 1991;179(1):55–9.
21. Horstman WG, Middleton WD, Melson GL, et al. Color Doppler US of the scrotum. Radiographics 1991; 11(6):941–57.
22. Chung JJ, Kim MJ, Lee T, et al. Sonographic findings in tuberculous epididymitis and epididymoorchitis. J Clin Ultrasound 1997;25:390–4.
23. Reddy NM, Gerscovich EO, Jain KA, et al. Vasectomy-related changes on sonographic examination of the scrotum. J Clin Ultrasound 2004;32(8): 394–8.

Ultrasonography of Hernias

Jared S. Burlison, MD, PhD, Michael R. Williamson, MD*

KEYWORDS

- Hernia • Ultrasonography • Bowel • Spigelian hernia

KEY POINTS

- Femoral hernias move from superior to inferior in the proximal thigh and are located adjacent to the femoral vein.
- Indirect hernias move obliquely, indirectly, from superiolaterally near the anterior superior iliac spine in an inferior medial direction toward the pubic symphysis.
- Direct hernias move directly from posterior to anterior in the medial part of the lower quadrants of the abdomen.
- Umbilical hernias occur anywhere within 2 to 3 cm of the center of the umbilicus.

 Videos of ultrasound technology being used on a range of hernias in different patients accompany this article at http://www.ultrasound.theclinics.com/

Ultrasound (US) evaluation of a possible hernia was seldom requested 20 years ago. Excluding umbilical and incisional hernias, we would receive approximately a half dozen requests per year for inguinal hernia evaluation. At present, we routinely perform US evaluation for all types of hernias (approximately 4–8 examinations per day at our institution). Our protocol requires that each of these examinations be evaluated in real time by a physician. Although many of our sonographers have become facile at these examinations, inadequate knowledge of the anatomy can lead to errors. The groin anatomy is complex and not easily understood. In addition, lack of fastidious scanning technique decreases the sensitivity of the examination. Therefore, the evaluation is initially performed by a sonographer, checked by a resident, and finally may be repeated by an attending. Cine clips can confirm and document the presence of hernias and are useful to the referring surgeon. It should be reemphasized that the hernia examination requires real-time participation by the physician. A well-trained sonographer can adequately perform these examinations, but only with enough prior physician supervised experience. Emergency room physicians often request hernia evaluation in the middle of the night. In this situation at our institution, it may not be possible for the examination to be repeated by a resident or attending. Therefore, it is essential that our sonographers be knowledgeable and capable of performing these examinations.

Pain in the lower quadrants and groin often poses a diagnostic challenge. With appendicitis, ovarian pathology, diverticular disease, and other colonic disorders in the differential diagnosis, we are often asked to evaluate for hernia when signs and symptoms are vague. Various musculoskeletal disorders such as rectus femoris muscle avulsions, sartorius muscle avulsions, iliopsoas injuries, and injuries to other pelvic and groin muscles may also produce symptoms that masquerade as a hernia.

Risk factors for hernia formation include congenital factors such as persistent processus vaginalis

Department of Radiology, The University of New Mexico, MSC 10 5530, 1 University of New Mexico, Albuquerque, NM 87131-0001, USA
* Corresponding author.
E-mail address: mwilliamson@salud.unm.edu

Ultrasound Clin 9 (2014) 471–487
http://dx.doi.org/10.1016/j.cult.2014.03.009

ultrasound.theclinics.com

in males or patent canal of Nuck in females; collagen abnormalities such as mucopolysaccharidoses, Ehlers-Danlos syndrome, Hunter-Hurler syndrome; family history; repeated pregnancies; obesity; surgical incisions; old age; poor muscle conditioning; peritoneal dialysis; ascites; and smoking. Frequent straining to urinate or defecate may also contribute.

A hernia is a fascial opening or defect through which tissues protrude from one anatomic compartment to another. Features of a hernia include the neck, defined as the size of the fascial defect, as well as the type and volume of the herniated contents (the hernia sac or the body of the hernia). The hernia sac is a diverticulum of peritoneum. The diverticulum contains tissues from the peritoneal cavity, usually fat and fluid, sometimes bowel, rarely other organs. Hernias may be reducible or irreducible, that is, the herniated contents can or cannot be returned to their normal anatomic compartment. Complications of small- or large-bowel herniation include luminal obstruction and vascular compromise (strangulation). There is almost always a small amount of fluid (peritoneal fluid) in the hernia sac.

Herniation may be exaggerated by maneuvers that increase intra-abdominal pressure such as the Valsalva maneuver, willful straining, or half sit ups (scanning while in an assisted half upright position). Imaging must be performed in both supine and standing positions. For example, many hernia examinations are in overweight and physically deconditioned patients who have poor abdominal muscle tone and cannot under any circumstance generate sufficient intra-abdominal pressure while supine. A complete examination cannot be performed if the patient cannot stand. However, there are occasional cases in which the hernia can only be seen with the patient supine.

The examination should be performed using a linear transducer (TD) with a wide field of view. Evaluating a large cross-sectional area is optimal as hernias are often identified several centimeters from where the patient indicates pain or symptoms. Therefore, it is important to evaluate the entirety of each cross section, as hernias are often initially seen at the corner or margin of an image. A variable-frequency TD with a range between 10 and 15 MHz is usually adequate for most hernia evaluations. A small percentage of obese patients require a lower-frequency TD for deeper penetration.

Hernias usually contain intraperitoneal or extraperitoneal fat. Extraperitoneal fat, also known as preperitoneal or properitoneal fat, lies between the peritoneal membrane and transversalis fascia, the deepest layer of the abdominal wall. However, US imaging cannot distinguish intraperitoneal from extraperitoneal fat. Although this limitation is usually inconsequential, it is important to understand that herniated intraperitoneal fat is often accompanied by bowel. As described earlier, herniated bowel is at risk for obstruction and/or strangulation, particularly if the hernia has a narrow neck. In the setting of a known hernia and acute abdominal pain, bowel ischemia should be considered since a delay in diagnosis and treatment can result in death. However, herniated fat can also produce pain if strangulated, an obviously less serious condition.

Therefore, detection of bowel within a hernia is of utmost importance. Bowel can be detected by the presence of peristalsis or intraluminal fluid levels, especially if fluid levels shift during the examination. Bowel gas within the herniated contents produces shadowing, and the combination of movement plus dirty shadows allows the diagnosis of bowel within the hernia with near certainty. Pressure and probing with the TD may aid in the detection of these features.

The US report should detail the sites and sides that were examined, that is, whether both spigelian and femoral hernia examinations, as well as direct and indirect hernia examinations, were performed and whether both right and left sides or just one side was examined. The size of the hernia sac and neck should be reported in 2 dimensions, which helps the surgeon determine the appropriate mesh size. The reducibility of the hernia should be commented on, as irreducible hernias are more likely to become strangulated. Finally, the contents of the hernia should be delineated, as the presence of bowel may necessitate surgical repair.

INGUINAL HERNIAS, THE QUICK VERSION

Before discussing the details of the US diagnosis of hernias, a short introduction to the 4 major types of inguinal hernias is given to familiarize the reader with each.

Indirect hernias protrude from superior-laterally at the anterior superior iliac spine in an inferior medial direction toward the pubic symphysis. These hernias always use the inguinal canal as their route and enter the groin indirectly from above.

Direct hernias are in the medial groin and protrude from posterior to anterior directly toward the US TD. They do not commonly use the inguinal canal as their route of travel.

Femoral hernias protrude inferiorly through the femoral canal, often into the medial thigh. The femoral canal is adjacent to and medial to the femoral vein.

Spigelian hernias protrude anteriorly along the linea semilunaris, usually in the lower abdominal wall. The linea semilunaris is the point where the rectus abdominis muscles meet the oblique muscles of the anterior abdominal wall.

WHO GETS HERNIAS AND WHY DO THEY GET THEM

Indirect hernias in infants and children occur because of a patent processus vaginalis (canal of Nuck in girls). The processus vaginalis is a diverticulum of peritoneum that extends down the inguinal canal. It should become obliterated after descent of the testicles. If the processus vaginalis remains patent, there is risk of protrusion of intraperitoneal contents, fat, and bowel, down the inguinal canal and, thus, formation of an indirect hernia. A patent processus vaginalis is found in about 20% of adult men. Not all of these develop a hernia.

Femoral hernias, spigelian hernias, and direct hernias are more influenced by the quality and strength of collagen.[1-3] Anything that decreases collagen strength increases the risk of hernia formation.

Type III collagen (immature) and type I collagen (mature) may exist in an abnormal ratio in patients with these types of hernias. An increase in the amount of type III collagen weakens connective tissues. This condition may occur not only on a congenital basis but also on an acquired basis in cigarette smokers.[4,5] Poor-quality collagen in cigarette smokers may explain their accelerated aging with increased skin wrinkling, poor wound healing, and increased incidence of abdominal aortic aneurysms.

Other factors are associated with hernia formation. In women, multiple pregnancies and the effects of estrogens on connective tissues are associated with hernias, especially femoral hernias. Patients who cough frequently or who breathe deeply often (such as patients with chronic obstructive pulmonary disease) increase intra-abdominal pressure and are predisposed to hernias.

INGUINAL HERNIAS
Pertinent Anatomy

An understanding of relevant groin anatomy is essential for evaluation of inguinal hernias by US (**Fig. 1**). Landmarks used during the examination include the femoral artery, the external iliac artery and vein, the deep inguinal ring as marked by the inferior epigastric artery where it arises from the external iliac artery, the spermatic cord (round ligament in women) as it courses through the inguinal canal, and the superficial and deep recurrent iliac arteries, 2 branch arteries arising from the external iliac artery (**Fig. 2**).[6-8]

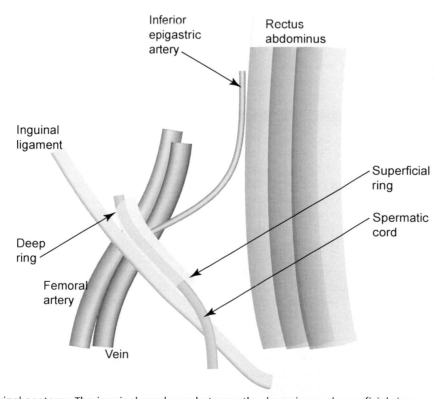

Fig. 1. Inguinal anatomy. The inguinal canal runs between the deep ring and superficial ring.

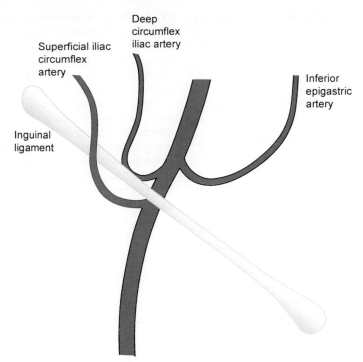

Fig. 2. Arterial branches from the iliac artery/femoral artery as it passes beneath the inguinal ligament in the groin. The inferior epigastric artery (also known as hypogastric artery) is the marker for the deep inguinal ring.

The origin of the inferior epigastric artery from the external iliac artery is the most important of these landmarks, as it indicates the entrance to the inguinal canal, the deep inguinal ring. The deep and superficial recurrent iliac arteries originate from the external iliac artery just distal to the inferior epigastric artery. The deep and superficial recurrent iliac arteries course laterally, whereas the inferior epigastric artery always courses medially from the external iliac. This relationship can thus be used to help locate the inferior epigastric artery and, thus, the deep ring.

For indirect and direct inguinal hernias, everything is centered on the inguinal canal (see Fig. 1). The inguinal canal is a tunnel extending from the deep inguinal ring above to the superficial inguinal ring below. The lateral wall of the tunnel is the inguinal ligament, the back or posterior wall is mainly transversalis fascia, the medial wall is transversalis fascia and transversus abdominis muscle plus internal oblique muscle, and the anterior wall is the aponeurosis of the external oblique muscle and the internal oblique muscle.[9] Through the inguinal canal passes the spermatic cord (round ligament). The spermatic cord can often be recognized by its linear striations coursing along the expected route of the inguinal canal. Within the spermatic cord are the vas deferens and deferential artery, the testicular artery and

venous plexus (pampiniform plexus), and the genital branch of the genitofemoral nerve (which supplies the cremaster muscle). The ilioinguinal nerve runs along the anterior side of the cord. This nerve supplies the external genitalia and the medial portion of the upper thigh. The indirect inguinal hernia comes down this tunnel from superior and lateral after entering at the deep ring. The direct hernia lies medial to this tunnel but may push through the back wall of the tunnel from behind.

An understanding of the course of the inferior epigastric artery is necessary to understand the location of the deep ring and also the anatomic areas where spigelian hernias may occur (see Fig. 2). The inferior epigastic artery is also known as the hypogastric artery. It branches from the external iliac artery and courses medially. It is the only significant medially directed branch from the iliac artery. This artery curves and runs superiorly along the back side of the abdominal wall posterior to the junction of rectus abdominis muscle and oblique muscles. If one can find the point where the inferior epigastric artery branches from the external iliac artery, one has found the deep ring. The deep ring cannot be seen, as it is collapsed closed, but its location is just anterior to the take off of the inferior epigastric artery.

The last part of the anatomy that is important to understanding hernia formation is the layers of the lower abdominal wall (**Fig. 3**). It is also important to be familiar with the term aponeurosis. An aponeurosis is a sheetlike fibrous tissue that allows for attachment of broad sheets of muscle. It is essentially a type of tendon that is broad and wide.

The layers of the anterior abdominal wall in the groin are as follows (from superficial to deep):

Skin
Camper fascia
Scarpa fascia
External oblique muscle and aponeurosis
Internal oblique muscle
Transversus abdominis muscle
Fascia transversalis
Preperitoneal tissue
Peritoneum

We are mainly concerned with the external oblique muscle and aponeurosis, internal oblique muscle, transversus abdominis muscle, and transversalis fascia. The peritoneum is important because it is a diverticulm of peritoneum that forms the hernia sac.

THE VARIOUS HERNIAS
Femoral Hernias

Femoral hernias occur adjacent, and usually posteromedially, to the femoral vein (**Fig. 4**). They are a protrusion inferiorly through the femoral ring (which is the entrance to the femoral canal).

Femoral hernias account for about 20% of hernias in women and about 5% of hernias in men. Pregnancy, especially, repeated pregnancy, leads to widening of the femoral canal because of increased abdominal pressure and increased laxity of connective tissues under the influence of hormones. These hernias occur 1 to 2 cm proximal to the point where the greater saphenous vein converges with the femoral vein. The hernia can be seen as a lobule of fat, sometimes with bowel, moving inferiorly as the patient strains or performs the Valsalva maneuver (**Figs. 5** and **6**, Videos 1 and 2). Femoral hernias are frequently irreducible and are at risk of strangulation, presumably because of the small diameter of the femoral canal resulting in a narrow hernia neck. The hernia sac may descend into the anterior medial thigh.

Indirect Hernias

Indirect hernias are said to be the most common groin hernia. The term indirect is somewhat of a misnomer because in the days before imaging, the surgeon would open the inguinal canal and the hernia sac could be seen entering the inguinal canal indirectly from above. All indirect hernias contain mesenteric fat; they may also contain bowel. Herniated contents enter the deep inguinal ring laterally and pass inferomedially down the inguinal canal toward the pubic symphysis and sometimes into the scrotum. By definition, the

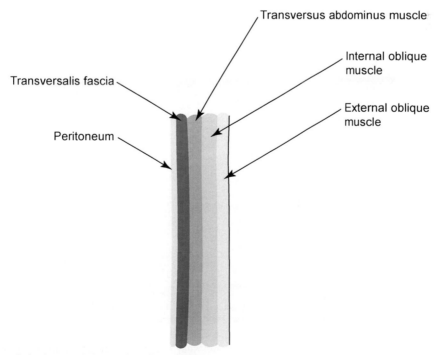

Fig. 3. Layers of the lower abdominal wall in profile.

Transversus abdominus muscle
Internal oblique muscle
External oblique muscle
Transversalis fascia
Peritoneum

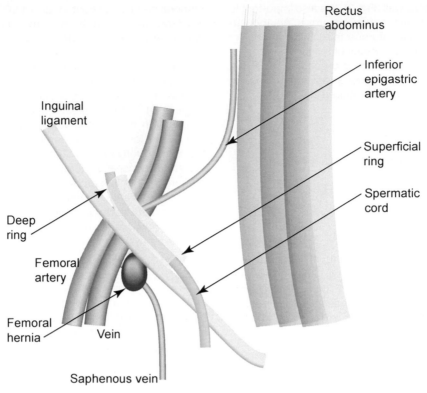

Fig. 4. Femoral hernia protruding inferiorly through the femoral canal medial to the femoral vein.

neck of the hernia is situated at the deep inguinal ring and the body of the hernia extends into the inguinal canal and/or scrotum (**Fig. 7**). The herniated, mobile fat courses anterior to the spermatic cord (**Figs. 8** and **9**, Videos 3 and 4), anterior to the origin of the inferior epigastric artery from the external iliac artery, and then moves inferomedially as the patient increases intra-abdominal pressure.

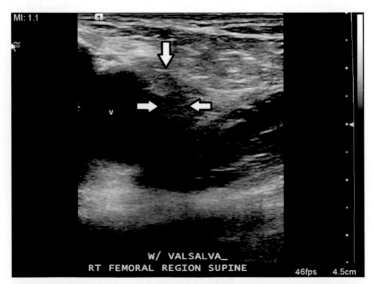

Fig. 5. Static image of femoral hernia with small amount of herniated fat marked by arrows. Transducer is oriented transversely to the adjacent femoral artery and vein near the level where the saphenous vein joins the femoral vein.

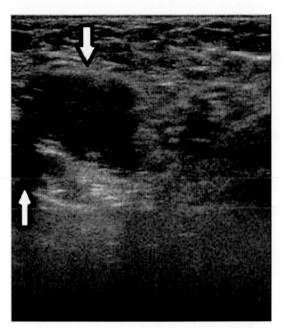

Fig. 6. Static image of hernia sac containing fat (*anterior arrow*). Hernia is alongside the femoral vein (*posterior arrow*).

US identification of this hernia may be difficult if the hernia does not reduce and remains static within the inguinal canal. In addition, a fat-containing indirect hernia may appear similar to the fat around it or can be mistaken for a spermatic cord lipoma.

Direct Hernias

A direct hernia has been called an old man's hernia because it is more common in elderly gentlemen with poor lower abdominal muscle tone. They are unusual in women. The name direct hernia originates from surgery because when the surgeon made an incision, the hernia protruded directly into the surgical field from posterior. It occurs in an area designated Hesselbach's triangle, which is an area of poor muscle convergence in the anterior abdominal wall. This area is inferior and medial in the abdominal wall near the pubic symphysis (**Fig. 10**). The musculature and fascia of Hesselbach triangle is reinforced by the conjoint tendon. The conjoint tendon is a convergence of internal oblique muscle, transversus abdominis muscle, and transversus abdominis aponeurosis near the pubic tubercle. A weakness or rent in this tendon has traditionally been blamed for many direct hernias, but that is currently debated. Instead,

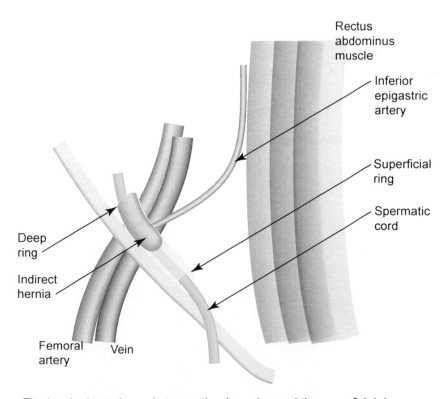

The inguinal canal runs between the deep ring and the superficial ring.

Fig. 7. Indirect inguinal hernia extending into inguinal canal.

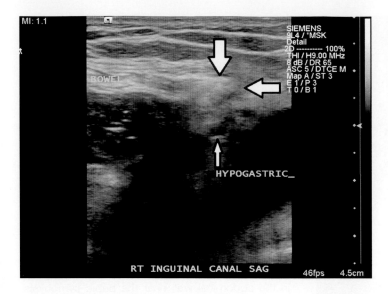

Fig. 8. Static image of an indirect inguinal hernia extending into the entrance to the deep ring anterior to the inferior epigastric artery. Indirect hernias always protrude anterior to the inferior epigastric artery moving from superiolateral to inferiomedial. This hernia protrudes only a short distance into the inguinal canal (*large arrows*). Transducer is parallel to the inguinal canal and inguinal ligament. Small arrow points to hypogastric artery (inferior epigastric artery).

weakness and/or tears in the transversus abdominis muscle and fascia may be the usual cause. Over time, intra-abdominal pressure pushes fat and/or bowel anteriorly through this area of thin musculature. This hernia moves in a posterior to anterior direction toward the TD as the patient strains or performs a Valsalva maneuver (**Figs. 11** and **12**, Videos 5 and 6). In contrast to indirect hernias, direct hernias occur medial to the origin of the inferior epigastric artery and deep inguinal ring and also are posterior to the spermatic cord (**Fig. 13**).

Some direct hernias can be confounding because they do not move in the expected posterior to anterior direction. They sometimes move obliquely between the layers of the abdominal wall, usually between the internal oblique and external oblique muscles, or alternately between the internal oblique and transversus abdominis muscles. Nevertheless, these hernias are classified as direct hernias.

Although the traditional definition of a hernia requires a rent in a fascial plane, in some cases a direct hernia does not obviously violate a fascial plane. Instead, weakness of the fascial layers of the Hesselbach triangle leads to extensive stretching and outward bulging, but there is no identifiable rent or tear in these layers. This condition should still be considered to represent a hernia, perhaps without an easily identifiable neck, and it requires surgical repair. At surgery there is usually a rent.

Direct hernias usually have a wide neck and reduce when the patient is supine, as gravity

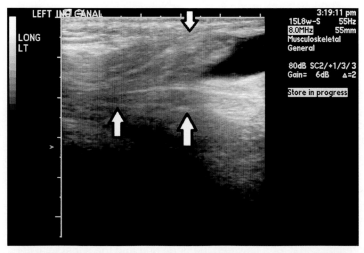

Fig. 9. Static image of indirect inguinal hernia (*arrows*) protruding down inguinal canal. Transducer is parallel to inguinal canal.

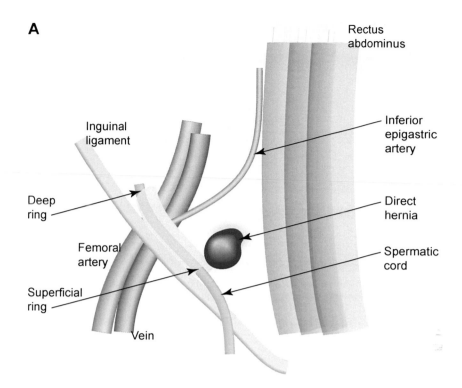

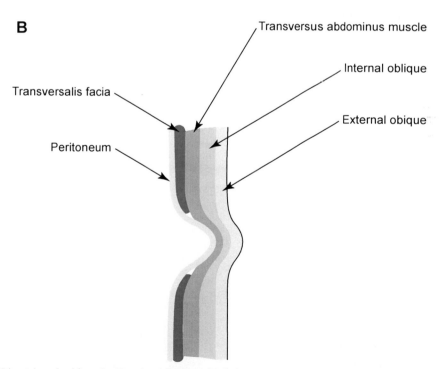

Fig. 10. (A) Direct inguinal hernia. Hernia sac protrudes from posterior to anterior toward the viewer. (B) Cross section of direct inguinal hernia showing a rent in trasversalis fascia.

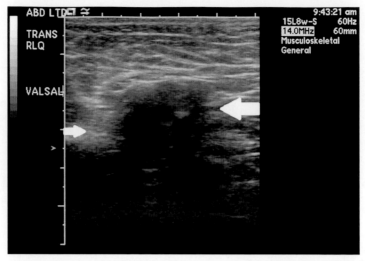

Fig. 11. Static image of direct inguinal hernia with hernia sac marked by large arrow and neck marked by small arrow. Neck is at level of the transversalis fascia. Transducer is perpendicular to long axis of patient's body in the medial lower quadrant.

displaces the contents back into the abdomen. These hernias do not generally strangulate and lead to bowel infarction, but they enlarge over time.

A small percentage of direct hernia sacs penetrate the back wall of the inguinal canal, which is transversalis fascia, and can enter the inguinal canal with the potential to protrude down the canal toward the scrotum.

Spigelian Hernia

This hernia occurs near the inferior epigastric artery through a defect in the aponeurosis of the internal oblique and transversus abdominis muscles, along the linea semilunaris (Fig. 14). The linea semilunaris is a membrane between the rectus abdominis and the oblique musculature. The fascial defect is usually lower in the abdomen where the inferior epigastric vessels penetrate the fascia and where the rectus abdominis is less broad. The spigelian hernia usually protrudes in a posterior-to-anterior direction (Fig. 15) but may take an oblique course between layers of the external and internal oblique muscles or alternatively between the internal oblique and transversus abdominis. Imaging along the abdominal wall at the junction between rectus abdominis muscles and the external and internal oblique muscles allows detection.

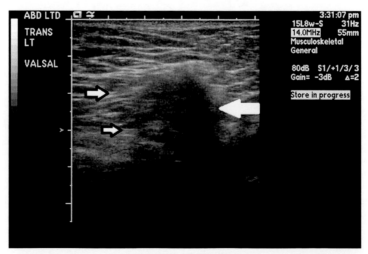

Fig. 12. Different patient with a direct inguinal hernia. Static image. Hernia sac is marked by large arrow. Small arrows mark echogenic fascial lines of the wall layers. Transducer is perpendicular to long axis of patient's body in the medial lower quadrant.

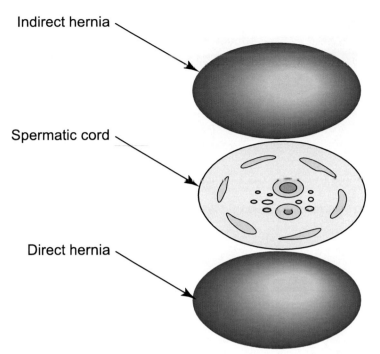

Fig. 13. Relationship of indirect and direct hernias to spermatic cord. Indirect is always anterior to cord and direct impinges upon the cord from behind. Often, the direct hernia is medial to inguinal canal and does not come in contact with the cord.

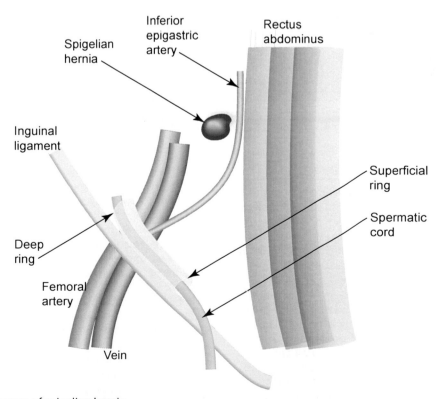

Fig. 14. Diagram of spigelian hernia.

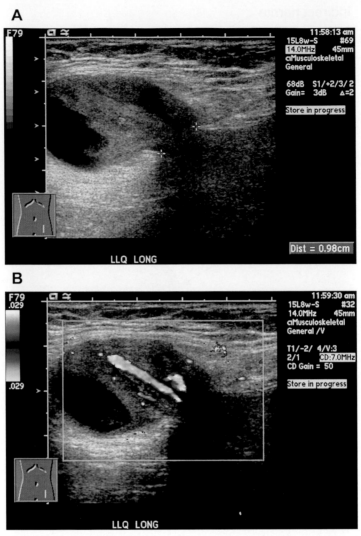

Fig. 15. (*A*) Spigelian hernia. Hernia sac protrudes anteriorly through the linea semilunaris at the junction between rectus abdominis and oblique muscles. (*B*) Color Doppler of spigelian hernia.

Umbilical and Periumbilical Hernias

Umbilical and periumbilical hernias occur in the vicinity of the umbilicus but may not occur directly in the deepest part of the umbilicus. They usually occur through the umbilical ring, which may become increased in size with advanced age or may be congenitally large in diameter. Therefore, one must move the TD around in a full 360° circumference centered on the umbilicus. Hernias can occur as far as 2 to 4 cm away from the deepest portion of the umbilicus. It is often difficult to examine the tissues directly behind the deepest portion of the umbilicus because of air within the umbilical crevice. Thorough visualization of the tissues and tissue planes behind the umbilicus is usually possible by completely filling the umbilicus

with scanning gel. Compaction of the gel with the TD usually displaces any remaining air bubbles. All patients, especially obese and poorly conditioned patients, should always be examined while standing, as they may not be able to adequately perform the Valsalva maneuver when supine. The hernia sac moves posterior to anterior, with some taking an oblique course (**Figs. 16** and **17**, Videos 7 and 8).

Umbilical hernias are common in infancy and childhood, probably because of failure of the whole midgut to return to the abdomen in early fetal life or possibly failure of round ligament (obliterated umbilical vein) to cross and reinforce the umbilical ring. Blacks have 8 times the incidence of whites and women have 5 times that of men.[10] Most adult umbilical hernias are actually

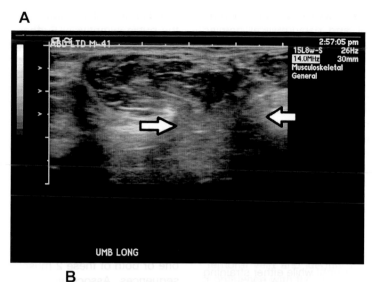

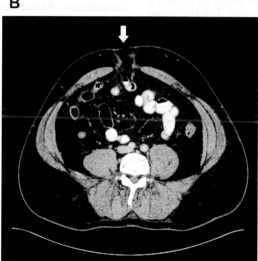

Fig. 16. (A) Umbilical hernia static image with neck marked by arrows. (B) Computed tomographic image of same patient (*arrow* marks hernia).

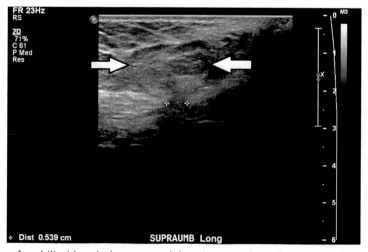

Fig. 17. Static image of umbilical hernia (*arrows* mark hernia sac and small crosses mark hernia neck).

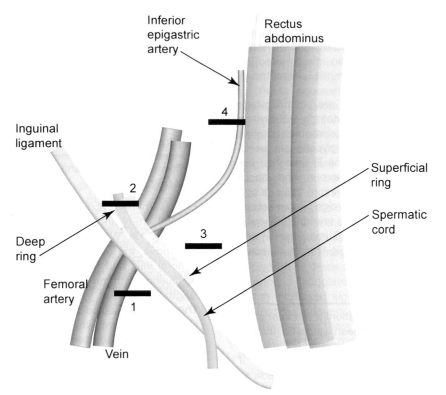

Fig. 19. Right inguinal anatomy with each line representing a different transducer position. Position 1 examines for a femoral hernia; position 2 examines for an indirect hernia; position 3 examines for a direct hernia; and position 4 examines for a spigelian hernia.

the TD is moved superiorly and inferiorly. Most direct hernias move in a posterior-to-anterior direction. As mentioned previously, some may seem to move in oblique or lateral planes.

7. The TD is next moved cephalad, following the path of the inferior epigastric artery, along the lateral margin of the rectus abdominis muscle (position 4, see **Fig. 19**). The patient is asked to strain or perform the Valsalva maneuver multiple times while the TD is moved up and down linea semilunaris. A spigelian hernia occurs at the junction between rectus abdominis and oblique muscles. The rectus abdominis junction with oblique musculature has a characteristic appearance and is easy to recognize.

8. Finally, the patient is asked to stand and the procedure is repeated.

It is tempting to skip the portion of the examination performed in the supine position and only do the examination with the patient standing. However, some hernias are only identified with the patient supine. In addition, anatomic landmarks are more easily identified with the patient supine. Because many of these patients are obese, protuberant fat often hangs into the scan field when the patient is upright. It may also be tempting to skip

the standing portion of the examination. A significant percentage of hernias is missed if only a supine examination is performed.

A controversy among surgeons is the question of whether to examine and repair both inguinal regions if bilateral hernias are found even though only one side is symptomatic. We currently examine only the requested (the symptomatic side) inguinal region unless the patient is clearly symptomatic on the opposite side. If a hernia is found, we then examine the other asymptomatic side, as our surgeons offer the patient a repair of both sides.

Accuracy of Ultrasound

The evaluation of sonography in adults with clinically equivocal features has been performed.[17] Surgery was used as the gold standard and sonography was compared with herniography. The results showed sonography to be 95% sensitive, 100% specific, positive predictive value 100%, and negative predictive value 50%. Sonography was superior to herniography.

SUPPLEMENTARY DATA

Videos related to this article can be found online at http://dx.doi.org/10.1016/j.cult.2014.03.009.

REFERENCES

1. Franz MG. Biology of hernia formation. Surg Clin North Am 2008;88:1–15.
2. Klinge U, Binnebosel M, Rosch R, et al. Hernia recurrence as a problem of biology and collagen. J Minim Access Surg 2006;2(3):151–4.
3. Zheng H, Binnebosel M, Mertens PR. Are collagens the culprits in the development of incisional and inguinal hernia disease? Hernia 2006;10(6):472–7.
4. Carnevali S, Nakamura Y, Mio T, et al. Cigarette smoke extract inhibits fibroblast-mediated collagen gel contraction. Am J Physiol 1998;274:L591–8.
5. Overbeek SA, Braber S, Folkerts G, et al. Cigarette smoke-induced collgen destruction; key to chronic neutrophilic airway inflammation? PLoS One 2013;8(10):e55612, 10, 1371.
6. Netter FH. Atlas of human anatomy. 4th edition. Philadelphia: Saunders; 2006.
7. Uflacker R. Atlas of vascular anatomy. Baltimore (MD): Williams and Wilkins; 1997.
8. Stavros AT, Rapp C. Dynamic ultrasound of hernias of the groin and anterior abdominal wall. Ultrasound Q 2010;26:135–69.
9. Nigam VK, Nigam S. Essentials of abdominal wall hernias. New Delhi (India): IK International Publishing House Pvt. Ltd; 2009. p. 24–9.
10. Ibid. p. 209.
11. Caudill P, Nyland J, Smith C, et al. Sports hernias: a systematic literature review. Br J Sports Med 2008;42:954–64.
12. Omar IM, Zoga AC, Meyers WC. Athletic pubalgia and "sports hernia": optimal MR imaging technique and findings. Radiographics 2008;28:1415–38.
13. Parra JA, Revuelta S, Farinas MC. Prosthetic mesh used for inguinal and ventral hernia repair: normal appearance and complications in ultrasound and CT. Br J Radiol 2004;77:262–5.
14. Brown CN, Finch JG. Which mesh for hernia repair? Ann R Coll Surg Engl 2010;92(4):272–8.
15. Furtschegger A, Sandbichler P, Egender G. Sonography in the postoperative evaluation of laproscopic inguinal hernia repair. J Ultrasound Med 1995;14:679–84.
16. Leber GE, Garb JL, Alexander AI, et al. Long term complications associated with prosthetic repair of incisional hernias. Arch Surg 1998;133:378–82.
17. Robinson P, Hensor E, Chapman AH. Inguinofemoral hernia: accuracy of sonography in patients with indeterminate clinical features. AJR Am J Roentgenol 2006;187:1168–78.

Ultrasonography of Tendons

Daniel B. Nissman, MD, MPH, MSEE[a],*, Nirvikar Dahiya, MD[b]

KEYWORDS

- Ultrasonography • Tendon • Tendinosis • Tenosynovitis • Shoulder • Ankle

KEY POINTS

- Tendon disease is common in the general population, particularly among athletes. Rotator cuff tears are very common in older age groups, as high as 50% for individuals in their 80s.
- Tendinosis refers to the chronic degeneration of the tendon resulting from overuse or age-related degeneration. Given the lack of inflammation in the chronic state, the term tendinitis should not be used.
- The combination of high-frequency ultrasound transducers and the superficial nature of most tendons make ultrasonography an ideal modality for the diagnosis of tendon disorders.
- Anisotropy is an important artifact of tendons to be avoided. Signal is lost when the probe is not exactly perpendicular to the tendon, and may simulate a tear.
- Ultrasonography and magnetic resonance imaging have equivalent accuracy for the diagnosis of rotator cuff tears.

Tendon disorders are a common cause of pain and loss of function.[1,2] Chronic tendon disorders are much more common than acute injuries, and are the result of overuse or age-related tendon degeneration. Athletes at all levels may develop tendon disorders as a result of too much exercise, improper mechanics, or both. Common chronic athletic tendon injuries include lateral epicondylosis (tennis elbow), proximal patellar tendinosis (jumper's knee), and Achilles tendinosis. Rotator cuff disease is the prime example of age-related tendon degeneration. Other activities and conditions may also lead to tendon disorders. Any repetitive motion continued for a long enough time can result in tendon-related disease, such as might be seen with repetitive work-related tasks or playing video games (Nintendinitis[3]). Certain systemic conditions are also associated with tendon disease, including diabetes[4,5] and rheumatoid arthritis.[6] Tendon ruptures often occur in the presence of some degree of tendon degeneration, particularly in the rotator cuff. Acute injuries are a relatively uncommon tendon disorder, mostly consisting of traumatic tendon ruptures and lacerations.

The development of high-frequency transducers, coupled with increasing cost pressures in the United States, has resulted in a resurgence of interest in musculoskeletal ultrasonography. The spatial resolution of clinical ultrasonography is on the order of 0.2 mm[7,8] whereas the spatial resolution of routine clinical magnetic resonance (MR) imaging is on the order of 0.3 mm.[7] The fibrillar structure of normal tendons is readily visualized with ultrasonography, whereas tendons are uniformly dark on MR imaging. Another advantage of ultrasonography over MR imaging is its dynamic nature, allowing one to stress structures in indeterminate situations. Finally, the superficial nature of most tendons in the body makes them particularly suited to ultrasonographic evaluation.

Disclosures: None.
[a] Musculoskeletal Imaging Section, Department of Radiology, University of North Carolina School of Medicine, 101 Manning Drive, CB# 7510, Chapel Hill, NC 27599-7510, USA; [b] Department of Radiology, Mayo Clinic, 5777 East Mayo Boulevard, Phoenix, AZ 85054, USA
* Corresponding author.
E-mail address: nissman@med.unc.edu

Ultrasound Clin 9 (2014) 489–512
http://dx.doi.org/10.1016/j.cult.2014.03.001

This article reviews the terminology and prevalence of tendon disorders, the physiology of tendons in health and disease, pertinent techniques of ultrasonography, and sonographic manifestations of tendon abnormalities, with emphasis on examples from the shoulder and ankle.

TERMINOLOGY

Tendinopathy is a general term encompassing all aspects of tendon disease, including abnormalities intrinsic to the tendon and abnormalities of the peritendinous tissues. Tendinosis is generally reserved for intrasubstance age-related and overuse-related tendon degeneration. Paratenonitis is a general term indicating an inflammatory process involving the peritendinous tissues, including the paratenon. Tenosynovitis more specifically refers to peritendinous inflammation in the presence of a synovial sheath.[9]

The term tendinitis is no longer descriptive of the underlying tendon disorder now referred to as tendinosis, and should no longer be used.[10] Although inflammation plays a role in the initial stages of tendon injury, it does not play a role in the chronic phase of tendinosis.

Calcium is not uncommonly found within tendons. When symptomatic an inflammatory response to the calcium is likely responsible for the symptoms, and the term calcific tendinitis can be used.[11] Asymptomatic calcium deposits are unlikely to have an inflammatory component, and the term calcific tendinosis can be used.

PREVALENCE OF TENDON DISORDERS

Data on the prevalence of tendinosis are greatest among athletes, with sparse data available on the population as a whole.[12] The lifetime prevalence of tendon disorders in athletes has been estimated to be between 30% and 50%.[1] Achilles tendinosis has a lifetime incidence of 5.9% in the general population, but may be as high as 50% in elite endurance athletes.[13] Patellar tendinosis has an overall prevalence among high-level athletes of 12%, but is particularly high among basketball and volleyball players at 40%.[14] Lateral epicondylosis has a prevalence of between 1% and 3%,[15] but may be as high as 35% among tennis players.[16] Based on physical examination alone, Ostor and colleagues[2] estimated that up to 85% of all shoulder pain is due to rotator cuff disease (tendinosis and tears).

The prevalence of rotator cuff tears is perhaps the best documented of all tendon disorders. Cadaver studies have reported a prevalence of rotator cuff tears of up to 40%.[17] Conducted in a Japanese mountain village, Yamamoto, and colleagues[18] performed one of the few population-based studies of rotator cuff tears, finding an overall prevalence of 20.7%, with 36% prevalence among symptomatic individuals and 16.9% in asymptomatic individuals. The incidence of rotator cuff tears increases with age. In the same study, 25.6% of individuals in their 60s had a cuff tear whereas 50% of individuals in their 80s had cuff tears.[18] Yamaguchi and colleagues[19] found that the average age of patients was 48.7 years for those with bilateral intact rotator cuffs, 58.7 years for those with a tear on only one side, and 67.8 years for those with bilateral rotator cuff tears. In patients with only one symptomatic shoulder, the chance of an asymptomatic contralateral cuff tear also increased with age, 35% for a patient in their 60s and 50% for a patient in their 80s. Tempelhof and colleagues[20] found that the prevalence of asymptomatic rotator cuff tears is common, at 23% in their study population as a whole, but very common, at 51%, in people older than 80 years.

Data on the incidence of acute tendon ruptures is sparse in comparison with data on tendinosis. The incidence of Achilles tendon ruptures ranges from 6 in 100,000 to 37 in 100,000.[21] Quadriceps and patellar tendon injuries are thought to be rare.[22] Over a 2-year period at a US Army base, 52 major tendon ruptures were reported (29 Achilles tendon, 12 patellar tendon, 7 pectoralis major tendon, and 4 quadriceps tendon), most of which occurred while playing basketball.[23] A rare, but important subgroup of knee extensor tendon tears is in the postoperative group; an incidence of 0.1% for quadriceps tendon tears has been reported in patients following total knee arthroplasty,[24] and 0.24% for patellar tendon tears in patients following anterior cruciate ligament reconstruction.[25] Incidence data on acute traumatic rotator cuff tears is lacking, but a recent review of demographic factors involving acute traumatic tears of the rotator cuff showed that they occur on average 10 years before tears in the setting of tendinosis.[26]

NORMAL TENDON ANATOMY

Tendon is a dynamic tissue composed of a highly ordered arrangement of collagen fibrils, noncollagenous matrix, and tenocytes that collectively transmit the contraction forces of muscle to bone.[27,28] Collagen fibrils are packed in a hierarchical series of bundles that support a matrix composed primarily of glycoproteins. Many of these glycoproteins, including a small amount of elastin, participate in the cross-linking of collagen fibrils that allows tendons some elasticity.

Tendons may stretch nearly 4% of their resting length before microtears are observed and nearly 8% of their resting length before macrotears are observed.[9] The collagen fibrils are composed predominantly of type I collagen along with small amounts of other collagen types.[9,27] Tenocytes, a form of fibroblast, are connected via gap junctions and act as mechanoreceptors. In response to the load stimuli they receive, the tenocytes direct the constant degradation and construction of the collagen fibrils and matrix.[29] While predominantly exposed to tensile stresses, tendons experience compressive stresses at sites where tendons deviate from a straight line in their normal course, such as that seen at the medial and lateral malleoli of the ankle. Although the function of the noncollagenous matrix is not well understood, the relative amount of the noncollagenous matrix is increased at sites of increased compressive stress, where it appears to resist mechanical compression.[30]

A thin connective tissue layer known as the epitenon invests the tendon unit as a whole. The first-order through third-order subunits of the collagen-bundling hierarchy are also invested by a similar connective tissue layer known as endotenon, which is in continuity with the epitenon. Normally there are few blood vessels and nerves in the epitenon and endotenon. No blood vessels or nerves are present in the tendon proper.

The paratenon is a thin fibrous connective tissue that surrounds the tendon, separated from the underlying tendon by loose areolar tissue. Numerous blood vessels and nerves are present in this layer. When a tendon is injured there is ingrowth of neovessels and nerve into the tendon, and when the tendon has healed these neovessels and nerves recede.[31]

At several sites in the body, tendons do not connect muscle to bone in a straight line, but deviate from a linear course during normal function. For example, the finger extensor and flexor tendons routinely bend to greater than 90°. To reduce friction from tendon movement over bony prominences and soft tissue–restraining structures, these tendons are surrounded by tendon sheaths lined with synovium. To prevent bow-stringing of the tendons during flexion and extension, particularly at the wrist and ankle, retinacula keep the tendons closely apposed to adjacent bone. In the fingers, the flexor tendons are kept close to bone by thin connective tissue rings called pulleys.

Like bone, tendons are able to remodel in response to applied stresses. When compared with an unloaded tendon, regular loading of a tendon results in a gradual remodeling of the tendon to be able to withstand greater applied forces.[9,27,28] As a result of this load responsiveness, an athlete's tendons will be able to withstand greater tensile forces than those of a sedentary person.

TENDON DISORDERS

Symptomatic tendon-related pathology is related either to the tendon, the peritendinous tissues, or both. Tendinosis, tendon tears, and tenosynovitis are discussed here.

Tendinosis

Tendinosis is primarily due to fatigue from chronic tendon overload. Though it is true that tendons are adaptable, at some point either the magnitude of loading or the frequency at which the tendon is loaded exceeds the ability of the tendon to properly remodel itself in a healthy fashion. Microtears occur when the mechanical limits of the tendon are exceeded. A multiphasic normal healing response begins with a brief inflammatory phase, followed by proliferative (weeks) and remodeling (weeks to months) phases.[31] The inflammatory phase is characterized by in-migration of inflammatory cells and neovascularity. The proliferative phase is characterized by the production of collagen and extracellular matrix, and the absence of inflammatory cells. During the remodeling phase, realignment of the newly created collagen fibers and matrix produced in the previous phase into an organized structure occurs. At the conclusion of the healing response, the neovessels will have receded from the tendon proper. Interrupting the healing phase with continued excessive loading of the tendon is likely to accelerate the transition to a chronic dysregulated tendon structure, perhaps by preventing entry into the remodeling phase. On the other hand, prolonged immobilization following injury is also not good for tendon health. The functional properties of tendon mobilized early after injury are greater than those that are immobilized; this difference is likely due to the remodeling stimulus from mechanical loading of the tendon.[9,27,28] Unfortunately, knowledge of the key details in the pathogenesis of tendinosis that would enable the design of optimal training programs to prevent tendinosis, or treatments to reverse tendinosis, remains unknown.

Histologic descriptions for 3 stages of tendinosis have been described.[32] In the earliest stage, the tendon enlarges because of an increase in the noncollagenous matrix, but without collagen fibril damage. Further enlargement in the next stage is due to continued derangement of the matrix, increasing collagen-fiber separation, appearance of abnormal tenocytes, and blood vessel ingrowth. The final stage is characterized by large-scale collagen fibril disruption, cell death, and marked blood vessel and nerve ingrowth. The first 2 histologic stages may be reversible.[32]

A variety of predisposing factors for the development of tendinosis have been described, including age,[12,19] genetics,[33] diabetes,[4,5] and fluoroquinolone use.[34] Of increasing interest is the role of the neural-mediated environment of the tendon.[31] Studies have shown that tendons deprived of their neuronal supply degrade despite an otherwise unchanged load environment, which may explain how diabetes and its associated neuropathy accelerates tendon degeneration. Other suggestive findings include greater incidence of rotator cuff tears in hemiplegic shoulders,[35] greater incidence of sciatica in patients with Achilles tendon ruptures,[36] and lack of normal proprioception in patients with lateral epicondylopathy.[37] A rich neurotransmitter environment exists both within and outside the tendon, which strikes a balance between proinflammatory and anti-inflammatory mediators. Aberrations in this balance may contribute to the development of tendinosis and the pain associated with tendinosis.[31]

Two forms of intratendinous mineralization occur: calcium hydroxyapatite deposition and intratendinous ossification. Hydroxyapatite deposition is a common radiographic finding particularly involving the rotator cuff, and arises in the setting of tendinosis.[38] When symptomatic, the pain associated with this usually self-limited disease is due to an inflammatory response secondary to the body's attempt to resorb the calcium deposit.[11] Percutaneous intervention occasionally is needed for intractable pain. Aside from the rotator cuff, this type of calcium deposition has also been described in other tendons including the pectoralis major, gluteus medius, and gluteus maximus tendons.[39] On the other hand, intratendinous ossifications that are commonly seen in the Achilles tendon are thought to be the result of enchondral ossification rather than hydroxyapatite deposition.[40]

Tendon Tears

Macroscopic tendon tears may be partial or complete. Although tears are often associated with abnormal tendons, as in tendinosis, normal tendons may also tear in certain circumstances. Acute ruptures may be the result of movements that greatly exceed the tensile limit of a tendon, common in athletic activities, or are due to lacerations, common in occupational activities. In the setting of tendinosis, complete tendon rupture usually begins as a partial tear that enlarges with time. A low-level traumatic event or an activity of daily living, such as reaching for something, may complete the tear. An important subset of tendon tears are longitudinal split tears, which commonly involve the peroneus brevis tendon. This type of tear is thought to be due to microinstability within the tendon sheath as it curves over a bony prominence, although the exact mechanism by which this tear is created has not been determined.[41]

Tenosynovitis

Tenosynovitis is usually the result of excessive friction in the tendon sheath, and is characterized by synovial hypertrophy, hyperemia, and pain. An associated tendon sheath effusion is common and may contain fibrinous material. Tenosynovitis is also associated with infection and the inflammatory arthritides, such as rheumatoid arthritis.

ULTRASONOGRAPHY OF TENDONS
Ultrasonography Technique

The superficial location of most tendons in the body makes them well suited for evaluation by ultrasonography. The high-resolution images generated by modern high-frequency linear ultrasound transducers (9 MHz and higher) allow one to see the fibrillar architecture of normal tendons. Unlike abdominal imaging whereby uniform contact with the ultrasound transducer is easy to obtain, tendons are often located on convexities, such as the Achilles tendon, or in concavities, such as the peroneal tendons (**Fig. 1**). When imaging on a convexity, the use of copious amounts of coupling gel are essential to minimize air-interface artifact. Alternatively, a stand-off pad can also be used. When imaging parts of the body with many bony prominences, such as around the ankle, the use of a small-footprint (hockey-stick) probe is useful. Holding the base of the transducer with the palm resting on the body provides stability and more controlled movements of the probe. Usually the closer the transducer is held to its scanning end, the more stable it is.

The ability to evaluate structures while moving them, either actively or passively, is one of the strengths of ultrasonography. The most common use is to stress a tendon when there is uncertainty about the presence of a complete rupture. Other uses would be to evaluate for peroneal tendon subluxation by forced eversion with dorsiflexion, and rotator cuff impingement can be evaluated by abducting the arm in various positions.

Proper positioning of the part being evaluated is essential to achieving a good examination.

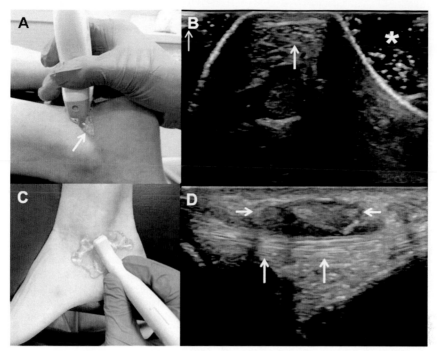

Fig. 1. Ultrasonographic imaging around convexities and concavities in the extremity. A copious amount of coupling gel is used to reduce the amount of air-interface artifact when the probe length is much longer than the width of the body part being imaged. (A) Probe position and "piled up" coupling gel (*arrow*) to obtain a transverse view of the Achilles tendon. (B) Resulting sonographic image. *Thick arrow*, posterior border of the Achilles tendon; *thin arrow*, artifact from air interface; *asterisk*, coupling gel. A small-footprint probe is used to achieve close contact with the skin around bony prominences. (C) Example of using the hockey-stick small-footprint probe to image the structures inferior to the lateral malleolus. (D) Resulting sonographic image. *Short arrows*, peroneus tendons; *long arrows*, calcaneofibular ligament.

The body part and perhaps the entire body may need to be moved when evaluating different aspects of the ankle. For example, a side-laying position is optimal for evaluation of the lateral ankle tendons, but a prone position would be best for evaluation of the Achilles tendon. Proper body mechanics of the sonographer cannot be overemphasized: minimizing strain on the examiner reduces the incidence of overuse disorders.[42] Often the examination can be performed from a seated position.

Proper labeling of images is extremely important, as one may not remember where or how an image was obtained when reviewing the images later. Unlike other forms of cross-sectional imaging, the relative position of structures and their identities are not always readily identifiable. Adding labels, such as medial, lateral, cephalic, and caudal, helps in orientation. The use of a standardized protocol is helpful when evaluating the structures of particular body parts. For example, the subscapularis and infraspinatus tendons in long axis can appear similar, with a "bird's beak" configuration at their insertions.

Ultrasonographic Appearance of Normal Tendons

The fibrillar pattern of normal tendons is readily visible with ultrasonography (**Figs. 2–4**). In long-axis view, this echotexture is characterized by alternating thin linear hyperechoic and hypoechoic bands. In the transverse view, tendon is characterized by numerous hyperechoic speckles in a field of relative hypoechogenic material. In all cases, the edges of the tendon are sharply marginated.

Sonographic anisotropy is an important and useful artifact associated with the study of tendons. When the insonation beam is not oriented at exactly 90° to the direction of fibers, the incoming ultrasound beam is not reflected directly back at the transducer but at an angle away from the transducer. The greater this angle is, the less signal is received, and the tendon appears

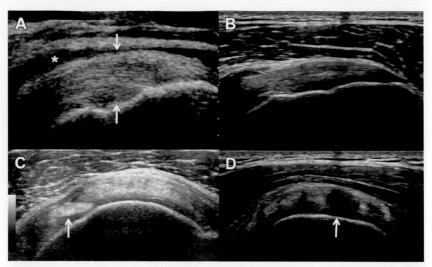

Fig. 2. Normal rotator cuff tendons. (*A, B*) Normal long-axis views of supraspinatus (*A*) and subscapularis (*B*) showing the beak-like shape of these tendons (*left side of image* is medial, *right side* is lateral). Relative hypoechogenicity of the subscapularis tendon at the insertion is due to anisotropy. *Arrows* show the superficial and deep borders of the supraspinatus tendon at the insertion. *Asterisk* indicates fluid in the subdeltoid bursa. (*C, D*) Normal short-axis views of the superior rotator cuff (*C*) and subscapularis (*D*) (*left side of image* is superior, *right side* is inferior). In *C*, the *arrow* points to the long head of biceps tendon within the rotator interval. In *D*, the multipennate pattern of subscapularis is characterized by multiple round hyperechoic regions on a background of relative hypoechogenicity. The hypoechoic interspaces (*arrow*) can be of variable size and may mimic tears.

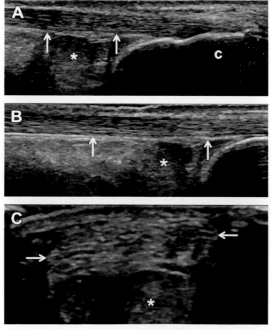

Fig. 3. Normal sonographic appearance of the Achilles tendon, which is characterized by a fibrillar pattern in long axis (*A, B*) and a speckled pattern in short axis (*C*). *Arrows*, tendon; *asterisk*, Kager fat pad; c, calcaneus.

hypoechoic or even anechoic.[43] Angles as small as 2° can result in a marked decrease in signal from the tendon.[44] When evaluating for a tear, it is essential to ensure that nonvisualization of the tendon is not due to anisotropy. Usually this can be achieved by tilting the transducer by small incremental amounts along the short axis or long axis of the transducer. Although anisotropy can be a pitfall for the inexperienced, there are times when the entire visualized field of view appears bright and speckled (usually when viewing tendons in the transverse projection). By tilting the transducer, one can locate the positions of tendons by observing the appearance of rounded hypoechoic areas. One can then verify the location of the tendon by placing the area of anisotropy in the center of the field of view and turning the transducer 90° to obtain the longitudinal view. Examples of anisotropy are given in **Fig. 5**.

Other structures with somewhat similar appearances are ligaments and nerves. Ligaments, like tendons, have a fibrillar echotexture and exhibit anisotropy (see **Fig. 1D**). Ligaments can be differentiated from tendons by anatomic location and by identifying both osseous attachments of a ligament. Nerves have a fascicular appearance with hypoechoic round structures against a general background of hyperechogenic fat, which also

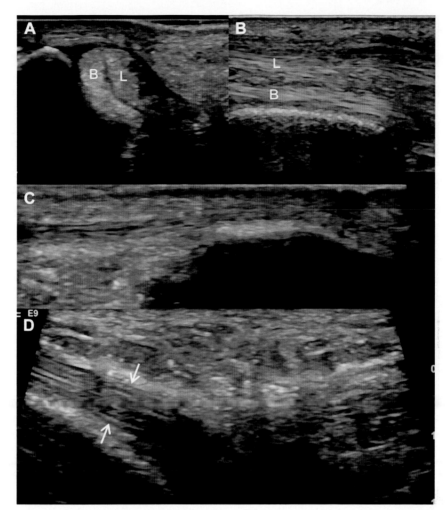

Fig. 4. Normal peroneus brevis and longus tendons. (*A*) Short-axis and (*B*) long-axis views of the normal peroneus brevis (B) and longus (L) tendons at the fibular tip. (*C*) Long-axis view of a normal peroneus brevis insertion at the base of the fifth metatarsal. (*D*) Long-axis view of a normal peroneus longus (*arrows*) as it dives deep just before its entry into the cuboid tunnel.

surrounds the nerve (**Fig. 6**). Nerves exhibit much less anisotropy than tendons.

Accuracy of Ultrasonography for the Diagnosis of Tendon Disorders

The accuracy of ultrasonography for tendon disorders is generally excellent. Most of the literature has focused on the accuracy of ultrasonography for rotator cuff tears. For the ankle there is a relative paucity of data, but the existing data still support ultrasonography as a diagnostic modality. For the following discussion, comparisons with MR imaging are emphasized.

Rotator cuff tears

MR imaging has been the mainstay of shoulder imaging in the United States for many years. MR imaging has the advantage of providing a complete evaluation of the shoulder soft tissue, including the glenoid labrum. The cross-sectional images depict anatomic relationships that are easy to understand, providing a clear link between abnormalities found and the relevant anatomy. A recent meta-analysis[45] has addressed the accuracy of shoulder ultrasonography, conventional MR imaging, and MR arthrography for rotator cuff abnormality whereby surgical correlation was the gold standard. All 3 techniques had similar sensitivities for full-thickness tears, but MR arthrography was slightly more specific. For partial-thickness tears, MR arthrography was both more sensitive and more specific than either of the other techniques; conventional MR imaging and ultrasonography were

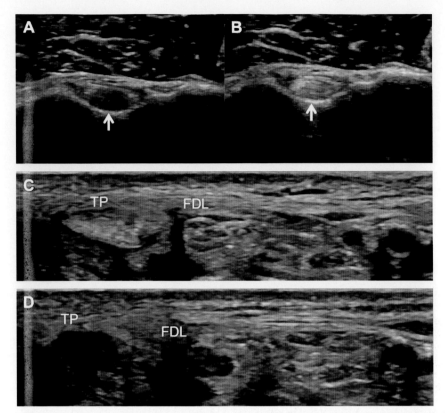

Fig. 5. Examples of anisotropy. (*A, B*) Long head of biceps tendon anisotropy. *Arrow* indicates bicipital groove. (*A*) Short-axis view obtained with the transducer not perfectly perpendicular to the tendon, showing a nearly anechoic oval within the bicipital groove. (*B*) Short-axis view obtained with the transducer perfectly perpendicular to the tendon, revealing a normal tendon within the bicipital groove. (*C, D*) Locating the tibialis posterior (TP) and flexor digitorum longus (FDL) in a bright complex-appearing field. (*C*) The TP is relatively easy to identify, but the location of FDL is not readily apparent. (*D*) The transducer has been tilted slightly to cause the normally hyperechoic appearance of TP and FDL to become hypoechoic. As the appearance of the rest of image has not changed, the location of FDL is easy to identify.

similar to each other, although a trend for increased sensitivity and specificity was noted in favor of ultrasonography. For full-thickness rotator cuff tears, MR imaging had sensitivity and specificity of 92.1% and 92.3%, compared with 92.3% and 94.4% for ultrasonography. For partial-thickness tears, MR imaging had a sensitivity and specificity of 63.6% and 91.7%, whereas sensitivity and specificity for ultrasonography were 66.7% and 93.5%. This meta-analysis echoes another meta-analysis with less stringent inclusion criteria, which also concluded that conventional MR imaging and ultrasonography had equivalent accuracy for rotator cuff abnormality.[46] A recent Cochrane review of the topic also found that the accuracy of MR imaging and ultrasonography for rotator cuff tears was equivalent.[47] Regarding accuracy of tear size in comparison with arthroscopy, Teefey and colleagues[48] found that ultrasonography and MR imaging were within 5 mm of actual tear size 87% and 80% of the time, respectively. Discrepant tear sizes were always present in the case of large rotator cuff tears, likely attributable to the difficulty of measuring on a curved surface.[48] Given the equivalence of ultrasonography with conventional MR imaging and the relative low cost of ultrasonography, the Society of Radiologists in Ultrasound issued a consensus statement on the imaging evaluation of shoulder pain, in which ultrasonography plays a central role.[49]

Ankle

The diagnostic performance of ultrasonography for the evaluation of tendon disorders around the ankle is excellent.[50] For example, in a study comparing ultrasonography with MR imaging using surgical correlation as the reference for the

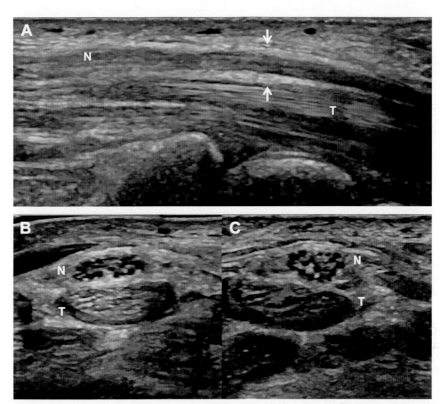

Fig. 6. Differentiating wrist flexor tendons from the median nerve. (A) Note the fibrillar pattern of the flexor tendons (T) and the more diffusely hypoechoic appearance of the median nerve (N) in the long-axis view. Nerves often have readily identifiable hyperechoic fat surrounding the tendon (arrows). (B, C) Short-axis views of the median nerve and the immediately subjacent flexor tendon with a view perpendicular to the tendon (B) and a slightly angled projection to the tendon (C). The median nerve (N) shows a hypoechoic fascicular pattern against a background of hyperechoic fat. By contrast, the tendon (T) is a characterized by bright speckles on a hypoechoic background. Owing to anisotropy, the appearance of the tendon in C is hypoechoic relative to the tendon in B. The appearance of the nerve is unaffected.

diagnosis of tendon abnormalities around the ankle, Rockett and colleagues[51] found a sensitivity and specificity of 100% and 89.9% for ultrasonography and 23.4% and 100% for MR imaging. For the detection of surgically created longitudinal tears in the tibialis posterior tendon, Gerling and colleagues[52] found the sensitivity and specificity of ultrasonography to be 69% and 81%, and 73% and 69% for MR imaging. In another study focusing on the clinical staging of tibialis posterior tendon dysfunction, ultrasonography and MR imaging were concordant in most cases, and in no case would there have been a difference in management.[53]

Operator Dependence

A frequently cited limitation of ultrasonography in general and shoulder ultrasonography in particular is operator dependence. Unlike MR imaging whereby a familiar cross-sectional depiction of the entire anatomy is provided in multiple planes, sonographic images only show a single thin projection wherever the ultrasound transducer is pointed. Skill in achieving standard views of the relevant structures while avoiding artifact, anisotropy in particular, takes time. Several articles have evaluated operator experience in the performance of shoulder ultrasonography.

Full-thickness rotator cuff tears are relatively easy to diagnose, even for those with limited experience. Some studies suggest that between 50 and 100 scans are necessary to become comfortable with making this diagnosis.[54] Partial-thickness tears are more challenging not just from an imaging perspective, but because there is often no arthroscopic correlate for intrasubstance tears. Most studies report modest accuracy at best for partial-thickness tears, with greater operator experience leading to somewhat increased accuracy.[55–57]

Ultrasonographic Appearance of Tendon Disorders

Tendinosis

The sonographic manifestations of tendinosis are:

- Enlargement of the tendon
- Focal hypoechoic areas
- Loss of the fibrillar pattern
- Calcification

Paralleling the histologic stages described earlier, the earliest manifestation of tendon degeneration is enlargement without fibril disruption. The hyperechoic fibrillar pattern should still be discernible in the early stages (**Fig. 7**). As tendinosis worsens, the tendon will usually continue to enlarge, but hypoechoic areas will develop to represent early areas of fibril disruption. Severe tendinosis will appear as marked enlargement with complete loss of the fibrillar pattern (**Fig. 8**). Focal anechoic areas on this background likely represent small interstitial tears. Calcifications appear as echogenic reflectors with posterior acoustic shadowing (**Fig. 9**).

Comparison with the contralateral, presumably normal side can be useful in indeterminate cases. There are times when tendon may appear hypoechoic because of other factors, including large distance from the probe or inability to obtain a true 90° insonation beam; comparison with the contralateral side may establish whether the appearance is more likely due to artifact rather than true abnormality.

Neovascularity can be observed with Doppler imaging. Blood flow entering the tendon can be observed with either color or power Doppler imaging. Power Doppler is more sensitive for low-level blood flow, but at the expense of direction information. In general, the presence of neovascularity is of greater use than knowledge of the direction of flow.

A secondary sign of tendinosis is cortical irregularity at the adjacent tendon-bone interface.[58,59] In the rotator cuff, cortical irregularity has been associated with rotator cuff tears.[58] Though not always present, this finding can be helpful in indeterminate cases.

Special case: achilles tendinosis Two primary patterns of Achilles tendinosis are observed, noninsertional (see **Fig. 7**) and insertional (**Fig. 10**). In the more common noninsertional form, the disease process is centered approximately 4 to 6 cm above the calcaneal insertion. Two possible

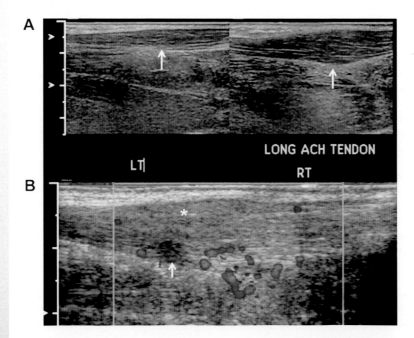

Fig. 7. Mild noninsertional Achilles tendinosis. Long-axis views of the right Achilles tendon show mild focal noninsertional enlargement (A), consistent with tendinosis, compared with the contralateral side. Arrows point to the deep border of the Achilles tendon. The fibrillar pattern is mostly preserved. Although overall there is a preserved fibrillar pattern, focal regions of hypoechogenicity and loss of the fibrillar pattern (B) are noted: Arrow, small focal hypoechoic area; asterisk, ill-defined area of enlargement and loss of the fibrillar pattern. Power Doppler shows neovascularity of the posterior aspect of the Achilles tendon in this region.

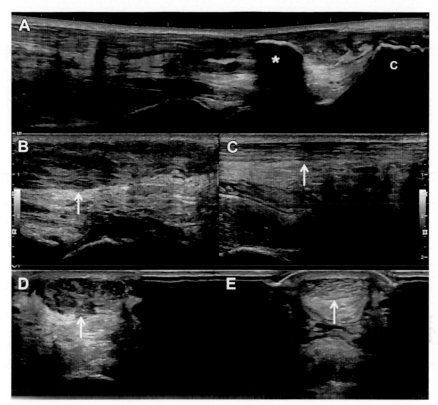

Fig. 8. Diffuse Achilles tendinosis. (*A*) Panoramic view of the Achilles tendon (*right side of image* is proximal, *left side* is distal). Note diffuse, but variable thickening of the tendon. *Asterisk*, intratendinous ossification; c, calcaneus. (*B, C*) Long-axis and (*D, E*) short-axis views of a diffusely enlarged tendon (*B, D*) with global hypoechogenicity and loss of the normal fibrillar pattern, consistent with severe tendinosis. The contralateral normal side (*C, E*) is shown for comparison. *Arrows* indicate posterior margin of the tendon.

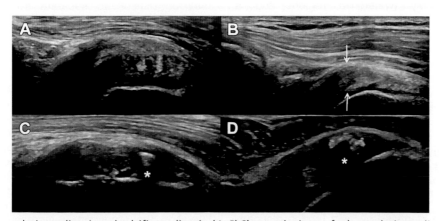

Fig. 9. Subscapularis tendinosis and calcific tendinosis. (*A, B*) Short-axis views of subscapularis tendinosis (*left side of image* is superior, *right side* is inferior). In *A*, subscapularis is diffusely thickened and the superior edge appears irregular because of edge artifact. In *B*, thickening of the tendon is isolated to the superior fibers (*arrows*), which is a common pattern of subscapularis tendinosis. (*C, D*) Long-axis views showing a focal hyperechoic structure with posterior acoustic shadowing (*asterisk*), consistent with calcium hydroxyapatite deposition. The adjacent tendon has a heterogeneous appearance consistent with tendinosis.

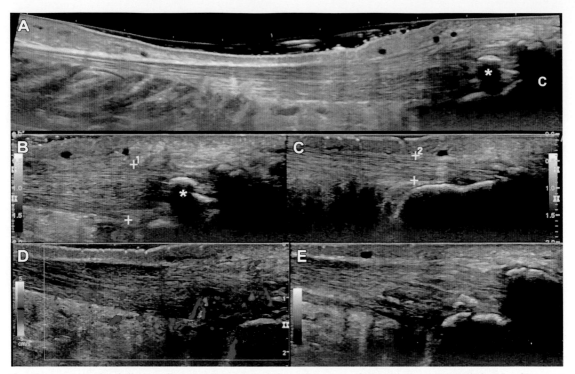

Fig. 10. Insertional Achilles tendinosis. (*A*) Panoramic long-axis view of the Achilles tendon (*left side of image* is proximal, *right side* is distal). Note the progressive enlargement of the tendon as it approaches the calcaneus (C). *Asterisk* indicates intratendinous ossification. (*B, C*) Long-axis view of the abnormal (*B*) tendon compared with the contralateral normal side (*C*). *Asterisk* indicates intratendinous ossification. (*D*) Color Doppler long-axis image shows marked intratendinous vascularity. (*E*) Long-axis view showing marked cortical irregularity at the attachment.

explanations for the susceptibility of this location to tendinosis include a relatively decreased vascular supply (watershed region) and a twisting/squeezing mechanism acting on the tendon in this region, owing to the way in which the constituent muscles attach to the tendon.[60] In the insertional form, an intrasubstance enthesophyte or heterotopic bone may be present.

Achilles tendinosis, like tendinosis elsewhere in the body, may or may not be associated with pain. Of note, most Achilles tendon ruptures occur in the setting of painless tendinopathy. In fact, the degree of tendon degeneration may be worse in tendons that ultimately rupture despite the lack of pain.[61]

Tears

Tears can be identified by overt tendon discontinuity, anechoic clefts, and contour abnormalities. In indeterminate cases, the tendon can be stressed to differentiate between complete ruptures and partial tears. **Figs. 11–13** show examples of long head of biceps tendon, Achilles

tendon, and tibialis anterior tendon tears. As tears often occur in the setting of tendinosis, small tears may be difficult to separate from advanced tendinosis.

Special case: rotator cuff tears The evaluation of the rotator cuff is complicated by the anatomy. The insertion of the supraspinatus, infraspinatus, and subscapularis tendons is broad, and the tendon curves as it approaches the attachment. The curvature introduces anisotropy directly at the bone interface, a common site for tears. Regarding the supraspinatus tendon, most of the tendon is concealed beneath the acromion. The Crass and modified Crass positions were developed to address the problem, whereby the length of the supraspinatus tendon visible lateral to the acromion is increased by introducing varying degrees of arm extension (**Figs. 14** and **15**).[62] In the case of subscapularis, the arm must be externally rotated to bring the tendon more anteriorly out from beneath the coracoid.

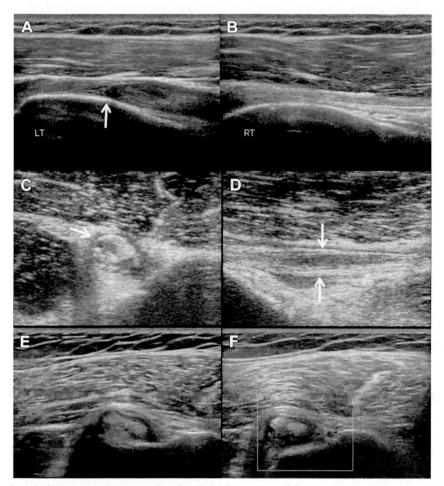

Fig. 11. Long head of biceps tendon tears. (*A, B*) Full-thickness tear of the long head of biceps tendon characterized by an anechoic cleft (*arrow*). The contralateral normal side (*B*) is shown for comparison. (*C*) Short-axis view of a partial-thickness tear with a small intrasubstance nearly anechoic defect (*arrow*). Long-axis view (*D*) shows the extent of the tear. *Arrows* indicate intact fibers on either side of the tear in this view. (*E, F*) Short-axis views of a longitudinal split tear. Near the transition from the intra-articular portion to the bicipital groove, the tendon has a biconcave (*E*) appearance, likely representing a step in the progression to a split tear. Somewhat more distal to the view in *E*, the tendon is split into two halves (*F*). The presence of color Doppler signal around the tendon indicates concomitant tenosynovitis.

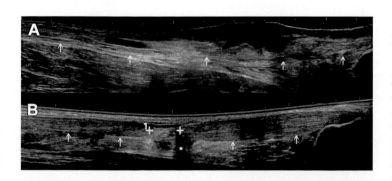

Fig. 12. Panoramic long-axis views of an Achilles tendon partial tear and full-thickness tear (*left side of image* is proximal, *right side* is distal). *Arrows* indicate posterior border of the tendon. (*A*) Partial tear. Note focal noninsertional fiber disruption and hypoechoic region in the superficial aspect of the tendon. Additional intrasubstance tear is noted more proximally. (*B*) Full-thickness tear. A complete noninsertional tear of a near uniformly thickened Achilles tendon is present with hyperechoic material (hemorrhage) interposed between the tendon edges. Fibrillar pattern is still discernible in the intact portions of the tendon. Anechoic streak/edge artifact (*asterisk*) is a useful indicator of a tear when present.

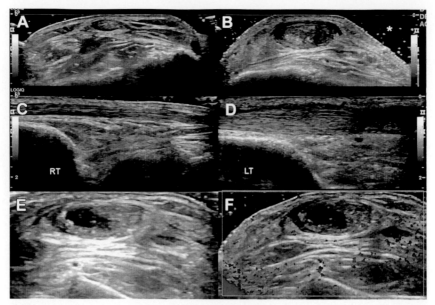

Fig. 13. Tibialis anterior tendinosis with partial tear. (*A, B*) Short-axis views of a normal (*A*) and an enlarged, heterogeneous-appearing (*B*) tibialis anterior tendon. The *asterisk* in B indicates coupling gel. (*C, D*) Long-axis views of a normal (*C*) and an enlarged (*D*) tibialis anterior tendon. (*E, F*) Short-axis views of an intrasubstance anechoic defect within the tendon consistent with a partial tear. Color Doppler image (*F*) shows no definite elevated vascularity.

Regarding tears involving other tendons, superior rotator cuff tears are primarily characterized by focal anechoic regions not attributable to anisotropy and architectural distortion. Complete tendon ruptures are easy to diagnose, as there is no tissue located between the deltoid muscle and the greater tuberosity. In the case of the supraspinatus tendon the free edge may still be visible, but is often retracted beneath the acromion. Full-thickness, partial-width tears can be similarly identified by a lack of tendon tissue between the greater tuberosity and the deltoid, but bordered on at least one side by intact tendon, which is often readily visible on the short-axis

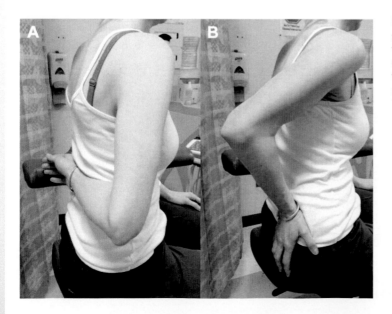

Fig. 14. Crass and modified Crass positions. (*A*) Crass position: marked internal rotation and mild extension of the arm. (*B*) Modified Crass position: mild internal rotation and marked extension of the arm.

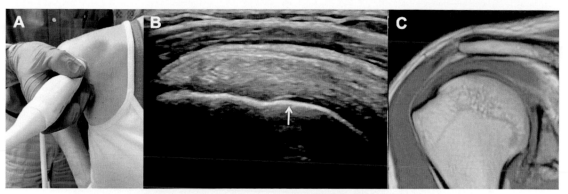

Fig. 15. Long-axis view of anterior superior rotator cuff in the modified Crass position. (*A*) Probe position for the long-axis view of the superior rotator cuff (supraspinatus and infraspinatus) in the modified Crass position. Note the anterior location of the rotator cuff in this position. (*B*) Long-axis view of the posterior supraspinatus tendon near the supraspinatus-infraspinatus junction. Note the hypoechoic appearance of the tendon adjacent to its insertion, owing to anisotropy. *Arrow* indicates normal cartilage interface. (*C*) Oblique coronal T1-weighted magnetic resonance (MR) image of the superior rotator cuff for correlation.

view. As the width of the tear becomes increasingly smaller, it becomes more difficult to make the diagnosis of a full-thickness tear. Once identified, the distance from the intra-articular long head of biceps tendon, found in the rotator interval, is helpful in allowing the referring clinician know which portion of the cuff is involved (**Fig. 16**).

Fig. 17 provides examples of full-thickness superior rotator cuff tears. A tear unique to the subscapularis tendon is a separation between the deep and superficial fibers adjacent to the bicipital groove into which the long head of biceps tendon subluxes (**Fig. 18**). Otherwise, subscapularis tears appear identical to superior rotator cuff tears.

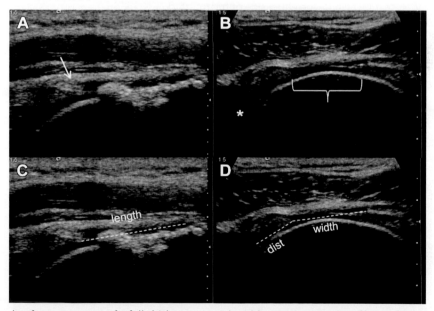

Fig. 16. Example of measurement of a full-thickness, partial-width superior rotator cuff tear. (*A*) Long-axis and (*B*) short-axis images. *Arrow,* lateral edge of the torn tendon; *asterisk,* long head of biceps tendon; *bracket,* extent of the full-thickness tear in short axis. Intact tendon is present both anterior (*left side of image*) and posterior (*right side of image*) to the tear. (*C*) The length of the tear measured on the long-axis view from the torn tendon edge to the lateral-most aspect of the tendon insertion (*dashed line*). For full-thickness, full-width tears, the length would represent the degree of retraction. (*D*) Measurement on the short-axis view. dist, the distance to the anterior edge of the tear from the biceps tendon; width, anterior-posterior width of the tear.

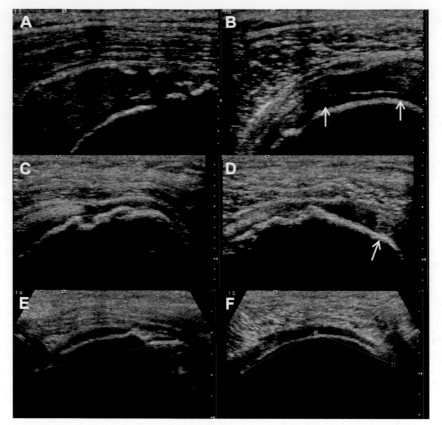

Fig. 17. Full-thickness tears of the superior rotator cuff. (A) Long-axis and (B) short-axis views of a full-thickness, partial-width tear. Note intact tendon on either side of the full-thickness tear on the short-axis view (arrows). Also note the bright cartilage interface. (C) Long-axis and (D) short-axis views of a full-thickness, near full-width tear. Note intact tendon in the posterior cuff (arrow). (E) Long-axis and (F) short-axis views of a full-thickness, full-width tear. No identifiable tendon is present, as the cuff has retracted beneath the acromion. The exact width of the tear is likely to be underestimated because the measurement is made on a curved surface.

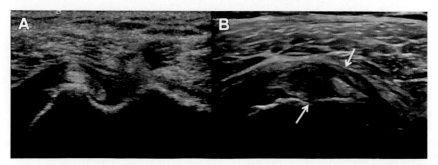

Fig. 18. Long head of biceps tendon subluxation. (A) Partial subluxation of the long head of biceps tendon out of the bicipital groove. Hypoechoic area within the tendon may represent focal tendinosis. (B) Subluxation of the long head of biceps tendon into the substance of a partially torn subscapularis tendon (arrows). The superficial and deep fibers of subscapularis have become separated adjacent to the bicipital groove. The superficial fibers remain in continuity with the transverse ligament.

Partial-thickness tears are described by their location: interstitial (intrasubstance), bursal-surface, or articular surface (Fig. 19). When present, a focal anechoic defect in the tendon is a primary sign of a partial tear. Contour deformities, a primary sign often associated with full-thickness tears, are generally not seen with partial tears unless the tear is large.

As the primary signs of anechoic regions with loss of the normal tendon architecture are not always observed with confidence, several secondary signs have been described to assist with the identification of rotator cuff tears (**Table 1**). Helpful secondary signs include cortical irregularity of the greater tuberosity, fluid within the subdeltoid bursa and bicipital tendon sheath, and a highly reflective cartilage interface (known as the cartilage interface sign or bare cartilage sign).[63] For differentiation of a full-thickness tear from either no tear or a partial tear, Jacobson and colleagues[63] found that the combination of greater tuberosity irregularity and bicipital tendon sheath effusion

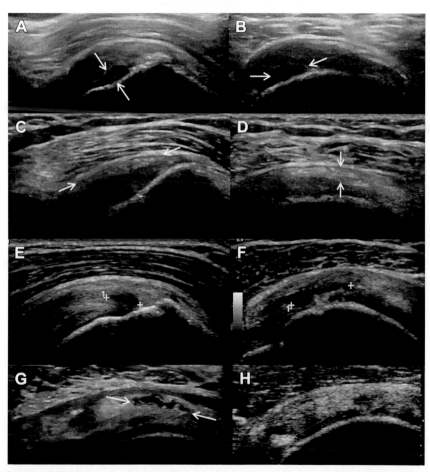

Fig. 19. Partial tears of the superior rotator cuff. (A) Long-axis and (B) short-axis views of an anterior supraspinatus articular surface tear (rim rent tear). Note the well-defined hypoechoic area (*arrows*) where there should be normal tendon. (C) Long-axis and (D) short-axis views of a bursal surface tear filled in by hyperechoic material (*arrows*), which may represent fat or blood. As the overall contour is preserved, one must recognize the hyperechoic region as abnormal to make the diagnosis. (E) Long-axis and (F) short-axis views of an intrasubstance insertional tear of the anterior superior rotator cuff. (G) Short-axis view of a small bursal surface tear (*arrows*) of the posterior cuff. (H) Short-axis view of a small intrasubstance tear likely at the supraspinatus-infraspinatus junction.

Table 1
Sonographic signs of rotator cuff tears

Signs	Image	Associated Pathology
Primary		
Anechoic defect		Tear, full-thickness or partial-thickness
Contour abnormality		Tear, full-thickness or large partial-thickness
Secondary		
Bony irregularity		Tendinosis Tear, full-thickness or partial-thickness
Cartilage interface sign		Tear, full-thickness or articular surface partial-thickness
Fluid in biceps tendon sheath and subdeltoid bursa		If tenosynovitis and bursitis are excluded, full-thickness tear can be considered
Hypoechoic area		Focal tendinosis or tear

Primary and secondary signs for the diagnosis of rotator cuff tears. When the primary signs are not observed with confidence, the secondary signs can help with diagnosis.

was the most useful, with sensitivity of 60% and specificity of 100% with a resultant positive predictive value of 100%. For the differentiation of any tear from no tear, the most specific signs were nonvisualization of the tendon and the cartilage interface sign (specificity of 100% for both). In this comparison, no particular combination had a diagnostic advantage over any of the single signs.

The rotator cuff muscles are an essential component of examination of a rotator cuff tendon, as muscle atrophy has a profound effect on treatment prognosis for tears.[64] The supraspinatus, infraspinatus, and teres minor muscles are scanned in cross section. Once a suitable supraspinatus muscle cross section is located, the transducer can be slid over the scapular spine to visualize the infraspinatus muscle. The teres minor is then visualized by moving the transducer slightly laterally. Normal muscle appears hypoechoic with echogenic central tendons (Fig. 20). Atrophic muscle has diminished bulk and appears hyperechoic (Fig. 21).

Tenosynovitis

Tenosynovitis is characterized by thickening of the lining of the tendon sheath as a result of edema and hyperemia. Often there is an accompanying effusion, which may have heterogeneous material within it. On the other hand, an effusion without debris or other findings of tenosynovitis is nonspecific; effusions involving intra-articular tendons such as the long head of biceps and flexor hallucis longus tendons may instead reflect an abnormality of the adjacent joint. Hyperemia is helpful when present on Doppler imaging, but its absence does not preclude inflammation. **Figs. 22–25** shows examples of tenosynovitis.

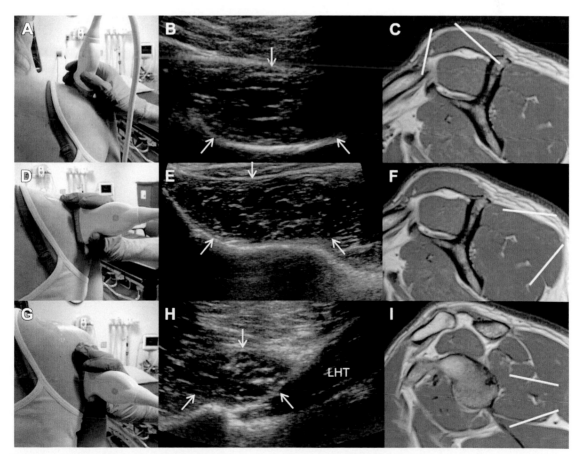

Fig. 20. Rotator cuff muscle evaluation. Probe positioning, sonographic appearance, and oblique sagittal T1-weighted MR imaging correlation of the rotator cuff muscles. For the sonographic images, the left side of the image is toward the head and the right side is toward the feet. *Arrows* indicate borders of the muscle. Angled white lines indicate relative probe position on the MR image. (*A–C*) Supraspinatus muscle. (*D–F*) Infraspinatus muscle. (*G–I*) Teres minor muscle. LHT, long head of triceps tendon (a useful landmark).

508

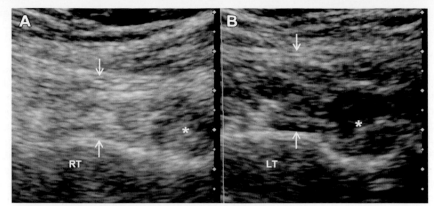

Fig. 21. Infraspinatus muscle atrophy. Note the diffusely hyperechoic appearance and decreased size of the infraspinatus muscle on the right (*A*) compared with the left (*B*). *Arrows*, superficial and deep edges of the infraspinatus muscle; *asterisk*, normal teres minor muscle.

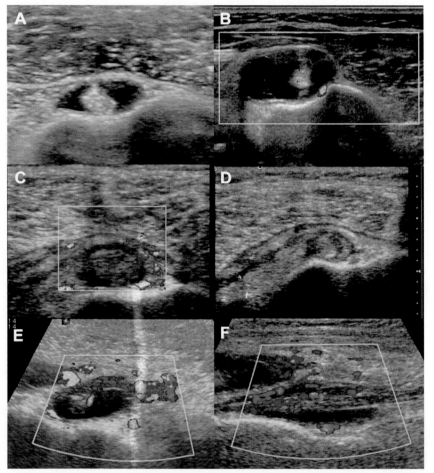

Fig. 22. Long head of biceps tenosynovitis. Tenosynovitis is characterized by 1 or more of the following: thickened hypoechoic sheath, increased vascularity, and effusion with or without echogenic debris. The presence of an effusion without debris and without other findings is insufficient to make the diagnosis of tenosynovitis. (*A*) Tendon sheath effusion, without inflammatory changes. Note the well-defined tendon sheath. (*B*) Large tendon sheath effusion with some associated vascularity, consistent with tenosynovitis. Large tense effusions can compress the surrounding vessels, decreasing the signal on color Doppler. (*C*) Enlarged hypoechoic tendon surrounded by a thickened sheath and a moderate amount of vascularity consistent with tendinosis and tenosynovitis. (*D*) Minimally enlarged tendon with hypoechoic, somewhat thickened sheath. (*E*) Short-axis and (*F*) long-axis views of a normal tendon surrounded by a moderate effusion, mildly thickened sheath, and a large amount of vascularity.

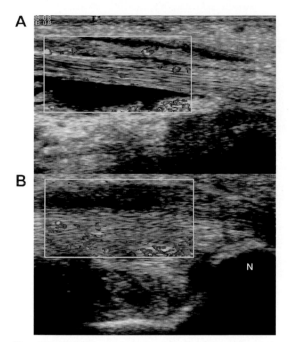

Fig. 23. Tibialis posterior tenosynovitis. Long-axis views of a normal tibialis posterior tendon surrounded by fluid. Color Doppler reveals associated vascularity. (*A*) Position between the medial malleolus and the navicular insertion. (*B*) At the navicular (N) insertion. The tibialis posterior tendon normally enlarges as it approaches the navicular insertion, and should not be confused with tendinosis.

SUMMARY

Tendon disorders range from asymptomatic degenerative changes, to inflammation of the peritendinous tissues, to rupture; these disorders are common as a group, particularly among athletes and the elderly. The high resolution of modern ultrasound equipment and the superficial location of most tendons in the body allow the spectrum of tendon abnormalities to be easily depicted with ultrasonography. Specific sonographic criteria for the diagnosis of tendinosis, tendon tears, and tenosynovitis exist, and are summarized in **Box 1**. Given the high prevalence of rotator cuff disease and the low cost of the shoulder ultrasonography examination relative to MR imaging, requests for shoulder sonography are likely to increase. It is therefore essential to become familiar with this examination. The ankle examination serves as a useful model for tendons in other parts of the body, both as a targeted examination and for the evaluation of very superficial structures.

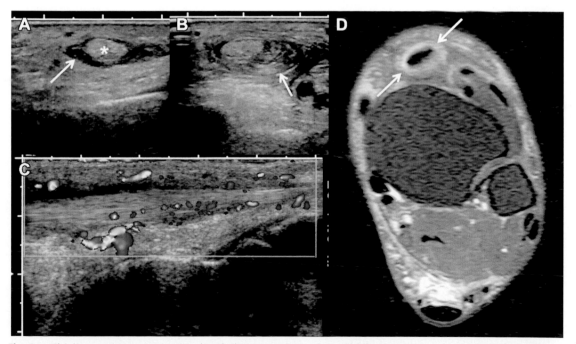

Fig. 24. Tibialis anterior tenosynovitis. (*A, B*) Short-axis views of the tibialis anterior tendon (*asterisk*) at different levels, showing a normal tendon surrounded by fluid (*A*) and echogenic debris (*B*). The *arrows* point to the tendon sheath. (*C*) Color Doppler long-axis view showing a normal tendon with marked adjacent vascularity. (*D*) Axial T1-weighted fat-suppressed postcontrast MR image from the same patient in *C* showing a normal-appearing tibialis anterior tendon surrounded by a thin layer of enhancement (*arrows*), consistent with tenosynovitis.

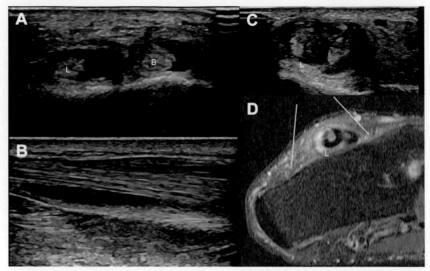

Fig. 25. Peroneus brevis and longus tendinosis and tenosynovitis. (*A*) Short-axis and (*B*) long-axis views of a mildly enlarged peroneus brevis (B) and longus (L) tendon distal to the lateral malleolus surrounded by fluid and heterogeneous material. (*C*) Short-axis view and (*D*) axial T2-weighted fat-suppressed MR image at approximately the same level, showing abnormal enlargement of the peroneal tendons surrounded by heterogeneous material. The MR image shows intrasubstance signal within the peroneus longus (L) tendon that extends to the tendon surface, suggesting a tear. Marked hypoechoic region in the peroneus longus on the sonographic image is the likely correlate. Angled lines indicate the approximate probe position able to achieve a sonographic view similar to that seen on the MR image.

Box 1
Sonographic findings of tendon disease. A summary of the sonographic findings in tendinosis, tendon tears, and tenosynovitis.

Tendinosis

  Primary

    Enlargement

    Hypoechoic

    Loss of fibrillary echotexture

    Calcifications

  Secondary

    Cortical irregularity at adjacent tendon-bone interface

Tears

  Anechoic cleft

  Architectural distortion

Tenosynovitis

  Thickened hypoechoic tendon sheath

  Effusion with debris

  Hypervascularity

REFERENCES

1. Kannus P. Tendons—a source of major concern in competitive and recreational athletes. Scand J Med Sci Sports 1997;7:53–4.

2. Ostor AJ, Richards CA, Prevost AT, et al. Diagnosis and relation to general health of shoulder disorders presenting to primary care. Rheumatology 2005; 44:800–5.

3. Brasington R. Nintendinitis. N Engl J Med 1990; 322(20):1473–4.

4. Abate M, Schiavone C, Salini V, et al. Occurrence of tendon pathologies in metabolic disorders. Rheumatology 2013;52:599–608.

5. Al-Homood IA. Rheumatic conditions in patients with diabetes mellitus. Clin Rheumatol 2013;32:527–33.

6. Grassi W, De Angelis R, Lamanna G, et al. The clinical features of rheumatoid arthritis. Eur J Radiol 1998;27(Suppl 1):S18–24.

7. Erickson SJ. High-resolution imaging of the musculoskeletal system. Radiology 1997;205:593–618.

8. Moran CM, Pye SD, Ellis W, et al. A comparison of the imaging performance of high resolution ultrasound scanners for preclinical imaging. Ultrasound Med Biol 2011;37(3):493–501.

9. Wang JH, Guo Q, Li B. Tendon biomechanics and mechanobiology—a minireview of basic concepts and recent advancements. J Hand Ther 2012;25: 133–41.

10. Maffulli N, Khan KM, Puddu G. Overuse tendon conditions: time to change a confusing terminology. Arthroscopy 1998;14(12):840–3.

11. Chiou HJ, Hung SC, Lin SY, et al. Correlations among mineral components, progressive calcification process and clinical symptoms of calcific tendonitis. Rheumatology 2010;49:548–55.

12. Maffulli N, Wong J, Almekinders LC. Types and epidemiology of tendinopathy. Clin Sports Med 2003;22:675–92.

13. Kujala UM, Sarna S, Kaprio J. Cumulative evidence of Achilles tendon ruptures and tendinopathy in male former elite athletes. Clin J Sport Med 2005; 15(3):133–5.

14. Lian OB, Engebretsen L, Bahr R. Prevalence of jumper's knee among elite athletes from different sports. Am J Sports Med 2005;33(4):561–7.

15. Smidt N, Assendelft WJ, van der Windt DA, et al. Corticosteroid injections for lateral epicondylitis: a systematic review. Pain 2002;96:23–40.

16. Pluim BM, Staal JB, Windler GE, et al. Tennis injuries: occurrence, aetiology, and prevention. Br J Sports Med 2006;40:415–23.

17. Tashjian RZ. Epidemiology, natural history, and indications for treatment of rotator cuff tears. Clin Sports Med 2012;31:589–604.

18. Yamamoto A, Takagishi K, Osawa T, et al. Prevalence and risk factors of a rotator cuff tear in the general population. J Shoulder Elbow Surg 2010; 19:116–20.

19. Yamaguchi K, Ditsios K, Middleton WD, et al. The demographic and morphological features of rotator cuff disease. J Bone Joint Surg Am 2006;88(8):1699–704.

20. Tempelhof S, Rupp S, Siel R. Age-related prevalence of rotator cuff tears in asymptomatic shoulders. J Shoulder Elbow Surg 1999;8(4):296–9.

21. Suchak A, Bostick G, Reid D, et al. The incidence of Achilles tendon ruptures in Edmonton, Canada. Foot Ankle Int 2005;26(11):932–6.

22. Bhargava SP, Hynes MC, Dowell JK. Traumatic patellar tendon rupture: early mobilisation following surgical repair. Injury 2004;35:76–9.

23. White DW, Wenke JC, Mosely DS, et al. Incidence of major tendon ruptures and anterior cruciate ligament tears in US Army soldiers. Am J Sports Med 2007;35(8):1308–14.

24. Dobbs RE, Hanssen AD, Lewallen DG, et al. Quadriceps tendon rupture after total knee arthroplasty. J Bone Joint Surg Am 2005;87A(1):37–45.

25. Benner RW, Shelbourne KD, Urch SE, et al. Tear patterns, surgical repair, and clinical outcomes of patellar tendon ruptures after anterior cruciate ligament reconstruction with a bone-patellar tendon-bone autograft. Am J Sports Med 2012;40:1834–41.

26. Mall NA, Lee AS, Chahal J, et al. An evidence-based examination of the epidemiology and outcomes of traumatic rotator cuff tears. Arthroscopy 2013;29(2):366–76.

27. Galloway MT, Lalley AL, Shearn JT. The role of mechanical loading in tendon development, maintenance, injury, and repair. J Bone Joint Surg Am 2013;95:1620–8.

28. Shepherd JH, Screen HR. Fatigue loading of tendon. Int J Exp Pathol 2013;94(4):260–70.

29. Banes AJ, Weinhold P, Yang X, et al. Gap junctions regulate responses of tendon cells ex vivo to mechanical loading. Clin Orthop 1999;367(Suppl): S356–70.

30. Thorpe CT, Birch HL, Clegg PD, et al. The role of non-collagenous matrix in tendon function. Int J Exp Pathol 2013;94(4):248–59.

31. Ackermann PW. Neuronal regulation of tendon homeostasis. Int J Exp Pathol 2013;94(4):271–86.

32. McCreesh K, Lewis J. Continuum model of tendon pathology—where are we now? Int J Exp Pathol 2013;94(4):242–7.

33. Scott A, Ashe MC. Common tendinopathies in the upper and lower extremities. Curr Sports Med Rep 2006;5:233–41.

34. Corrao G, Zambon A, Bertu L, et al. Evidence of tendinitis provoked by fluoroquinolone treatment. Drug Saf 2006;29(10):889–96.

35. Yi Y, Shim JS, Baek SR, et al. Prevalence of the rotator cuff increases with the weakness in hemiplegic shoulder. Ann Rehabil Med 2013;37(4):471–8.

36. Maffulli N, Irwin AS, Kenward AG, et al. Achilles tendon rupture and sciatica: a possible correlation. Br J Sports Med 1998;32(2):174–7.

37. Juul-Kristensen B, Lund H, Hansen K, et al. Poorer elbow proprioception in patients with lateral epicondylitis than in healthy controls: a cross-sectional study. J Shoulder Elbow Surg 2008;17: 72S–81S.

38. Flemming DJ, Murphey MD, Shekitka KM, et al. Osseous involvement in calcific tendinitis: a retrospective review of 50 cases. AJR Am J Roentgenol 2003;181:965–72.

39. Chan R, Kim DH, Millett PJ, et al. Calcifying tendinitis of the rotator cuff with cortical bone erosion. Skeletal Radiol 2004;33:596–9.

40. O'Brien EJ, Frank CB, Shrive NG, et al. Heterotopic mineralization (ossification or calcification) in tendinopathy or following surgical tendon trauma. Int J Exp Pathol 2012;93(5):319–31.

41. Raikin SM, Elias I, Nazarian LN. Intrasheath subluxation of the peroneal tendons. J Bone Joint Surg Am 2008;90:992–9.

42. Roll SC, Evans KD, Hutmire CD, et al. An analysis of occupational factors related to shoulder discomfort in diagnostic medical sonographers and vascular technologists. Work 2012;42:355–65.

43. Fornage BD. The hypoechoic normal tendon. A pitfall. J Ultrasound Med 1987;6(1):19–22.

44. Connolly DJ, Berman L, McNally EG. The use of beam angulation to overcome anisotropy when viewing human tendon with high frequency linear array ultrasound. Br J Radiol 2001;74:183–5.

45. de Jesus JO, Parker L, Frangos AJ, et al. Accuracy of MRI, MR arthrography, and ultrasound in the diagnosis of rotator cuff tears: a meta-analysis. AJR Am J Roentgenol 2009;192:1701–7.

46. Dinnes J, Loveman E, McIntyre L, et al. The effectiveness of diagnostic tests for the assessment of shoulder pain due to soft tissue disorders: a systematic review. Health Tech Assess 2003;7(29):1–166.

47. Lenza M, Buchbinder R, Takwoingi Y, et al. Magnetic resonance imaging, magnetic resonance arthrography and ultrasonography for assessing rotator cuff tears in people with shoulder pain for whom surgery is being considered. Cochrane Database Syst Rev 2013;9:1–137.

48. Teefey SA, Rubin DA, Middleton WD, et al. Detection and quantification of rotator cuff tears: comparison of ultrasonographic, magnetic resonance imaging, and arthroscopic findings in seventy-one consecutive cases. J Bone Joint Surg Am 2004; 86A(4):708–16.

49. Nazarian LN, Jacobson JA, Benson CB, et al. Imaging algorithms for evaluating suspected rotator cuff disease: Society of Radiologists in Ultrasound Consensus Conference Statement. Radiology 2013;267(2):589–95.

50. Jacobson JA. Musculoskeletal ultrasound: focused impact on MRI. AJR Am J Roentgenol 2009;193: 619–27.

51. Rockett MS, Waitches G, Sudakoff G, et al. Use of ultrasonography versus magnetic resonance imaging for tendon abnormalities around the ankle. Foot Ankle Int 1998;19(9):604–12.

52. Gerling MC, Pfirrmann CW, Farooki S, et al. Posterior tibial tendon tears: comparison of the diagnostic efficacy of magnetic resonance imaging and ultrasonography for the detection of surgically created longitudinal tears in cadavers. Invest Radiol 2003;38(1):51–6.

53. Nallamshetty L, Nazarian LN, Schweitzer ME, et al. Evaluation of posterior tibial pathology: comparison of sonography and MR imaging. Skeletal Radiol 2005;34(7):375–80.

54. Alavekios DA, Dionysian E, Sodl J, et al. Longitudinal analysis of effects of operator experience on accuracy for ultrasound detection of supraspinatus tears. J Shoulder Elbow Surg 2013;22: 375–80.

55. O'Connor PJ, Rankine J, Gibbon WW, et al. Interobserver variation in sonography of the painful shoulder. J Clin Ultrasound 2005;33(2):53–6.

56. Le Corroler T, Cohen M, Aswad R, et al. Sonography of the painful shoulder: role of the operator's experience. Skeletal Radiol 2008;37(11):979–86.

57. Rutten MJ, Jager GJ, Kiemeney LA. Ultrasound detection of rotator cuff tears: observer agreement related to increasing experience. AJR Am J Roentgenol 2010;195:W440–6.

58. Levin D, Nazarian LN, Miller TT, et al. Lateral epicondylitis of the elbow: US findings. Radiology 2005;237:230–4.

59. Jiang Y, Zhao J, van Holsbeeck MT, et al. Trabecular microstructure and surface changes in the greater tuberosity in rotator cuff tears. Skeletal Radiol 2002;31:522–8.

60. Lesic A, Bumbasirevic M. Disorders of the Achilles tendon. Curr Orthop 2004;18:63–75.

61. Tallon C, Maffulli N, Ewen SW. Ruptured Achilles tendons are significantly more degenerated than tendinopathic tendons. Med Sci Sports Exerc 2001;33(12):1983–90.

62. Crass JR, Craig EV, Feinberg SB. The hyperextended internal rotation view in rotator cuff ultrasonography. J Clin Ultrasound 1987;15(6):416–20.

63. Jacobson JA, Lancaster S, Prasad A, et al. Fullthickness and partial-thickness supraspinatus tendon tears: value of US signs in diagnosis. Radiology 2004;230:234–42.

64. Gladstone JN, Bishop JY, Lo IK, et al. Fatty infiltration and atrophy of the rotator cuff do not improve after rotator cuff repair and correlate with poor functional outcome. Am J Sports Med 2007;35(5): 719–28.

Joint Ultrasound

Diana Gaitini, MD

KEYWORDS

- Musculoskeletal imaging • Ultrasonography • Joints • Anatomy • Bursitis
- Ultrasound-guided procedures

KEY POINTS

- Joint ultrasound indications are rapidly expanding because of the technological improvements of modern equipments, high availability, and low cost compared with sophisticated imaging techniques.
- Proper operator skills and high-resolution transducers are demanded.
- Color and power Doppler examinations are recommended in every joint study; static imaging of joints should be followed by a dynamic examination.
- Ultrasound is limited in the diagnosis of intra-articular anatomy and pathologic processes that are hidden by bone structures.
- Ultrasound findings in an inflamed joint are nonspecific.
- Ultrasound guidance allows precise and time-saving performance of diagnostic and therapeutic procedures.

 Video of a Cine loop showing the moving air bubbles in real-time accompanies this article at http://www.ultrasound.theclinics.com/

INTRODUCTION

Ultrasound is rapidly becoming the first-line modality for examination in the field of musculoskeletal imaging. Advanced ultrasound technology has increased imaging resolution, even at a higher level than magnetic resonance. The ability of Doppler imaging to evaluate vascularity and dynamic examination in real time and its low cost, and high availability are clear advantages over computed tomography (CT) and magnetic resonance imaging (MRI).[1,2] Reliable diagnoses and proper therapeutic interventions may be achieved through knowledge of ultrasound principles, techniques of examination, and ultrasound anatomy and abnormalities, and experience in scanning and performance of interventional procedures. Joint imaging and ultrasound-guided interventional procedures should follow the guidelines and general consensus published in the literature.[3–5] The article describes the normal anatomy and scanning technique of joints, as the first step to perform an effective ultrasound evaluation, followed by pathologic ultrasound findings and ultrasound-guided joint procedures.

ULTRASOUND TECHNOLOGY

Broadband high-resolution linear array transducers (7–15 MHz) provide enough penetration for the examination of large joints with an excellent resolution. A 3- to 9-MHz frequency is needed for a deeper penetration in a larger patient, at the expense of lower resolution.[6–8] Small field of view hockey stick–shaped transducers are ideal for evaluating small superficial joints and performing dynamic maneuvers.

Spatial compound sonography obtains information from several different angles of insonation and combines them to produce a single image, reducing speckle and improving definition of

The author has nothing to disclose.
Unit of Ultrasound, Department of Medical Imaging, Rambam Health Care Center and Bruce Rappaport Faculty of Medicine, Israel Institute of Technology, Ha'aliya 8, POB 9602, 31096 Haifa, Israel
E-mail address: d_gaitini@rambam.health.gov.il

Ultrasound Clin 9 (2014) 513–524
http://dx.doi.org/10.1016/j.cult.2014.03.004
1556-858X/14/$ – see front matter © 2014 Elsevier Inc. All rights reserved.

tissue planes, thus improving image quality on musculoskeletal ultrasound.[9]

Extended-field-of-view imaging technology allows display of large anatomy and the full extent of an abnormality, showing its relationship with adjacent structures over long distances and curved surfaces.[10]

Color and power Doppler systems allow the detection of low velocity flow in small vessels to correlate hyperemic changes with structural joint abnormalities.[11]

Ultrasound contrast media injection (after switching the machine to contrast menu, which has a low mechanical index and inversion recovery harmonics to optimize the microbubble response) has allowed the evaluation of microvasculature perfusion, leading to encouraging results in imaging arthritis and other rheumatologic conditions.[12]

SCANNING TECHNIQUE

Examination technique depends on the different joints, but as a rule of thumb, a 4-side B-mode scan is recommended, covering the joint from anterior, lateral, medial, and posterior sides. Color and power Doppler imaging are useful for showing the vascular anatomy. Dynamic maneuvers are functional tests to visualize joints during real-time examination.

NORMAL ANATOMY

Joint anatomy is adapted to specific functional requirements and varies among joints. Synovial joints are the most commonly examined with ultrasound. They are composed of the articulating bone surfaces covered by hyaline articular cartilage and the joint capsule, inserting marginally into the cortical bone and periosteum. The articular cartilage is seen as a hypoechoic smooth linear band over a regular hyperechoic line corresponding to the subchondral bone. Cartilage thickness may be accurately measured on ultrasound. The joint capsule and the peripheral boundaries of the cartilage and fibrous capsule, the so-called bare areas, are lined by a synovial membrane (**Fig. 1**). The synovial membrane is too thin to be visible. The capsule is reinforced by ligaments inserted just above the joint line. The joint capsule and ligaments appear hyperechoic. Similar to tendons, the ligaments are anisotropic; care should be taken to place the transducer as parallel as possible to avoid artifactual hypoechogenicity, which could mimic an abnormality.

Intra-articular fibrocartilaginous structures (such as menisci in the knee, the labrum in the hip and

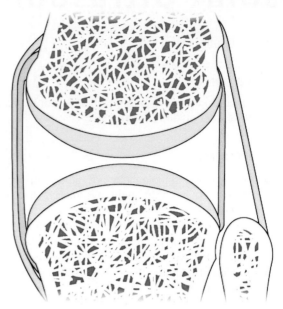

Fig. 1. Synovial joint anatomy, schematic drawing. Articular cartilage (*green*) covering the adjacent bone plates (*white*) and joint capsule (*brown*), which inserts beyond the articular cartilage. Note the articular cartilage different thicknesses from loading and weight-bearing demands. Ligaments (*gray*), either adjacent to the fibrous capsule (on the tibia side) or at a certain distance (on the fibular side), act to reinforce and stabilize the joint. A synovial membrane invests the joint cavity and the bone between the articular cartilage boundaries and the capsule insertion (bare area). Fibrocartilaginous structures and fat pads are void of synovial lining.

shoulder, the triangular fibrocartilage in the wrist, and the volar and plantar plates in hand and foot), intra-articular ligaments, fad pads (such as the Hoffa pad behind the patellar tendon and the elbow pads); and the synovial fluid in the joint space, act as shock absorbers and increase the congruence of the articular surfaces.[13] The fibrocartilaginous structures are homogeneously hyperechoic and adherent to the bone or joint capsule. Because of their deep position in the joint, they can only be partially evaluated. Intrajoint ligaments are invisible on ultrasound because of overlapping bones. Fat pads are hyperechogenic structures (**Fig. 2**).

JOINT ABNORMALITIES
Joint Effusion

Ultrasound is highly sensitive, although not specific, in detecting joint fluid that may indicate a joint problem. Different types of synovial effusion (traumatic, inflammatory, infectious, or neoplastic) are not definitively differentiated based on their

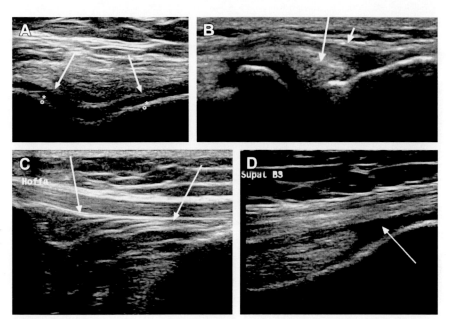

Fig. 2. Ultrasound anatomy of a synovial joint. Knee joint. (A) Normal hypoechoic hyaline cartilage (arrows) covering the hyperechoic subchondral bone (asterisks and circles). (B) Fibrocartilage lateral meniscus (long arrow) attached to the articular capsule. Lateral collateral ligament reinforcing the capsule (short arrow). (C) Hoffman fat pad (Hoffa) (arrows). (D) Anechoic synovial fluid (arrow) in the suprapatellar bursa (Supat BS).

ultrasound appearance (**Fig. 3**). Noninfectious nonhemorrhagic fluid is anechoic or may contain scattered echoes caused by proteins, fibrin, crystals, or cellular debris. Synovial inflammation or infection may appear as an irregularly thickened synovium with hypoechoic or echogenic fluid.[14] Hemarthrosis may be highly echoic in the acute phase. Lipohemarthrosis appears as a fat-fluid level, because of echogenic fat over hypoechogenic blood, and can be considered highly suspicious of intra-articular fracture.[15]

Rheumatoid Arthritis

Rheumatoid arthritis is a chronic inflammatory joint disease of unknown origin affecting primarily the small hand and proximal interphalangeal joints, sparing the distal interphalangeal joints. The early diagnosis of synovitis is an indication to initiate adequate therapy. Synovial hyperemia is the first symptom, followed by edema and swelling of the synovium and joint effusion. Hypertrophy of the synovial membrane leads to progressive damage of the articular cartilage, joint surface, and subchondral bone, with formation of subchondral cysts and erosions, ligament and capsular tearing, joint instability, and deformities. The hallmark of rheumatoid arthritis is the bilateral symmetric involvement of more than 3 joints. Ultrasound can estimate the amount of cartilage destroyed and detect joint space abnormalities and the

presence of loose bodies, seen as hypoanechoic "rice bodies" a few millimeters in size (**Fig. 4**).[16,17] Hypervascular pannus may be easily diagnosed on color Doppler, which has proved to be even more sensitive than MRI in detecting synovitis. Contrast-enhanced ultrasound seems to be an effective means to assess the activity of the disease.

Seronegative (Rheumatoid Factor–Negative) Arthropathies

Psoriasis arthritis is a chronic disorder with significant joint damage that asymmetrically affects mainly the distal interphalangeal joints. Ultrasound can assess synovitis, entesitis, and tenosynovitis (**Fig. 5**). Ankylosing spondylitis affects large joints, leading to joint narrowing, subchondral sclerosis, and synovitis. Reiter arthritis is more prevalent in the distal lower extremities, leading to new bone deposition. Inflammatory bowel disease arthritis commonly affects the knee and ankle and is transitory and nondestructive.

Septic Arthritis

Septic arthritis is a rapidly destructive monoarticular process, involving the large joints. Ultrasound detects early joint effusion, before cartilage destruction, as a low-level echoes effusion and thickened synovial walls. Hyperechoic effusion with debris and septations may also be found

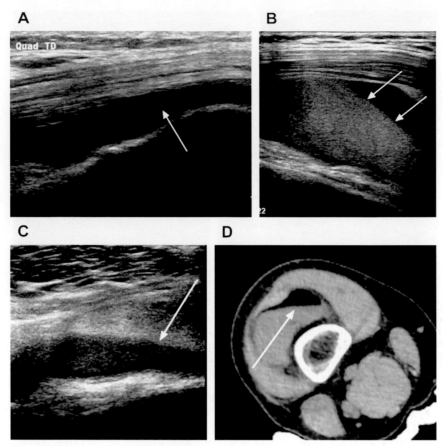

Fig. 3. Joint effusion. Suprapatellar knee recess. (*A*) Anechoic fluid in the suprapatellar bursa (*arrow*), which may be related to mechanical or inflammatory conditions. (*B*) Hyperechoic hemorrhagic fluid with a fluid-fluid level (*arrows*). (*C*) Lipohemarthrosis, fatty-fluid level composed of an echogenic fat layer over hypoechogenic blood (*arrow*). (*D*) Computed tomography correlation showing the fatty-fluid level (*arrow*) from the hypodense fat over the isodense blood.

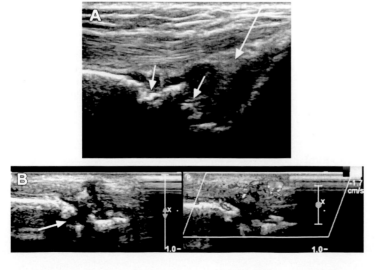

Fig. 4. Rheumatoid arthritis. (*A*) Bone erosions (*short arrows*), hypoechoic thickened synovium (*long arrow*), and synovial effusion at the dorsal wrist. (*B*) Split scan at the third finger proximal interphalangeal joint. Bone erosions on gray scale (*arrow, left slot*) and hypervascular synovial pannus on color Doppler (*right slot*) are shown. Note the low velocity scale on color Doppler (1.7 cm/s) to increase the flow sensitivity of small vessels.

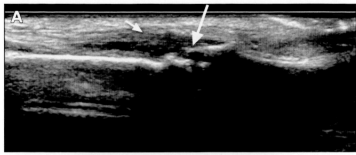

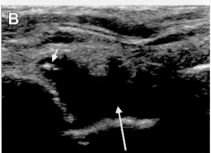

Fig. 5. Psoriatic arthritis. (*A*) Destruction of the articular surfaces (*long arrow*) and extensor tendon tenosynovitis (*short arrow*), at first toe interphalangeal joint. (*B*) Proliferative lesion of bone (*short arrow*) and joint effusion (*long arrow*) in anterior tibiotarsal joint.

(**Fig. 6**). On dynamic examination with probe compression, echoes swirling into the fluid may be seen. Color and power Doppler show hyperemia in hypertrophic synovium and para-articular tissues. Fluid aspiration is needed to confirm infection.

Osteoarthritis

Osteoarthritis is a degenerative process of the articular cartilage and bone margins, comprising a heterogeneous group of disorders, and is the most widespread form of joint disease in the western world.[18] Aging, genetic factors, local joint injuries, obesity, muscle weakness, chronic underuse, and repetitive overuse are some factors that contribute to the development of osteoarthritis. Osteoarthritis initially affects the articular cartilage, causing edema, followed by fibrillation, clefts, ulcerations, and, in several forms, cartilage loss. The subchondral bone shows sclerosis, cysts (geodes), and marginal osteophytes. Intra-articular loose bodies from detached cartilage or bone fragments may activate new cartilage or bone formation. Ultrasound is seldom used to diagnose osteoarthritis. Diagnosis is based on clinical and radiographic evaluation. Ultrasound may show articular cartilage thinning and irregularity, bone osteophytes, and abnormalities in soft tissue (**Fig. 7**),[19] and is helpful in guiding intra-articular injections.

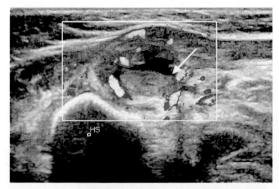

Fig. 6. Septic arthritis. Fluid-pus level (*arrow*) in the right subacromial-subdeltoid bursa in a 2-month infant. Hyperemia in synovial lining is seen on color Doppler. HS, humeral shaft.

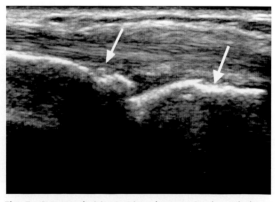

Fig. 7. Osteoarthritis. Erosive changes in the subchondral bone at the dorsal wrist (*arrows*).

Deposition Arthropathies

Arthropathies developing from microcrystalline deposition in synovium, articular cartilage, and para-articular soft tissues lead to chronic synovitis with intermittent acute flares. Gout (caused by crystals of monosodium urate deposition); chondrocalcinosis or pseudogout (caused by calcium pyrophosphate dihydrate [CPPD] crystal deposition), and hydroxyapatite deposition disease (HADD) (caused by deposition of calcium phosphate crystals), are deposition arthropathies.[20] Gout typically affects the first metatarsophalangeal joint and pseudogout affects the knee, but any joint may be involved. Ultrasound findings in an inflamed joint are not specific, sharing the presentation of acute synovitis, namely joint effusion, para-articular edema, and hyperemia. On ultrasound, hyperechogenic deposits can be seen on articular cartilage and on tendons, close to the bone insertion (**Fig. 8**).

Trauma

Traumatic injuries affecting joints can lead to osteochondral fractures. Degenerative osteoarthritis, osteochondromatosis, and neuropathy may follow joint fractures with progressive joint derangement.[21] Ultrasound examinations may show irregularities at the joint surface, involving the articular cartilage and the hyperechoic line of the subchondral bone. Intra-articular loose bodies, representing osseous, cartilaginous, or combined fragments released in the joint cavity, may be seen and even displaced when applying transducer pressure (**Fig. 9**). Fibrocartilaginous tears, such as of the meniscus in the knee, labrum in the shoulder, and triangular fibrocartilage in the wrist, can only be partially seen on ultrasound because of their position in close contact with the bones.[22] Fibrocartilaginous tears may be indirectly inferred from the presence of parameniscal

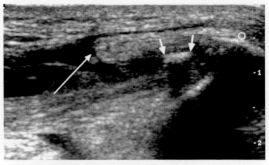

Fig. 9. Osteochondral fracture. After a complete tear of the quadriceps tendon (*arrow*) and patellar dislocation (*circle*), an osteochondral loose body is seen in the suprapatellar recess (*small arrows*), surrounded by synovial fluid or blood.

and paralabral cysts that derive from synovial fluid extruded through a tear, displacing the capsule into the surrounding tissue (**Fig. 10**). Tears of ligaments around joints can be seen with ultrasound. An acute torn ligament appears swollen and hypoechoic; a partially torn ligament is seen as continuous (**Fig. 11**), whereas a totally torn ligament is discontinuous, with a hypoechoic intrasubstance cleft or retracted free ends (**Fig. 12**). With a chronic partial tear, the ligament remains thick and calcifications may occur. Dynamic maneuvers under ultrasound are useful in diagnosing partial tears. Widening of the joint space may be seen under stress because of loss of normal tightness of the torn ligament.[23]

Masses

Synovial space-occupying lesions, such as pigmented villonodular synovitis, lipoma arborescence, synovial osteochondromatosis, and hemangioma, may be seen in patients referred for ultrasound because of a painful or swollen joint and decreased range of motion, mainly involving

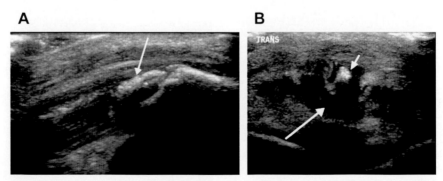

Fig. 8. Deposition arthropathy. (*A*) Calcifying tendinitis. Calcium hydroxyapatite deposits in quadriceps tendon at the patellar insertion (*arrow*). (*B*) Chondrocalcinosis. Hyperechogenic deposits of calcium pyrophosphate dehydrate (*short arrow*) and joint effusion (*long arrow*) in suprapatellar bursa.

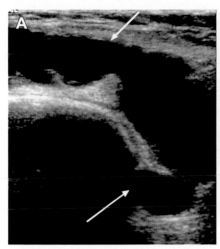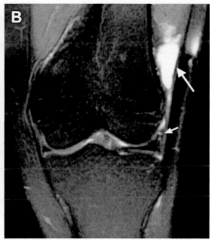

Fig. 10. Parameniscal cyst associated with fibrocartilaginous tears. (A) An irregular cyst with internal septa was detected, adjacent to the lateral meniscus (*arrows*). (B) Magnetic resonance imaging correlation. A lateral meniscal cleft (*short arrow*) and meniscal cyst (*long arrow*) on MRI of the knee.

the knee. Pigmented villonodular synovitis is considered either a chronic inflammatory process or a benign neoplasm.[24] Ultrasound findings in the diffuse type show the presence of a diffusely finger-like thickened synovium and, in the focal type, show an irregular intrajoint mass associated with joint effusion and synovial hyperemia on Doppler color (Fig. 13).[25] Lipoma arborescence is a rare monoarticular disorder, characterized by focal fat-containing synovial proliferation. Ultrasound shows an hyperechogenic mass from the presence of fat, seen as villous tree-shaped projections of the synovium, with intermittent joint effusion (Fig. 14). Synovial osteochondromatosis is a benign condition, characterized by proliferation of synovial chondral or osteochondral nodules that are later released within the joint cavity. Synovial chondromatosis is a primary disease, and must be differentiated from other causes of secondary chondromatosis. Ultrasound shows thickened synovium with hypoechoic nodules that may calcify (Fig. 15). Synovial hemangioma is a rare benign tumor. On ultrasound, hypoechoic tissue with fluid-filled areas is seen, occasionally with slow flow on Doppler color. Magnetic resonance imaging is pathognomonic, with marked hyperintense areas on T2-weighted imaging and after gadolinium injection.[26]

ULTRASOUND-GUIDED PROCEDURES

Interventional procedures under ultrasound guidance related to joints, both for diagnostic and therapeutic purposes, range from simple and commonly performed ones, such as fluid aspiration and steroid injection in joints or para-articular tissues, to more complex ones, such as needle biopsy of space-occupying lesions and removal

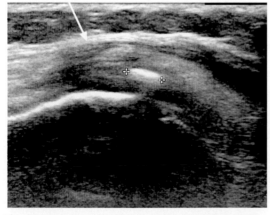

Fig. 11. Acute partial ligament tear. A swollen and hypoechoic medial collateral ligament is seen (*arrow*) from a twisting injury of the knee. The hyperechogenic line (*cursors*) represents an osteochondral fracture.

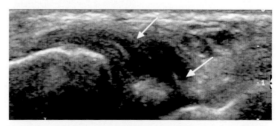

Fig. 12. Complete ligament tear. Anterior talofibular ligament tear at left ankle. A hematoma fills in the gap between the free ends (*arrows*).

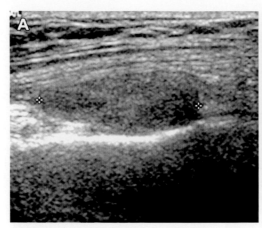
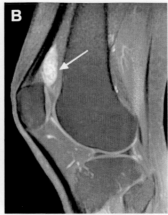

Fig. 13. Pigmented villonodular synovitis. (*A*) Hypoechoic oval mass (*cursors*) at the suprapatellar recess. (*B*) Magnetic resonance imaging of the knee shows an intensely enhanced lesion in the suprapatellar recess (*arrow*) on T1-weighted imaging with gadolinium.

of foreign bodies.[27–29] Patients are required to sign an informed consent after being informed of the procedure steps, benefits, and risks. Ultrasound examination of the target joint is performed to localize the lesion and plan the best path of approach. The skin is disinfected and a sterile sheath with a hole over the area of interest is placed. A sterile set of instruments and a sterile cover for the probe are used (**Fig. 16**). Local anesthesia is injected at the point of puncture. Applying a freehand approach, the needle is advanced under continuous ultrasound control. With the long-axis approach, the needle is detected as a bright straight echo with posterior reverberations, and the needle tip is seen as a strong echo with a posterior acoustic shadow. With the short-axis approach, just the needle tip is visualized into the target (**Fig. 17**). Arthrocentesis is indicated when substantial fluid is found in a symptomatic joint, and should be routinely performed in patients with monoarthritis (**Fig. 18**). Synovial fluid analysis for leucocytes, fluid culture, and microcrystals can lead to the diagnosis of septic arthritis, gout, and chondrocalcinosis. Drainage of soft tissue collections can be precisely performed under ultrasound guidance. Large Baker cysts may be evacuated to release pressure and pain (**Fig. 19**). Injection procedures using a mixture of lidocaine and steroid within joint cavities and tendon sheaths are better performed under ultrasound guidance than blindly, especially in small or deeply localized joints (**Fig. 20**, Video 1). Precise location of the needle is essential to avoid intratendonal or periarticular soft tissue injections that may lead to corticosteroid-induced tendon necrosis and rupture or necrosis of subcutaneous tissues. After

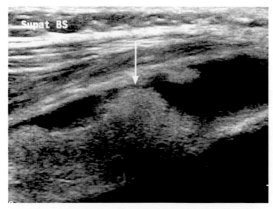

Fig. 14. Lipoma arborescence. Hyperechogenic tree-shaped intra-articular mass in the knee (*arrow*), surrounded by fluid.

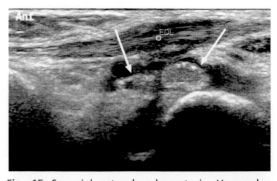

Fig. 15. Synovial osteochondromatosis. Hyperechogenic nodules with foci of calcifications surrounded by fluid are detected at the anterior recess of the ankle (*arrows*). Signs of tenosynovitis in the extensor digitorum longus (EDL) tendon running above the lesions.

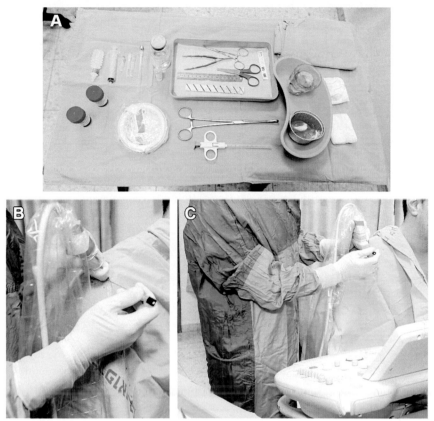

Fig. 16. Preparation for an ultrasound-guided interventional procedure. (*A*) Strict aseptic technique includes sterile instruments, sterile gel, local anesthesia, sterile needles for fluid aspiration and therapeutic drug injection, and sterile tubes. (*B, C*) Ultrasound guided needle insertion is shown, using sterile skin, wrapped sterile probe, and sterile gloves.

injection, the needle should be washed with injection of saline before removal to avoid spreading corticosteroid into the soft tissue along the needle path. Tumor biopsy of soft tissue and lytic areas in bone tumors under ultrasound guidance allows precise location of the needle, avoiding areas of necrosis and large tumor vessels (**Fig. 21**).[30] Large core biopsies are performed with a 14- to 18-gauge needle in a biopsy gun, whereas for fine-needle aspiration biopsies, an 18- to 22-gauge needle is

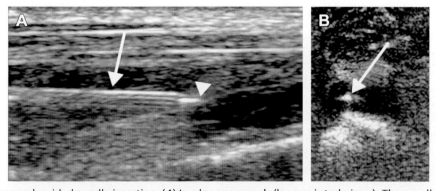

Fig. 17. Ultrasound-guided needle insertion. (*A*) In-plane approach (long-axis technique). The needle is advanced at an angle relative to the ultrasound beam, allowing visualization of the whole shaft, which is seen as a bright straight echo (*arrow*), and the needle tip, seen as a bright short echo (*arrowhead*). (*B*) Out-of-plane approach (short-axis technique). The needle is advanced parallel to the probe, which is tilted continuously to visualize the needle tip. The needle tip is seen as a single bright dot (*arrow*).

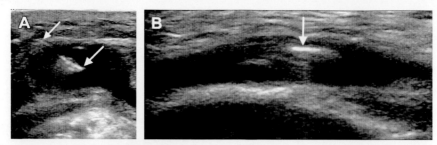

Fig. 18. Arthrocentesis. (*A*) In-plan approach. The needle shaft is seen as a bright straight line with the needle tip in the fluid-filled subacromial subdeltoid bursa (*arrows*). (*B*) Septic arthritis of hip. Drainage of anterior recess fluid under ultrasound guidance (*arrow*), performed using an out-of-plane approach.

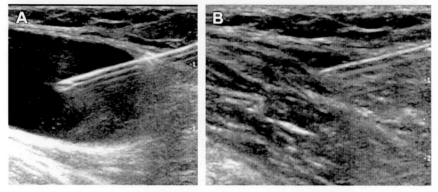

Fig. 19. Drainage of a large Baker cyst. (*A*) A 20-gauge spinal needle is placed under ultrasound guidance using a posterior approach to evacuate fluid and release intracystic pressure and pain. (*B*) Complete cystic drainage at the end of the procedure.

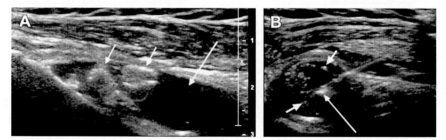

Fig. 20. Injection procedure. (*A*) Fluid (*long arrow*) and free foreign bodies (*short arrows*) are seen in the inferior recess of the subacromial subdeltoid bursa on longitudinal scan. (*B*) A mixture of lidocaine and corticosteroid is injected under ultrasound guidance on transverse scan. Diffusion of the drugs into the joint can be seen as a hyperechoic filling because of air bubbles in the fluid (*short arrows*) surrounding the needle tip (*long arrow*).

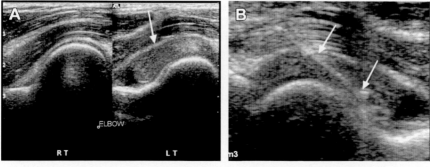

Fig. 21. Tumor biopsy. (*A*) Intra-articular oval mass in left anterior elbow joint (*arrow*). In a split image, the normal contralateral elbow is shown for comparison. (*B*) A core needle was placed into the intra-articular mass under ultrasound guidance (*arrows*) and fired by a Tru-Cut biopsy gun, The histologic diagnosis was pigmented villonodular synovitis.

used. Close collaboration with tumor surgeons is key in applying a correct approach, ensuring that the needle path is within the planned area of tumor resection. Removal of foreign bodies under ultrasound assistance may be performed using a forceps inserted through a small incision in the skin, following the precise localization of the foreign body. Ultrasound-guided regional anesthesia is increasingly used for anesthetic blocks of the brachial plexus in the upper limb, psoas compartment block, pudendal nerve block, and femoral, lateral femoral cutaneous, and obturator nerve blocks in the lower limb.[31,32] Ultrasound-guided interventions are also performed for the treatment of conditions such as amputation stump neuromas, Morton neuroma in the forefoot, and carpal tunnel syndrome, and for the aspiration of ganglia. Percutaneous treatment of calcifying tendinitis, particularly at the rotator cuff, relies on puncturing the calcification into fragments and aspirating the calcium.

SUPPLEMENTARY DATA

Video related to this article can be found online at http://dx.doi.org/10.1016/j.cult.2014.03.004.

REFERENCES

1. Jacobson JA. Fundamentals of musculoskeletal ultrasound. Philadelphia: Saunders/Elsevier; 2007.
2. Bianchi S, Martinoli C. Ultrasound of the musculoskeletal system. Berlin, New York: Springer; 2007.
3. AIUM Practice Guideline for the Performance of a Musculoskeletal Ultrasound Examination. Guideline developed in conjunction with the American College of Radiology (ACR), the Society for Pediatric Radiology (SPR), and the Society of Radiologists in Ultrasound (SRU). American Institute of Ultrasound in Medicine. 2012. Available at: www.aium.org/resources/guidelines.
4. European Society of Musculoskeletal Radiology (ESSR). Musculoskeletal ultrasound: technical guidelines. Insights Imaging 2010;1:99–141.
5. Naredo E, Bijlsma JW, Conaghan PG, et al. Recommendations for the content and conduct of European League Against Rheumatism (EULAR) musculoskeletal ultrasound courses. Ann Rheum Dis 2008;67:1017 22.
6. Jacobson JA. Shoulder US: anatomy, technique and scanning pitfalls. Radiology 2011;260:6–16.
7. Gaitini D, Militianu D, Nachtigal A, et al. Shoulder. In: Dogra V, Gaitini D, editors. Musculoskeletal ultrasound with MRI correlations. Stuttgart (Germany), New York: Thieme; 2010. p. 337–9.
8. Gaitini D. Shoulder ultrasonography: performance and common findings. J Clin Imaging Sci 2012;2:38.
9. Lin CD, Nazarian LN, O'Kane PL, et al. Advantages of real time spatial compound sonography of the musculoskeletal system versus conventional sonography. AJR Am J Roentgenol 2002;171:1629 31.
10. Lin EC, Middleton WD, Teefey SA. Extended field of view sonography in musculoskeletal imaging. J Ultrasound Med 1999;18:147–52.
11. Gaitini D. Introduction to color Doppler ultrasound. In: Wortsman X, Jemec G, editors. Dermatologic ultrasound with clinical and histologic correlations. New York: Springer; 2013. p. 3–14.
12. Claudon M, Tranquart F, Evans DG, et al. Advances in ultrasound. Eur Radiol 2002;12:7–18.
13. Zamorani MP, Valle M. Bone and joint. In: Bianchi S, Martinoi C, editors. Ultrasound of the musculoskeletal system. Berlin, Heidelberg (Germany): Springer; 2007. p. 189–331.
14. Wilson DJ. Soft tissue and joint infection. Eur Radiol 2004;14:64–71.
15. Bianchi S, Zwass A, Abdelwahab IF, et al. Sonographic evaluation of lipohemarthrosis: clinical and in vitro study. J Ultrasound Med 1995;14:279–82.
16. Taouli B, Guermazi A, Sack K, et al. Imaging of the hand and wrist in RA. Ann Rheum Dis 2002;61:867–9.
17. Martini G, Tregnaghi A, Bordin T, et al. Rice bodies imaging in juvenile idiopathic arthritis. J Rheumatol 2003;30:2720–1.
18. Felson DT. An update on the pathogenesis and epidemiology of osteoarthritis. Radiol Clin North Am 2004;42:1–9.
19. Grassi W, Filipuchi E, Farina A. Ultrasonography in osteoarthritis. Semin Arthritis rheum 2005;34:19–23.
20. Clement JP IV, Kassarjian A, Palmer WE. Synovial inflammatory process in the hand. Eur J Radiol 2005;56:307–18.
21. Bianchi S, Martinoli C. Detection of loose bodies in joints. Radiol Clin North Am 2000;37:536–9.
22. Azzoni R, Cabitza P. Is there a role for sonography in the diagnosis of tears of the knee menisci? J Clin Ultrasound 2002;30:472–6.
23. Brasseur JL, Morvan G, Godoc B. Dynamic ultrasonography. J Radiol 2005;86:1804–910.
24. Mukhopadhyay K, Smith M, Hughes PM. Multifocal PVNS in a child followed over 25 years. Skeletal Radiol 2006;35:539–42.
25. Middleton WD, Patel V, Teefey SA, et al. Giant cell tumors of the tendon sheath: analysis of sonographic findings. AJR Am J Roentgenol 2004;183:337–9.
26. Okahashi K, Sugimoto K, Iwai M, et al. Intra-articular synovial hemangioma: a rare cause of knee pain and swelling. Arch Orthop Trauma Surg 2004;124:571–3.
27. Hadduck TA, van Hosbeeck MT, Girish G, et al. Value of ultrasound before joint aspiration. AJR Am J Roentgenol 2013;201:W453–9.
28. Cardinal E, Chhem RK, Beauregard CG. Ultrasound-guided interventional procedures in the

musculoskeletal system. Radiol Clin North Am 1998;
36:597–604.

29. Adler RS, Sofka CM. Percutaneous ultrasound-guided injections in the musculoskeletal system. Ultrasound Q 2003;19:3–12.

30. Gil-Sanchez S, Marco-Domenech SE, Irurzun-Lopez J, et al. Ultrasound-guided skeletal biopsies. Skeletal Radiol 2001;30:615–9.

31. Jandrasits O, Likar R, Marhofer P, et al. The use of ultrasonography for regional anesthetic techniques: upper extremity blockades. Acta Anaesthesiol Scand 1998;24:48–51.

32. Kiechmail L, Entner T, Kapral S, et al. Ultrasound guidance for the psoas compartment block: an imaging study. Anesth Analg 2002;93: 477–81.

Ultrasonography of Peripheral Nerves
Anatomy and Pathology

Bianca Bignotti, MD[a],*, Alberto Tagliafico, MD[b],
Carlo Martinoli, MD[a]

KEYWORDS

- Peripheral nerve • Ultrasonography • Anatomy • Pathology

KEY POINTS

- High-resolution ultrasonography (US) allows swift evaluation of peripheral nerves of the upper and lower extremities.
- Peripheral nerves are characterized by fascicular echotexture, made up of alternated bands of hypoechoic fascicles and hyperechoic epineurium.
- High-resolution US provides morphologic information regarding a variety of nerve abnormalities, including entrapment syndromes, traumatic injuries, polyneuropathies, and neurogenic masses.
- US can improve clinical decision making regarding conservative or surgical treatment.
- US is an important complement to clinical and electrophysiology for the diagnostic assessment of patients with peripheral neuropathies.

INTRODUCTION

Peripheral nerve imaging is an important complement to clinical and neurophysiologic assessment in the evaluation of peripheral nerves. For this assessment, ultrasonography (US) and magnetic resonance (MR) imaging represent the techniques of choice. Conventional MR and its promising techniques, such as MR neurography, diffusion tensor imaging, and fiber tractography,[1] are especially recommended for the settings of deep nerve or central diseases but are not always available and need a long acquisition time. US is the first-choice imaging technique for the assessment of peripheral nerves: it is a low-cost, widely available technique that allows dynamic imaging and evaluation of the entire segment of a nerve during one examination,[1] but it requires a long learning curve and anatomic competence.

ANATOMY AND US TECHNIQUE

The internal structure of the peripheral nerves consists of myelinated and nonmyelinated nerve fibers. Each nerve fiber is embedded in an intimate connective tissue sheath, the endoneurium. Fibers are banded together in nerve fascicles, which are surrounded by the interfascicular perineurium, which consists of perineurial cells and collagen. Nerve fascicles are then bounded by the outer epineurium, which represents the nerve sheath.[2] Nerves differ from each other in size and the number of fascicles.

US images of peripheral nerves correlate considerably with nerve structure (**Fig. 1**), showing, during a long-axis scan, a characteristic fascicular appearance because of the parallel course of nerve fascicles, which look like hypoechoic bands, alternated with hyperechoic bands related to the

Funding sources: no funding sources.
Conflict of interest: no conflict of interest.
[a] Radiology Department, DISSAL, Università di Genova, Via Pastore 1, Genova 16132, Italy; [b] Department of Experimental Medicine, DIMES, Università di Genova, Largo R. Benzi 8, Genova 16132, Italy
* Corresponding author.
E-mail address: bignottibianca@gmail.com

Ultrasound Clin 9 (2014) 525–536
http://dx.doi.org/10.1016/j.cult.2014.03.006

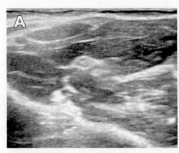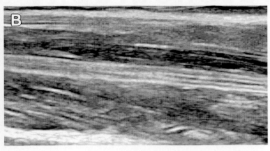

Fig. 1. (*A*) Short-axis scan and (*B*) long-axis scan showing the normal US appearance of a peripheral nerve. Note the characteristic fascicular pattern of the peripheral nerve.

epineurium; a short-axis scan shows the nerve as an oval or round structure with hypoechoic rounded fascicles surrounded by hyperechoic areas of connective tissue.[3]

The analogous hyperechoic appearances of the epineurium and the perineural fat make the nerve contour difficult to define.

Peripheral nerves are mobile structures, and during US dynamic examination, they can slip over the surface of an artery, tendon, or muscle. Nerves are less susceptible to anisotropy than tendons, so tilting the probe does not change the appearance of the nerve.[3]

Deep technical skills and anatomic knowledge are necessary for a good scanning technique. US of peripheral nerves requires a linear high-frequency (center frequency >10 MHz) transducer. A US scan begins in the short axis and proceeds by moving the transducer proximally and distally, using an elevator technique, to assess the entire course of the nerve.[3] In particular, it is important to evaluate the size, shape, and texture of the nerve and the appearance of adjacent structures. Longitudinal US evaluation of the nerve is subsequently performed. It is then possible to perform a dynamic examination, which can show nerve instability or compression in relation to muscle contraction or movement of the joints.

US can show nerves that are in a superficial position and are not covered by bone structures; however, it cannot visualize deep nerves or a nerve course under bony structures, such as cranial nerves, nerve roots exiting in the dorsal, lumbar, and sacral spine, sympathetic chains, and the splanchnic nerves in the abdomen.

ANATOMIC VARIANTS

The importance of anatomic variants of peripheral nerves is related to the patient's symptoms and the surgical treatment plan.

The most frequent variant found in clinical practice is the bifid median nerve at the wrist,[4,5] which consists of 2 contiguous bundles of fascicles within the carpal tunnel (**Fig. 2**).

The bifid median nerve can be associated with the persistent median artery, which originates from the ulnar artery at the proximal forearm and passes close to the median nerve throughout the forearm and carpal tunnel. This accessory artery can also occur with a normal nerve.

Nerve variants also include an unusual course, such as the C5 root, which runs in front of the anterior scalene muscle.[6]

There are several extrinsic abnormalities that may determine nerve compression. An example is the supracondylar process, which may occur with Struthers ligament, which inserts on the medial epicondyle of the distal humerus, forming an osteofibrous tunnel, in which the median nerve and brachial artery pass and may predispose to entrapment syndrome. Moreover, there are several anomalous muscles that may entrap a nerve; for example, the chondroepitrochlearis and the anconeus epitrochlearis may both cause compression of the ulnar nerve, respectively, at the axilla and at the elbow.[7] The Gantzer muscle is an accessory head of the flexor pollicis longus that can determine entrapment of the anterior interosseous nerve in the proximal forearm.[7] A proximal tendon and a distal muscle bell characterize

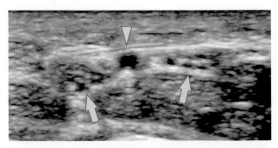

Fig. 2. Grayscale transverse US image of the bifid median nerve. Note the 2 contiguous bundles of fascicles (*arrows*) within the carpal tunnel. *Arrowhead*, persistent median artery.

reversed palmaris longus; it can predispose to carpal or Guyon tunnel syndrome caused by excess muscle tissue at the level of the wrist.[7] The median nerve can also be compressed at the level of the carpal tunnel by the palmaris profundus. This muscle arises from the flexor digitorum superficialis or the distal radius and ulna, passes through the carpal tunnel, and inserts into the flexor retinaculum. The nerve and the tendon may occasionally share the sheath (musculus concomitants nervi mediani).

The accessory abductor digiti minimi constitutes the roof of the Guyon tunnel; when it is hypertrophied, it may determine ulnar compression.[7] Patients with tarsal tunnel syndrome may present with flexor digitorum accessorius longus that crosses the tarsal tunnel close to the tibial nerve.[8]

Moreover, nerve instability may be predisposed by congenital absence of the retinacula at the osteofibrous tunnels. Dynamic examination can show an anterior dislocation of the ulnar nerve over the medial epicondyle in the case of nerve instability; it may occur with a snapping triceps syndrome, a displacement of a hypertrophied medial head of the triceps muscle.[9]

COMPRESSIVE NEUROPATHY

Entrapment syndrome is usually determined by chronic or dynamic compression of nerves in fibro-osseous or fibromuscular tunnels, caused by their rigid wall or related to the presence of a space-occupying lesion, such as accessory muscles, ganglia, or osteophytes; other causes of compression along the nerve course are less common. Entrapment syndrome determines motor and sensory disturbances caused by ischemia, Wallerian degeneration, and fibrosis of the nerve. For this condition, neurophysiologic studies and MR can also be helpful.[10,11] US is particularly useful to define the exact point of compression with evidence of tunnel anatomy and delineation of nerve morphology. Depending on US evaluation, entrapment syndrome can be divided into 3 main classes:

- Class 1 includes large nerves such as the median, ulnar, peroneal, and tibial nerve, which are easily visualized by US with a probe frequency up to 13 MHz. Morphologic alterations and nerve cross-sectional area (CSA) are defined with high performance, similar to MR imaging.
- Class 2 includes small nerves with caliber less than 2 mm, such as the posterior and anterior interosseous, muscolocutaneous, sural, and distal divisional branches of large nerves. Their assessment requires high-resolution

US (probe frequency ≤18 MHz) and includes only pattern recognition, because low nerve diameter prevents CSA definition. We consider high-resolution US superior to MR imaging because US can differentiate small nerves from vessels. Often, there are no denervation changes because of the sensory nature of distal nerve branches, and this is the main disadvantage of MR imaging.
- Class 3 include nerves are not well detected by US because of their deep course or interposing bone, which is independent from nerve caliber; some examples are the inferior calcaneal nerve, which is small, and a large nerve such as the sciatic nerve in its intrapelvic course. US cannot assess these nerves directly but can give information about denervation changes in muscles, even if US is not as accurate as MR imaging in early detection (intramuscular extracellular edema).

US shows characteristic features of compressive neuropathy at the level of the entrapment site, identifying the exact point of compression at which the nerve is flattened; proximal to this point, the nerve appears swollen.[12] The steep transition between the flattened and swollen segment is called the notch sign. The early phase of compression includes nerve enlargement caused by intraneural edema and venous congestion, and increased water content, which determines axon loss (axonotmesis)[13]; nerve CSA and the severity of electromyographic findings correlate positively.[14] There may be no fascicular pattern with hypoechoic nerve echotexture, as a result of swelling of the fascicles and loss of echogenicity of the epineurium; this appearance is more severe in long-standing compression.[12] Doppler imaging could be positive because of intraneural hyperemia. In carpal tunnel syndrome (CTS), Doppler signal seems to correlate with disease severity.[15] Long-standing compression leads to intraneural fibrosis, which tends to determine irreversible nerve function damage, which could remain after decompressive surgery.[16]

US assessment of compressive neuropathies includes calculation of the CSA for class 1 nerves or maximum cross-sectional diameter for class 2 nerves. The CSA is calculated with the indirect method using calibers and applying the ellipse formula (transverse diameter × anteroposterior diameter × π/4) or with the direct method using manual tracing and automated calculation of the area.[17] This parameter should be calculated from the outer margin of the hypoechoic fascicles, excluding the outer epineurium, where the nerve appears maximally enlarged, with the most severe alteration in echotexture. It is important to maintain the probe perpendicular to the long axis of the nerve to avoid variability in the CSA calculation. Gender, weight, body mass index, and race can affect the cutoff of nerve CSA.[18]

Using the regional approach, the most frequent sites of nerve entrapment in the upper and lower extremities that can be assessed with US are described in the following sections.

Shoulder

At this level, the most frequent entrapment syndromes involve the suprascapular nerve and the axillary nerve. Suprascapular neuropathy may be determined by stretching injuries, ligament abnormalities, overuse or a space-occupying mass along the nerve course. Denervation changes depend on the level of entrapment: if the nerve is compressed in the supraspinous fossa, both the supraspinatus and infraspinatus muscles are affected, whereas only the infraspinatus muscle is involved if the nerve is compressed at the spinoglenoid notch. The most frequent causes of suprascapular neuropathy are paralabral cysts associated with tears of the posterior glenoid labrum.[19,20] These cysts are often large (>3 cm) and extend into the spinoglenoid or suprascapular notches, causing nerve compression and muscle denervation. Standard US examination of the rotator cuff may lose large cysts because of their deep position. However, when visible, a paralabral cyst appears as an oval hypoechoic lesion with well-defined margins, fixed in position and shape during arm movements; a US scan may also show the continuity of the cyst with the lesion of the posterior labrum; moreover, it can guide percutaneous needle aspiration to decompress the nerve.[21]

Because of its small size and deep position, the axillary nerve can be visualized by US, with the arm elevated, because it runs across the quadrilateral space close to the glenohumeral joint.[22] The most frequent causes of axillary neuropathy are stretching injures and stenosis of the quadrilateral space by fractures, fibrous bands, or inferior paraglenoid cysts.[23] Specific muscle atrophy can be verified by comparing muscles thickness with the infraspinatus muscle or the contralateral healthy side.[24]

Elbow

Ulnar neuropathy may occur both in the proximal and distal tunnel as a result of several causes, such as bony abnormalities (eg, medial osteophytes), enlarged tunnel floor (joint capsule and posterior band of the medial collateral ligament), and space-occupying masses (eg, accessory muscles).

In the early phase of cubital tunnel syndrome, clinical and electrophysiologic diagnosis may be difficult[25]; in cubital tunnel syndrome, a US scan shows a fusiform hypoechoic swelling of the nerve with loss of the fascicular pattern, and an ulnar nerve CSA greater than 10 mm^2 is considered pathologic with a sensitivity of 95% to 100%.[26] Moreover, US dynamic examination with elbow flexion can show nerve impingement, such as for a hypertrophied medial head of triceps.

US evaluates the posterior interosseous nerve at the radial tunnel, and in cases of neuropathy, it can assess nerve impingement against the fibrous arcade or visualize an oval enlargement in the middle of the tunnel.[27] A fibrous band, fan-shaped recurrent radial vessels (leash of Henry), or a closed passage within the supinator are the most frequent causes of posterior interosseous syndrome. Focal nerve swelling in the middle-distal tunnel may also be related to stretching trauma.

The anterior interosseous neuropathy, or Kiloh-Nevin syndrome, is commonly caused by anchor compression: over the elbow, when the fascicles are still included in the median nerve, by a supracondylar bony spur and ligament of Struthers; in the forearm, where the median and the anterior interosseous nerve run in a deep position, passing through the tendinous connection between the humeroulnar and the radial heads of the flexor digitorum superficialis muscle. The most common causes of Kiloh-Nevin syndrome include compression by an extrafibrous band or by anomalous muscles in the forearm (eg, Gantzer muscle). US examination cannot evaluate this small and deep nerve directly, but it can help in the diagnosis by excluding the presence of a mass and assessing the atrophy of muscles supplied by this nerve (flexor pollicis longus, flexor digitorum profundus for the index and middle finger and the pronator quadratus).[28]

Wrist

Although the prevalence of CTS is high, there is no gold standard for its diagnosis. In addition to the diagnostic features of clinical presentation, electrodiagnostic testing, and treatment response, US is crucial to assess the size and morphologic alteration of the median nerve[29] and to identify anatomic variants (eg, bifid median nerve) and space-occupying masses (eg, ganglion cysts) (Fig. 3). Nerve size is based on CSA measurement. Cutoff values range from 9 mm^2 to 13 mm^2 without a definite threshold value, even if many studies consider it to be greater than 10 or 11 mm^2 at the level of the carpal tunnel inlet.[30]

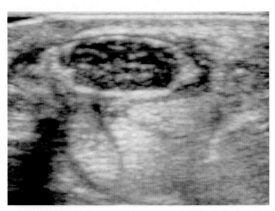

Fig. 3. Grayscale transverse US image of the carpal tunnel in a case of CTS: the median nerve appears markedly swollen and with loss of the normal fascicular pattern.

A comparison between the CSA of the median nerve at the level of the wrist and in a more proximal position is an alternative method to diagnose CTS. Recently, a wrist/forearm ratio of the median nerve CSA was proposed.[31] The CSA is calculated at the level of the distal wrist and 12 cm proximally in the forearm. A wrist/forearm ratio of more than 1.4 has 100% sensitivity for detecting CTS.[31] Others measure the proximal CSA of the median nerve at the level of the proximal third of the pronator quadratus muscle.[32] A difference (ΔCSA) between the 2 measurements of 2 mm² or more has a sensitivity of 99% and a specificity of 100% for a diagnosis of CTS.[32] An analogous procedure can be obtained with CSA measurement of the radial and ulnar branches of the bifid median nerve.[33–37]

Ulnar nerve entrapment rarely occurs in the Guyon canal (Fig. 4). A space-occupying mass (ie, pisotriquetral ganglia, ulnar artery pseudoaneurysms, accessory abductor digiti minimi muscle)[12] may compress the ulnar nerve proximal to

its division (zone 1) or distal to it, involving therefore only one of its terminal branches, the superficial sensory (zone 2) or deep motor (zone 3). The main US landmark of the Guyon canal is the pisiform; the ulnar nerve is appreciated between this bone and the ulnar artery. A dynamic scan allows evaluation of both the sensory branch, which runs superficial to the hamate hook, and the motor branch, which runs in the medial side of the hamate. In the case of acute or chronic (cyclist palsy) compression, the ulnar nerve is pressed against the hamate hook, and the ulnar artery may collapse (hypothenar hammer syndrome).

Hip

US assessment of neuropathy around the hip is limited because of the intrapelvic deep position of the nerves, for which MR imaging is the imaging of choice. However, US could evaluate entrapment syndromes that involve the lateral femoral cutaneous nerve and the femoral nerve in their superficial course.

Lateral femoral cutaneous nerve entrapment at the level of the inguinal ligament determines the so-called meralgia paresthetica, characterized by sensory disorder and numbness in the anterolateral thigh. A US transverse scan may show change in nerve size, especially a fusiform enlargement, which occurs more frequently proximal to the inguinal ligament (Fig. 5).[38,39]

US assessment of the femoral nerve is possible only in the infra-inguinal area, because of its proximal deep position and its distal multiple division with branches smaller than 1 mm. In the lacuna musculorum, the femoral nerve presents an average 22.7 mm² of CSA.[40] Femoral neuropathy at this level is usually caused by space-occupying masses, such as acetabular ganglia or giant iliopsoas bursitis.

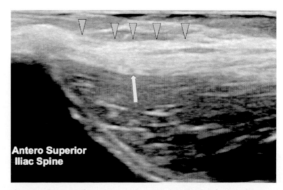

Fig. 5. Grayscale transverse US image of the lateral femoral cutaneous nerve (arrow) at the level of the inguinal ligament (arrowheads), in the proximity of the anterior-superior iliac spine. Normal appearance.

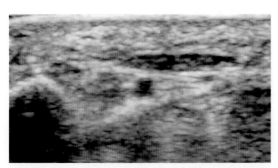

Fig. 4. Grayscale transverse US image of the ulnar nerve at the level of the Guyon canal: normal appearance.

Knee

Peroneal nerve entrapment, which can involve both the common peroneal nerve or one of its branches, may be caused by anatomic accessory structures (eg, enlarged peroneus longus aponeurosis), by postural, dynamic, or idiopathic start (eg, habit of crossing legs), by a space-occupying mass (eg, tibiofibular ganglia), by trauma (eg, fractures), or iatrogenic causes. US assessment of peroneal neuropathy may be characterized by nerve enlargement adjacent to the fibular neck or more proximal to it (**Fig. 6**).[41]

Ankle and Foot

Tibial neuropathy at this level (tarsal tunnel syndrome) causes a sly clinical presentation correlated with the exact site of nerve compression, such as paresthesia or burning pain on the plantar side of the foot, which can irradiate into the toes. The most frequent causes of tarsal tunnel syndrome are bone and joint diseases (eg, spurs, deltoid ligament sprains), space-occupying masses (eg, ganglion cysts) and congenital deformities of the foot; US examination shows compression of the tibial nerve,[42] which usually appears normal (**Fig. 7**).

The deep peroneal nerve can be compressed when it passes under the inferior retinaculum; it is crossed by the extensor hallucis longus and, more distally, by the extensor hallucis brevis. Deep peroneal neuropathy (anterior tarsal tunnel syndrome) can also be determined by midtarsal osteophytes.

The superficial peroneal nerve runs in the lateral leg between the peroneus longus and the extensor digitorum longus muscles. Then, it crosses the crural fascia and becomes superficial almost 10 to 12.5 cm proximal to the lateral malleolus.[43] Repetitive or acute forces at the level of fascia

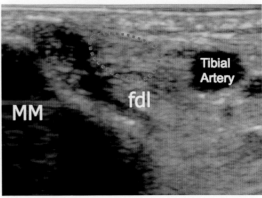

Fig. 7. Grayscale transverse US image of the tibial nerve (*traced line*) at the level of the tarsal tunnel showing a normal US appearance of the nerve. fdl, flexor digitorum longus; MM, medial malleolus.

crossing (eg, inversion ankle sprain) may cause superficial peroneal neuropathy, which is characterized by sensory symptoms along the nerve course.[44] US detects focal nerve enlargement associated with a thickened fascia.

In Morton neuroma, US sensitivity ranges between 85% and 98%.[45] US shows a focal rounded hypoechoic mass (**Fig. 8**) and a distended intermetatarsal bursa.[45,46]

POLYNEUROPATHIES
Inherited Disorders

Charcot-Marie-Tooth (CMT) disease (hereditary motor and sensory neuropathy or peroneal muscular atrophy) includes a large group of inherited conditions that involve the peripheral nervous system.[47] There is a demyelinating (CMT-1) and axonal (CMT-2) form. CMT-1 involves all peripheral nerves and is characterized by general slowing of conduction velocity on electrophysiology and by the onion bulb appearance on

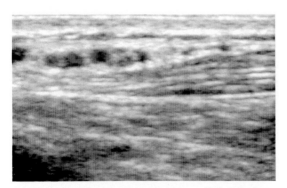

Fig. 6. Grayscale transverse US image of the common peroneal nerve adjacent to the fibular head showing mild enlargement of nerve fascicles compatible with entrapment syndrome.

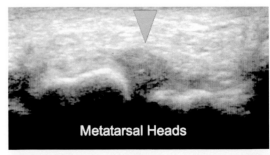

Fig. 8. Grayscale transverse US image of a Morton neuroma (*arrowhead*), which appears as a focal hypoechoic mass located between the heads of the second and third metatarsal bone.

histology caused by Schwann cell hypertrophy.[48] On US evaluation, the nerves are particularly enlarged but with a preserved echotexture.[49,50] CMT-2 includes more different forms with only moderate enlargement of nerves.[45]

Hereditary neuropathy with liability to pressure palsies is characterized by segmental demyelination and tomaculous myelin sheath swelling caused by trivial trauma.[51] US detects fusiform nerve enlargement and fascicular swellings (sausage-shaped) along the course of the nerves.[51]

Immune-Mediated Polyneuropathies

The dysimmune polyneuropathies include acute inflammatory demyelinating polyradiculoneuropathy (Guillain-Barré syndrome), chronic inflammatory demyelinating polyradiculoneuropathy (CIDP), and multifocal motor neuropathy (MMN).[52]

Chronic demyelination of peripheral nerves and their roots with onion bulb formation characterizes CIDP. It could evolve in secondary axonal loss. In correlation with conduction blocks in electrophysiologic studies, US shows segmental swelling of the affected nerve[53] and individually swollen fascicles, both in enlarged and thinned segments.[54]

Guillain-Barré syndrome is an acute polyneuropathy characterized by immune-related damage of myelin. In 80% of cases, mild evolution occurs with rapid recovery. However, in 20% of cases, there is axonal damage and a remyelination process is crucial for recovery. The most effective treatment includes intravenous immunoglobulin and plasmapheresis within the first week of onset of symptoms. US has been suggested to show some abnormalities in the early stage of this polyneuropathy, when electrophysiology may give mild results.[50] US findings include focal enlargement of the nerve or the single fascicle, which may be surrounded by nonaffected fascicles.[55] Moreover, US detects nerve dimension response to treatment (reduction in size) before any neurophysiologic improvement.[55]

MMN is a pure motor neuropathy that is characterized by motor conduction blocks and normal sensory response on electrophysiology. US can show multifocal nerve enlargement.[56]

In patients with acromegaly, the main nerve trunks in the extremities are involved. US shows diffuse nerve enlargement caused by intraneural edema, without changing the fascicular echotexture.[57]

Deposition Disease

Amyloid arthropathy is related to long-term hemodialysis treatment and multiple myeloma. It may be associated with CTS caused by amyloid deposition in the tunnel that compresses the median nerve.[58]

Leprosy

Hansen disease is an infectious disease that affects skin and peripheral nerves, representing the most diffuse neuropathy worldwide. Acute neuritis may occur with a high grade of pain, and US can assess the nerve damage, including nerve enlargement and loss of the fascicular pattern with thickened epineurium,[59,60] which usually occurs near the osteofibrous tunnels, and in particular in proximity to the cubital tunnel. Abnormalities are amplified in acute neuritis recurrence.[59] Intense intraneural hyperemia seen by the Doppler technique may predict the beginning of acute neuritis. In these cases, immediate treatment with corticosteroids is recommended.[59] Moreover, US can guide needle biopsy as an alternative to open nerve biopsy.[61]

TRAUMATIC INJURIES

This group of nerve diseases includes penetrating trauma and stretching and contusion injuries.

There are 3 main groups of nerve fiber injury: neuroapraxia (block of nerve conduction without morphologic alterations), axonotmesis (axon and myelin sheet breakage without damage in the nerve connective tissue framework, which allows axonal regeneration), and neurotmesis (interruption of nerve fascicles and epineurium, which needs surgical treatment). The Sunderland nerve injury classification includes class 1, neuroapraxia; class 2, mild axonotmesis; class 3, severe axonotmesis (ie, axon interruption with undamaged perineurium and epineurium); class 4, severe axonotmesis (ie, axon interruption with only the epineurium remaining intact); and class 5, neurotmesis (ie, complete nerve transection).[62] US cannot recognize class 1 and 2 injuries. In class 3, US detects nerve enlargement with a preserved fascicular pattern. In class 4, US shows an alteration in the nerve caliber with loss of fascicular echotexture. Focal nerve enlargement may correspond to a high grade of axon loss. In class 5, nerve stubs are retracted and it could be difficult in US examination to differentiate severe axonotmesis from neurotmesis.

Penetrating Injuries

In penetrating injury, the nerve can be partially or completely transected. In complete nerve transection, US detects terminal neuroma as a hypoechoic oval mass in continuity with the nerve extremity.[63] Terminal neuroma may also help to recognize dislocated nerve ends and the exact site of damage, especially in small nerve injury. Neuroma may sometimes present an irregular margin because of surrounding tissue or scar tissue adhesion.[63] Connective tissue may be positioned between the near nerve ends simulating a partial tear. In partial transection, a fusiform neuroma may develop in continuity with the nerve, which may involve both preserved and transacted fascicles. US has a high negative predictive value for excluding structural nerve lesions. US may help the treatment decision, especially for minor nerve injury or nerve impingement by fracture, fibrous tissue, or orthopedic devices, when the patient cannot undergo MR imaging. US measurements include the gap between the 2 nerve ends and the neuroma length; these measurements are important for surgical treatment, which could include implant of an appropriate tube of hydrogel between the nerve ends to facilitate proximal nerve regeneration.[64]

Stretching Injuries

In strain injuries with complete laceration, US assesses nerve discontinuity and possible retraction of nerve ends.[65] In the acute setting, US determines nerve damage when MR imaging may be difficult because of local soft tissue edema and hemorrhage. In severe trauma without laceration, US may detect a fusiform hypoechoic enlargement without a fascicular pattern, indicating a neuroma. The brachial plexus is frequently involved in stretching injuries after car accidents. Nerves are particularly susceptible to stretching when they cross the fasciae. In mild stretching injuries, such as burners, US may be normal.

Contusion Trauma

Nerves running above bony surfaces are particularly exposed to external pressure and contusion trauma.[66] Imaging is not always necessary because it could be a reversible condition. US may be useful in cases of repeated minor trauma. US assessment of nerve contusion includes fusiform hypoechoic enlargement of the nerve with swollen fascicles and thickened epineurium.

The Postoperative Nerve

Iatrogenic trauma includes stretching or compressive injury, direct needle trauma, and chemical damage.[67] US can show the status of a postoperative nerve, which includes intraneural edema and hyperemia and possible formation of scar.

In partial transection, surgical treatment includes nerve decompression and intraneural scar elimination; however, some preserved fascicles may be damaged directly or by a new close scar.

In complete transection, nerve reconstruction depends on the end-to-end distance. If this gap is short, the reconstruction consists of anastomosis between nerve extremities; if the gap is greater than 5 mm, a nerve graft is needed (eg, created from the sural nerve). US shows sutures in the perineurium and epineurium as an intraneural hyperechoic spot with comet-tail artifact.

US shows a fusiform thickening of the nerve in the site of the anastomosis, but prominent bulging may indicate inadequate nerve end unification and postoperative neuroma.[67] A postoperative scar may envelop the nerve, and it could be difficult to differentiate from surrounding fibrosis. A long-axis scan may help in showing nerve continuity beyond the scar.

BRACHIAL PLEXOPATHIES

The brachial plexus is formed by the ventral branches of C5, C6, C7, C8, and T1. The roots of the nerve run from the foramina to the interscalene triangle. The roots form 3 main trunks: the upper trunk (roots of C5-C6), middle trunk (roots of C7), and lower trunk (roots of C8-T1). At the level of the supraclavicular region, each trunk divides into anterior and posterior divisions. The divisions merge in many connections, forming the secondary trunks or cords: the lateral cord (formed by the anterior division of the upper and middle trunks), the medial cord (formed by the anterior division of the lower trunk), and the posterior cord (formed by the posterior divisions of each trunk). The cords continue as peripheral nerves: the axillary and radial nerves (from the posterior cord), the musculocutaneous and part of median nerve (from lateral cord), and the ulnar nerve (from the medial cord).

There are 3 main clinically relevant spaces along the nerve course: the interscalene triangle, the costoclavicular space, and the retropectoralis minor space.

Scanning Technique

US can show normal brachial plexus nerves.[68] The main landmarks are bones (roots), muscles (trunks), and vessels (divisions and cords). US assesses the level of nerve roots because the posterior tubercle of C7 is absent.[69] At the interscalene triangle, the most superficial nerve belongs to C5 and the deepest to C8. In the supraclavicular space, the cords can be identified in the posterior aspect of the subclavian artery. US cannot assess the brachial plexus in the costoclavicular space because of the interposition of the clavicle. More distally, in the retropectoralis minor space, the nerves run around the axillary artery.[68]

Traumatic Plexopathies

These plexopathies occur in 5% of high-velocity motor vehicle accidents. Trauma can involve all brachial plexus nerves (complete injury) or only some nerves (incomplete injury). Trauma involving only some nerves is divided into upper (C5, C6 ± C7) or lower (C8, T1 ± C7). Moreover, injuries are also classified as preganglionic or postganglionic (extraforaminal). Treatment planning needs early evaluation of the length and severity of injury.[70] First, preganglionic injuries must be excluded with MR imaging, because of the poor outcome and lack of treatment. If preganglionic lesions are excluded, US can assess brachial plexus lesions outside the spinal canal, offering an alternative to MR imaging. US evaluation includes the identification of a lesion, its site, and the level of nerve involvement. Moreover, US may confirm or exclude nerve transection.[71]

Neurogenic Thoracic Outlet Syndrome

This condition often occurs with neurovascular compression at the interscalene triangle and the costoclavicular space, which cannot be evaluated with US. In patients with supernumerary cervical ribs, US may show nerve division impingement with the rib during stress tests.

Parsonage-Turner Syndrome

MR is the imaging method of choice for the assessment of shoulder girdle muscles involved in this brachial neuritis.

Tumors and Postradiation Imaging

Brachial plexus tumors include primary and secondary tumors. Primary tumors include schwannomas and neurofibromas. In metastasis, US may detect a well-defined solid hypoechoic mass with irregular margins that surround the nerve,[71] but sometimes, tumors may not appear as a clear mass. US is not able to differentiate metastasis from postradiation effects.

NERVE TUMORS AND TUMORLIKE LESIONS
Neurogenic Histotypes (Schwannoma and Neurofibroma)

The most common benign nerve tumors are schwannoma (neurinoma) and neurofibroma. They can be asymptomatic. They may occur as isolated lesions or in association with neurofibromatosis type 1 (NF1). Treatment of these lesions is different: schwannoma is usually removed

without permanent nerve damage, whereas neurofibroma needs transection of the nerve. A US pathognomonic feature is a soft tissue mass in continuity with the nerve.[72] A rim of fat can be found as a triangular echogenic cap at the proximal and distal poles of the mass. US alone cannot truly differentiate schwannomas from neurofibromas. Schwannomas appear as a spherical mass that arises from an individual fascicle and compresses the uninvolved fascicles in the periphery of its bulk (Fig. 9).[72] Neurofibromas appear as a fusiform mass intimately associated with the nerve; US may show the target sign, a hyperechoic fibrous center surrounded by a hypoechoic rim of myxomatous tissue.[72] There are 3 classes of neurofibroma: localized, diffuse, and plexiform.[72]

Malignant peripheral nerve sheath tumors (MPNST) are rare. About 20% to 50% of patients with MPNST have NF1. Malignant transformation must be suspected if there are new symptoms or enlargement of a mass in patients with NF1. MPNST do not present a specific US appearance. Compared with benign tumors, they tend to be larger (>5 cm), with indistinct margins and high vascular flow on Doppler imaging. Sometimes, they show internal bleeding and necrotic areas.

Intraneural perineurioma is a benign tumor that usually involves the sciatic nerve, or its branches, in young people. Its US appearance is specific, showing as a fusiform enlargement with preserved fascicular pattern.

Nonneurogenic Masses

Nerves may be affected by nonneuronal masses, which can infiltrate or join them. These masses include lipomas, paragangliomas, hemangiomas, lymphomas, extrinsic soft tissue neoplasms, and ganglion cysts.[73]

Fibrolipomatous hamartoma presents at birth or childhood and usually involves the median nerve or other nerves of the upper limb. It may be associated with macrodystrophia lipomatosa. US detects

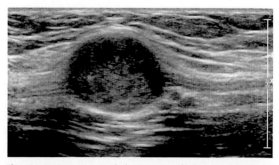

Fig. 9. Nerve tumor (schwannoma): longitudinal US image obtained over a median nerve schwannoma.

hypoechoic enlarged fibrotic neural fascicles separated by echogenic fat.[73]

Intraneural ganglia most frequently involve the common peroneal nerve. US shows a lobulated anechoic mass close to the fibular neck. Muscle atrophy and increased echogenicity of the anterior compartment of the leg may occur. Intraneural ganglia do not present a fibrous capsule.

Traumatic neuroma (stump or amputation neuromas) capsules occur in complete or partial nerve injuries. US can show the degree of nerve damage in the acute setting,[74] frequently a hypoechoic fusiform mass in continuity with the nerve proximal to the injury.

REFERENCES

1. Kermarrec E, Demondion X, Khalil C, et al. Ultrasound and magnetic resonance imaging of the peripheral nerves: current techniques, promising directions, and open issues. Semin Musculoskelet Radiol 2010;14:463–72.

2. Stewart JD. Peripheral nerve fascicles: anatomy and clinical relevance. Muscle Nerve 2003;28: 525–41.

3. Martinoli C, Bianchi S. In: Bianchi S, Martinoli C, editors. Ultrasound of the musculoskeletal system. Berlin: Springer-Verlag; 2007.

4. Propeck T, Quinn TJ, Jacobson JA, et al. Sonography and MR imaging of bifid median nerve with anatomic and histologic correlation. AJR Am J Roentgenol 2000;175:1721–5.

5. Gassner EM, Schocke M, Peer S, et al. Persistent median artery in the carpal tunnel: color Doppler ultrasonographic findings. J Ultrasound Med 2002;21:455–61.

6. Martinoli C, Gandolfo N, Perez MM, et al. Brachial plexus and nerves about the shoulder. Semin Musculoskelet Radiol 2010;14:523–46.

7. Martinoli C, Perez MM, Padua L, et al. Muscle variants of the upper and lower limb (with anatomical correlation). Semin Musculoskelet Radiol 2010;14: 106–21.

8. Sammarco GJ, Stephens MM. Tarsal tunnel syndrome caused by flexor digitorum accessorius longus. J Bone Joint Surg Am 1990;72:453–4.

9. Jacobson JA, Jebson PJ, Jeffers AW, et al. Ulnar nerve dislocation and snapping triceps syndrome: diagnosis with dynamic sonography–report of three cases. Radiology 2001;220:601–5.

10. Spratt JD, Stanley AJ, Grainger AJ, et al. The role of diagnostic radiology in compressive and entrapment neuropathies. Eur Radiol 2002;12:2352–64.

11. Subhawong TK, Wang KC, Thawait SK, et al. High resolution imaging of tunnels by magnetic resonance neurography. Skeletal Radiol 2012;41: 15–31.

12. Martinoli C, Bianchi S, Gandolfo N, et al. US of nerve entrapments in osteofibrous tunnels of the upper and lower limbs. RadioGraphics 2000;20: 199–217.

13. Powell HC, Myers RR. Pathology of experimental nerve compression. Lab Invest 1986;55:91–100.

14. Ziswiler HR, Reichenbach S, Vögelin E, et al. Diagnostic value of sonography in patients with suspected carpal tunnel syndrome: a prospective study. Arthritis Rheum 2005;52:304–11.

15. Ghasemi-Esfe AR, Khalilzadeh O, Vaziri-Bozorg SM, et al. Color and power Doppler US for diagnosing carpal tunnel syndrome and determining its severity: a quantitative image processing method. Radiology 2011;261:499–506.

16. Mondelli M, Filippou G, Aretini A, et al. Ultrasonography before and after surgery in carpal tunnel syndrome and relationship with clinical and electrophysiological findings. A new outcome predictor? Scand J Rheumatol 2008;37:219–24.

17. Alemán L, Berná JD, Reus M, et al. Reproducibility of sonographic measurements of the median nerve. J Ultrasound Med 2008;27:193–7.

18. Thoirs K, Williams MA, Cert G, et al. Ultrasonographic measurements of the ulnar nerve at the elbow. J Ultrasound Med 2008;27:737–43.

19. Tung GA, Entzian D, Stern JB, et al. MR imaging and MR arthrography of paraglenoid labral cysts. AJR Am J Roentgenol 2000;174:1707–15.

20. Martinoli C, Bianchi S, Prato N, et al. US of the shoulder: non-rotator cuff disorders. Radio-Graphics 2003;23:381–401.

21. Hashimoto BE, Hayes AS, Ager JD. Sonographic diagnosis and treatment of ganglion cysts causing suprascapular nerve entrapment. J Ultrasound Med 1994;13:671–4.

22. Loomer R, Graham B. Anatomy of the axillary nerve and its relation to inferior capsular shift. Clin Orthop Relat Res 1989;243:100–5.

23. Chautems RC, Glauser T, Waeber-Fey MC, et al. Quadrilateral space syndrome: case report and review of the literature. Ann Vasc Surg 2000;14: 673–6.

24. Brestas PS, Tsouroulas M, Nikolakopoulou Z, et al. Ultrasound findings of teres minor denervation in suspected quadrilateral space syndrome. J Clin Ultrasound 2006;34:343–7.

25. Campbell WW. Guidelines in electrodiagnostic medicine. Practice parameter for electrodiagnostic studies in ulnar neuropathy at the elbow. Muscle Nerve 1999;8:171–205.

26. Yoon JS, Walker FO, Cartwright MS. Ultrasonographic swelling ratio in the diagnosis of ulnar neuropathy at the elbow. Muscle Nerve 2008;38: 1231–5.

27. Chien AJ, Jamadar DA, Jacobson JA, et al. Sonography and MR imaging of posterior interosseous

nerve syndrome with surgical correlation. AJR Am J Roentgenol 2003;181:219–21.

28. Martinoli C, Bianchi S, Pugliese F, et al. Sonography of entrapment neuropathies in the upper limb (wrist excluded). J Clin Ultrasound 2004;32:438–50.

29. Buchberger W, Judmaier W, Birbamer G, et al. Carpal tunnel syndrome: diagnosis with high-resolution sonography. AJR Am J Roentgenol 1992;159:793–8.

30. Hobson-Webb LD, Padua L, Martinoli C. Ultrasonography in the diagnosis of peripheral nerve disease. Expert Opin Med Diagn 2012;6:457–71.

31. Hobson-Webb LD, Massey JM, Juel VC, et al. The ultrasonographic wrist-to-forearm median nerve area ratio in carpal tunnel syndrome. Clin Neurophysiol 2008;119:1353–7.

32. Klauser AS, Halpern EJ, Zordo De, et al. Carpal tunnel syndrome assessment with US: value of additional cross-sectional area measurements of the median nerve in patients versus healthy volunteers. Radiology 2009;250:171–7.

33. Klauser AS, Halpern EJ, Faschingbauer R, et al. Bifid median nerve in carpal tunnel syndrome: assessment with US cross-sectional area measurement. Radiology 2011;259:808–15.

34. Moran L, Perez M, Esteban A, et al. Sonographic measurement of cross-sectional area of the median nerve in the diagnosis of carpal tunnel syndrome: correlation with nerve conduction studies. J Clin Ultrasound 2009;37:125–31.

35. Miwa T, Miwa H. Ultrasonography of carpal tunnel syndrome: clinical significance and limitations in elderly patients. Intern Med 2011;50:2157–61.

36. Meys V, Thissen S, Rozeman S, et al. Prognostic factors in carpal tunnel syndrome treated with a corticosteroid injection. Muscle Nerve 2011;44:763–8.

37. Tagliafico A, Pugliese F, Bianchi S, et al. High-resolution sonography of the palmar cutaneous branch of the median nerve. AJR Am J Roentgenol 2008;191:107–14.

38. Tagliafico A, Serafini G, Lacelli F, et al. Ultrasound-guided treatment of meralgia paresthetica (lateral femoral cutaneous neuropathy): technical description and results of treatment in 20 consecutive patients. J Ultrasound Med 2011;30:1341–6.

39. Aravindakannan T, Wilder-Smith EP. High resolution ultrasonography in the assessment of meralgia paresthetica. Muscle Nerve 2012;45:434–5.

40. Gruber H, Peer S, Kovacs P, et al. The ultrasonographic appearance of the femoral nerve and cases of iatrogenic impairment. J Ultrasound Med 2003;22:163–72.

41. Peer S, Kovacs P, Harpf C, et al. High-resolution sonography of lower extremity peripheral nerves: anatomic correlation and spectrum of disease. J Ultrasound med 2002;21:315–22.

42. Vijayan J, Therimadasamy AK, Teoh HL, et al. Sonography as an aid to neurophysiological studies in diagnosing tarsal tunnel syndrome. Am J Phys Med Rehabil 2009;88:500–1.

43. Canella C, Demondion X, Guillin R, et al. Anatomic study of the superficial peroneal nerve using sonography. AJR Am J Roentgenol 2009;193:174–9.

44. Johnston EC, Howell SJ. Tension neuropathy of the superficial peroneal nerve: associated conditions and results of release. Foot Ankle Int 1999;20:576–82.

45. Quinn TJ, Jacobson JA, Craig JG, et al. Sonography of Morton's neuromas. AJR Am J Roentgenol 2000;174:1723–8.

46. Hughes RJ, Ali K, Jones H, et al. Treatment of Morton's neuroma with alcohol injection under sonographic guidance: follow-up of 101 cases. AJR Am J Roentgenol 2007;188:1535–9.

47. Dyck RJ, Chance P, Lebo R, et al. Hereditary motor and sensory neuropathies. In: Dyck PJ, Thomas PK, editors. Peripheral neuropathy. 3rd edition. Philadelphia: Saunders; 1993. p. 1094–136.

48. Sereda M, Griffiths I, Pühlhofer A, et al. A transgenic rat model of Charcot-Marie-Tooth disease. Neuron 1996;16:1049–60.

49. Martinoli C, Schenone A, Bianchi S, et al. Sonography of median nerve in Charcot-Marie-Tooth disease. AJR Am J Roentgenol 2002;178:1553–6.

50. Zaidman CM, Al-Lozi M, Pestronk A. Peripheral nerve size in normals and patients with polyneuropathy: an ultrasound study. Muscle Nerve 2009;40:960–6.

51. Hooper DR, Lawson W, Smith L, et al. Sonographic features in hereditary neuropathy with liability to pressure palsies. Muscle Nerve 2011;44:862–7.

52. De Sousa EA, Chin RL, Sander HW, et al. Demyelinating findings in typical and atypical chronic inflammatory demyelinating polyneuropathy: sensitivity and specificity. J Clin Neuromuscul Dis 2009;10:163–9.

53. Granata G, Pazzaglia C, Calandro P, et al. Ultrasound visualization of nerve morphological alteration at the site of conduction block. Muscle Nerve 2009;40:1068–70.

54. Taniguchi N, Itoh K, Wang Y, et al. Sonographic detection of diffuse peripheral nerve hypertrophy in chronic inflammatory demyelinating polyradiculoneuropathy. J Clin Ultrasound 2000;28:488–91.

55. Almeida V, Mariotti P, Veltri S, et al. Nerve ultrasound follow-up in a child with Guillain-Barré syndrome. Muscle Nerve 2012;46:270–5.

56. Beekman R, van den Berg LH, Franssen H, et al. Ultrasonography shows extensive nerve enlargements in multifocal motor neuropathy. Neurology 2005;65:305–7.

57. Tagliafico A, Resmini E, Nizzo R, et al. Ultrasound measurement of median and ulnar nerve cross-sectional area in acromegaly. J Clin Endocrinol Metab 2008;93:905–9.

58. Ferrara MA, Marcelis S. Ultrasound examination of the wrist. J Belge Radiol 1997;80:78–80.

59. Martinoli C, Derchi LE, Bertolotto M, et al. US and MR imaging of peripheral nerves in leprosy. Skeletal Radiol 2000;29:142–50.

60. Visser LH, Jain S, Lokesh B, et al. Morphological changes of the epineurium in leprosy: a new finding detected with high-resolution sonography. Muscle Nerve 2012;46:38–41.

61. Lolge SJ, Morani AC, Chaubal NG, et al. Sonographically guided nerve biopsy. J Ultrasound Med 2005;24:1427–30.

62. Sunderland S, editor. Nerve injuries and their repair: a critical appraisal. New York: Churchill Livingstone; 1991.

63. Chiou HJ, Chou YH, Chiou SY, et al. Peripheral nerve lesions: role of high-resolution US. RadioGraphics 2003;23:E15.

64. Belkas JS, Munro CA, Shoichetb MS, et al. Peripheral nerve regeneration through a synthetic hydrogel nerve tube. Restor Neurol Neurosci 2006;23:19–29.

65. Peer S, Bodner G, Mairer R, et al. Examination of postoperative peripheral nerve lesions with high-resolution sonography. AJR Am J Roentgenol 2001;177:415–9.

66. Toth C. Peripheral nerve injuries attributable to sport and recreation. Phys Med Rehabil Clin N Am 2009;20:77–100.

67. Peer S, Harpf C, Willeit J, et al. Sonographic evaluation of primary peripheral nerve repair. J Ultrasound Med 2003;22:1317–22.

68. Demondion X, Herbinet P, Boutry N, et al. Sonographic mapping of the normal brachial plexus. AJNR Am J Neuroradiol 2003;24:1303–9.

69. Martinoli C, Bianchi S, Santacroce E, et al. Brachial plexus sonography: a technique for assessing the root level. AJR Am J Roentgenol 2002;179:699–702.

70. Songcharoen P. Management of brachial plexus injury in adults. Scand J Surg 2008;97:317–23.

71. Tagliafico A, Succio G, Serafini G, et al. Diagnostic performance of ultrasound in patients with suspected brachial plexus lesions in adults: a multicenter retrospective study with MRI, surgical findings and clinical follow-up as reference standard. Skeletal Radiol 2013;42:371–6.

72. Abreu E, Aubert S, Wavreille G, et al. Peripheral tumor and tumor-like neurogenic lesions. Eur J Radiol 2013;82:38–50.

73. Gruber H, Glodny B, Bendix N, et al. High-resolution ultrasound of peripheral neurogenic tumors. Eur Radiol 2007;17:2880–8.

74. Cartwright MS, Chloros GD, Walker FO, et al. Diagnostic ultrasound for nerve transection. Muscle Nerve 2007;35:796–9.

Index

Note: Page numbers of article titles are in **boldface** type.

Moving?

Make sure your subscription moves with you!

To notify us of your new address, find your **Clinics Account Number** (located on your mailing label above your name), and contact customer service at:

Email: journalscustomerservice-usa@elsevier.com

800-654-2452 (subscribers in the U.S. & Canada)
314-447-8871 (subscribers outside of the U.S. & Canada)

Fax number: 314-447-8029

Elsevier Health Sciences Division
Subscription Customer Service
3251 Riverport Lane
Maryland Heights, MO 63043

*To ensure uninterrupted delivery of your subscription, please notify us at least 4 weeks in advance of move.

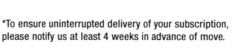

ELSEVIER

CPI Antony Rowe
Eastbourne, UK
November 03, 2014